# Pain Clinic Manual

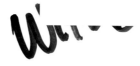

Edited by

**Simon J. Dolin** MB BS, FRCA, PhD
*Consultant in Pain Management*
*King Edward VII Hospital, Midhurst, and*
*St Richard's Hospital, Chichester, UK*

**Nicholas L. Padfield** MB BS, FRCA
*Consultant in Anaesthesia and Pain Management*
*Greenwich District Hospital, London, and*
*King Edward VII Hospital, Midhurst, UK*

**Jane A. Pateman** MB BS, FRCA
*Consultant in Anaesthesia*
*Royal Sussex County Hospital, Brighton, UK*

With a Foreword by
**Douglas Justins**
*Pain Management Centre*
*St Thomas's Hospital, London, UK*

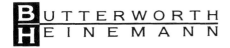

Butterworth-Heinemann
Linacre House, Jordan Hill, Oxford OX2 8DP
A division of Reed Educational and Professional Publishing Ltd

Ɋ A member of the Reed Elsevier plc group

OXFORD  BOSTON  JOHANNESBURG
MELBOURNE  NEW DELHI  SINGAPORE

First published 1996
Reprinted 1997

**British Library Cataloguing in Publication Data**
A catalogue record for this book is available from
the British Library

**Library of Congress Cataloguing in Publication Data**
A catalogue record for this book is available from
the Library of Congress

ISBN 0 7506 2036 6

Typset by BC Typesetting, Bristol
Printed in Great Britain

# Contents

**Part 4  Common Pain Problems**

**Part 5  Palliative care**

# Contributors

**Brendan Amesbury** MRCGP
Medical Director, St Wilfrid's Hospice, and Consultant in Palliative Medicine, St Richard's Hospital, Chichester, UK

**Rosalind C. Bacon** MBBS, FRCA
Registrar, St George's Hospital, London, UK

**Jonathan Bell** FRCS
Registrar in Orthopaedic Surgery, St George's Hospital, London, UK

**Caroline J. Fairley** MB BS, FRCA
Senior Registrar in Anaesthesia, St George's Hospital, London, UK

**Nicholas M. Girdler** JP, BSc, BDS, MIBiol, CBiol, FDSCRCSEng, FFDRCSIrel
Consultant Senior Lecturer in Dental Sedation, University of Newcastle Dental School and Hospital, Newcastle upon Tyne, UK

**Jane M. Green** BSc, AfBPsS
Chartered Clinical Psychologist, Pain Clinic, St Richard's Hospital, Chichester, UK

**John H. Hughes** MB BS, FRCA
Consultant in Anaesthesia and Pain Management, South Cleveland Hospital, Middlesbrough, Cleveland, UK

**Paul M. Jameson** MB BS, FRCA
Senior Registrar in Anaesthesia, St George's Hospital, London, UK

**Joel Kent** MD
Fellow in Anesthesiology and Pain Management, University of Maryland Medical System, Baltimore, Maryland, USA

**Lewis Marshall** MB BS (W Aust), MPH
Coordinator of Infectious Diseases Control, Health Department, Perth, Australia

**Joseph P. O'Dwyer** MB, BAO, MRCP, FRCA
Consultant in Anaesthesia and Pain Relief, Worthing and Southlands
Hospitals, Worthing, UK

**Nigel E. S. Payne** MB BS, FRCA
Consultant in Anaesthesia, Royal Surrey County Hospital, Guildford, UK

**Martin G. Ridley** MB, MRCP
Consultant Physician, Department of Rheumatology, St Richard's
Hospital, Chichester, UK

**Elizabeth J. Roberts** BM, FRCA
Consultant in Anaesthesia, Critical Care Directorate, Queen Mary's
Hospital, Sidcup, UK

**Lee J. Taylor** FRCS
Consultant Orthopaedic Surgeon, St Richard's Hospital, Chichester, UK

**John E. Williams** MB BS, FRCA
Senior Registrar in Anaesthesia, Nuffield Department of Anaesthesia, John
Radcliffe Hospital, Oxford, UK

# Foreword

This is a timely book which reflects the considerable experience and enthusiasm of a predominantly young group of contributors whose refreshing approach to the subject is not encumbered by some of the traditional concepts handed down by previous generations. The last 25 years have witnessed major advances in our understanding of the basic mechanisms of pain and in the therapeutic options available to manage patients with chronic pain. The authors do not make unrealistic therapeutic claims and admit that management remains difficult for a significant group of patients. Unfortunately the new insights into the pathophysiology of pain have not always resulted in improvement of the clinical management of every category of chronic pain. One major advance has been the adoption of a biopsychosocial perspective, rather than the rigid, traditional, mechanistic, disease model which was employed for centuries and this book certainly emphasises the need to consider the whole patient and his environment.

Over the centuries the management of pain has been based on theories which were sometimes wonderfully bizarre. The technological and pharmacological advances of the last few decades have encouraged the proliferation of more and more therapies. Many of these have a strong theoretical base in contemporary scientific knowledge but there are still some new treatments for which a rational explanation is awaited. The wide diversity in the approaches to management has, in some cases, led to a sharp polarisation of clinicians into apparently opposing camps. The problem arises most commonly when a particular therapist adopts a theory of unitary causation for chronic pain and then proceeds to apply a single therapy to every patient whom he encounters. The interventionists and the behaviourists can be equally guilty in this respect. A classic example of the theory of unitary causation was during the so-called 'era of the disc' when intervertebral disc prolapse was regarded as the cause of all back pain with the result that many unwarranted discectomies were performed. The present authors have tried to present a wide range of therapeutic options wherever appropriate.

The most likely situation is that, for any particular therapy, there will be a very specific and well defined group of patients who will benefit, and equally a group of patients in whom such a therapy is inappropriate. Although we know many of the questions we do not have the answers when it comes to a critical appraisal of pain therapies. Those of you who are embarking upon a career in pain management will have to carry on the enormous task of evaluating the scientific evidence for all the existing therapies. This is the age of evidence based medicine and the work of evaluating pain management has commenced already. The chapters in this book will help to highlight those areas in which doubts exist about the efficacy and indications for various treatments. Many experts would state that the gold standard for the evaluation of any therapy is the randomized controlled trial. Such trials are sadly lacking in the world of chronic pain.

The management of chronic pain remains a much neglected activity in many parts of the world. The Royal College of Anaesthetists, The Association of Anaesthetists and the Pain Society have begun to tackle the provision and organisation of pain management services, as well as the training of doctors in non-acute pain relief, in the United Kingdom. Organisation such as the International Association for the Study of Pain are attempting to educate policy making bodies and the public on a global scale so that the provision of services for chronic pain is beginning to receive high priority in some places.

This book will serve as an ideal resource for any doctor involved in the management of patients with chronic pain. As a consequence of the current pace of change in the basic and applied sciences relating to pain I would expect to see new editions of this book in the near future but before taking up their pens afresh the authors should be congratulated on completing this first volume.

**Douglas Justins**
Consultant in Pain Management and Anaesthesia
Pain Management Centre
St Thomas's Hospital
London, UK

1

# The pain clinic

**S. J. Dolin**

## Reasons for existence

Pain is usually a symptom of an underlying condition that needs diagnosis and treatment. This statement is generally true with conditions of recent onset (acute) or conditions that are progressive. However in many patients pain may continue once a diagnosis has been made and treatment of the underlying condition completed. Also there are some conditions where a diagnosis has been made but treatment is only palliative rather than curative. Further there are a number of patients who continue to experience pain even though no diagnosis can be made. These patients suffer from chronic pain, i.e. pain lasting a long time ($\chi\rho o\nu o\sigma$ = period of time). Chronic pain is no longer giving useful information, in contrast to acute pain, and it is deemed reasonable to treat pain on a symptomatic basis. Because chronic pain patients cover most medical specialties there arose a need to establish a team who had a special interest in treating the most difficult cases of chronic pain. This development has been widely welcomed by other medical specialties.

Although Bonica[1] advocated the establishment of multidisciplinary pain clinics in the 1950s, it was only in 1961 that the first modern pain treatment centre was set up at the University of Washington. In the 1970s pain clinics became more widely established with further input from the ideas of Fordyce[2] and Sternbach.[3] They established the principle of pain treatment using a multidisciplinary approach. This approach allows simultaneous treatment of physical, emotional, behavioural, vocational and social aspects of pain in a more effective way, ideally at less expense. Since then pain clinics have spread throughout the world and are now in the mainstream of health care delivery. Pain clinics have grown up in parallel with palliative care services for the terminally ill and there is much common ground between them. The growth of pain clinics has also paralleled the growth of anaesthesia as a specialty and the interest amongst groups of anaesthetists in clinical areas outside the operating theatre. The involvement of anaesthetists was an extension of their role in postoperative pain relief and regional analgesia. Anaesthesia was not the only specialty with an early interest in chronic pain but the majority of specialists willing to devote time to this clinical area have been anaesthetists and this trend still persists.

## Role of pain clinics

The role of the pain clinic can be summed up as follows:

- decrease subjective pain experience
- increase general level of activity
- decrease drug consumption
- return to employment or full quality of life
- decrease further use of health care resources

An important additional function of pain clinics is education. Patients should be taught about the difference between acute and chronic pain. Misconceptions about the nature of the pain and its significance may need to be dispelled. Patients may arrive in the pain clinic having had many opinions from doctors as well as other health professionals. They may have been given variable information and much disinformation on the way. The message from the pain clinic should be that, while the pain may not be curable, it should be treatable and that there are many ways in which patients can take responsibility for their pain and learn to live with it. Much of the aim of pain clinics is to do with reducing disability and maladaptive coping styles. The primary goal is to improve the patient's level of functioning while decreasing as much as possible the frequency and intensity of pain. It is important that the educational message should be consistent within the team, and it is helpful if the message is reinforced at every turn. Education not only applies to patients but also to other staff within the hospital and also to referring doctors. It does take considerable time and effort to communicate with colleagues about what the pain clinic is capable of and also what the operating philosophy is within the clinic. One of the important functions of the pain clinic is to terminate the cycle of perpetual specialist referral.

Teaching is also an important role of pain clinics. Undergraduates do not tend to spend time in pain clinics, or indeed in acute pain control, and there has been criticism of this. Some medical schools have now started to address this problem. Most teaching is postgraduate and pain therapy is now seen as an important part of training by the College of Anaesthetists. Teaching at any level by other disciplines remains unstructured at present.

There is a great need for good research in the field of chronic pain. The need is for randomized clinic trials to assess different modes of therapy. This is as true in the field of pharmacology as it is in physiotherapy and nerve blocks. Much of the currently accepted mode of activity within the pain clinic is poorly supported by definitive clinical trials. The psychologists have been an exception in this field, with many published studies supporting the role of psychological therapies in chronic pain.[4]

## Referral patterns

Referral numbers and patterns will vary enormously between pain clinics. The question is whether pain clinics should take patients on a primary, secondary or even tertiary referral basis. This will be determined in part by the nature of the pain condition and in part by the expertise available within the clinic. Some conditions such as postherpetic neuralgia will be readily diagnosed by the general practitioner and will be suitable for primary referral. For many conditions an initial diagnostic work-up is essential. Given the wide spectrum of medical conditions the initial diagnostic work-up may need to be done by orthopaedic surgeons, rheumatologists, neurologists, gynaecologists, general physicians, general surgeons, neurosurgeons, thoracic surgeons, maxillofacial surgeons, to name a few. While some of these may work closely or be integral to the pain clinic, it is likely that most referrals will need to go through the diagnostic work-up in other clinics and then come to the pain clinic as a secondary referral.

There is a need for regional referral centres that take tertiary referral from other pain clinics. This is especially so when sophisticated or invasive techniques are being considered. It may be that some centres with neurology and neurosurgery services will offer expertise unavailable elsewhere. It may also be appropriate to have expensive facilities such as residential pain management programmes concentrated at one centre rather than trying to reproduce such facilities on a smaller local scale.

There will also be referrals from the local hospice or terminal care facility if this is not part of an integrated service. These referrals will tend to be at short notice and will need prompt assessment and intervention. While it will only be a small minority of patients whose pain cannot be controlled by the palliative care physicians, the techniques available within the pain clinic are usually highly effective at gaining rapid pain control in this situation.

## Staff required[5-7]

Current management of chronic pain embodies the concept that patients with complex pain problems are best served by a team of specialists with different health care backgrounds. Many different practice styles are used in achieving the coordination of services and specialists. Solo practitioners may use referrals to other specialists in their area. Larger practices may permit several specialists to work in the same premises. Pain clinics in larger hospitals may have extensive programmes involving specialists with every possible interest as well as inpatient services. The broad expertise available in a multidisciplinary team allows consideration of emotional, psychological, familial and occupational consequences of the patients' pain.

The specialties involved in pain management are psychology, psychiatry, neurology, neurosurgery, anaesthesia, rehabilitation medicine, palliative care physicians, rheumatology and physiotherapy. There will need to be a director of the pain clinic and this is most often but not necessarily an anaesthetist. Input from occupational therapy, dietary specialists and vocational rehabilitation will also be useful. Dedicated nursing staff are essential to the running of an effective pain clinic. Office support personnel such as a business manager, receptionist and secretarial staff as well as good access to medical records are essential contributors to the team. The actual mix of personnel will vary between pain clinics depending on patient demand and available funding.

The International Association for the Study of Pain[8] has published guidelines called *Desirable Characteristics for Pain Treatment Facilities*. Pain treatment facilities have been categorized as follows:

- multidisciplinary pain centres, to include representatives of two medical specialties together with a psychiatrist or psychologist and offer full diagnostic and therapeutic services for outpatient, inpatient and emergency care. The centre should be part of a major health science education or research organization and should be actively engaged in research and education.
- multidisciplinary pain clinics which will have identical facilities to the multidisciplinary pain centre but need not teach or research or be part of a major health science education or research organization.
- the pain clinic must interact with at least three physicians of different specialties, one of whom must be a psychiatrist or psychologist. It must have both diagnostic and therapeutic facilities and provide emergency care.
- modality-oriented clinics use only one treatment modality such as nerve blocks or acupuncture.

Actual staffing levels vary enormously between pain clinics. It is not clear what constitutes the ideal staffing ratio per head of population. Proposals for two consultant sessions (one outpatient, one procedure-based) for every 250 000 head of population have been made.[9] However, those who work on this basis still find themselves overwhelmed with referrals and develop waiting lists. This figure also does not take account of other specialists, therapists, nurses and administrative staff needed within the pain clinic.

## Facilities required

Just as dedicated staff are essential to the continuity of patient care and building up teamwork, so a dedicated facility is also essential. The biggest challenge for pain clinics is often acquiring enough space to allow for efficient handling of the flow of patients through the clinic. A fixed locus of operation is ideal for outpatient visits, medical consultations, trans-cutaneous electrical nerve stimulation (TENS) clinics, group sessions for education, psychological or physical therapies, and inpatient stay. A conference room for regular team meetings is helpful, as is a staff lounge area. There must be sufficient space for reception and secretarial services as well as storage space for equipment. The treatment area must allow for access to X-ray screening when needed and have adequate monitoring devices, oxygen, suction and ready access to resuscitation facilities. The ability to do some procedures under general anaesthesia is essential. A biplane fluoroscope with a C-arm and memory is generally sufficient for imaging purposes, although some more sophisticated facilities include carbon fibre floating tables. A well-staffed recovery area is also essential.

Inpatient services are expensive in time and resources and must be limited to relatively few patients. Inpatient care can be an excellent option for those requiring drug detoxification to more appropriate medications, extensive psychological or behavioural therapy, or therapies involving extended administration of drugs via complex routes, e.g. epidural or intrathecal. Inpatient care may also be essential when outpatient care has failed and for those who may need temporary removal from a detrimental home environment to enable therapies to be more effective.

## Funding

Sources of funding are various. In publicly funded hospitals pain clinics will have an annual contract to treat a certain number of patients and be given an agreed budget to achieve this contract. The size of the contract and the staff and facilities provided will need to be agreed on an annual basis with the purchasers of the health service. Additional contracts for further work may be obtained if the pain clinic can provide a service at a price that is attractive to other purchasers outside the local hospital. More recently a number of general practitioners now hold their own budgets and they are free to purchase pain clinic services as needed. However, not all of the pain clinic services may be on the list from which general practitioners can purchase, so this avenue of funding may be limited. Specialized units such as residential pain management programmes or those with special expertise may get referral from other pain clinics on an extracontractual referral basis. The funding for these referrals will generally come from the purchasers of the referring hospital. National tertiary referral centres may need to depend largely on such referrals.

Private insurance companies are generally willing to cover patients for some, but not all, pain clinic treatments. Most insurance companies prefer to pay for treatments such as nerve blocks but are often unwilling to pay for clinical psychology or inpatient rehabilitation.

## Value of pain clinics

With the increasing cost of health care it is essential that pain clinics justify the money spent on them. The benefits of pain clinic treatment are not simply limited to the subjective perception of patients but also extend to objective behavioural variables such as return to work and decreased use of the health care system. It is increasingly important that pain clinics audit their outcomes in the widest sense.

## Suggested algorithm

Figure 1.1 shows possible paths that a patient may take through the pain clinic at St Richard's Hospital, Chichester.

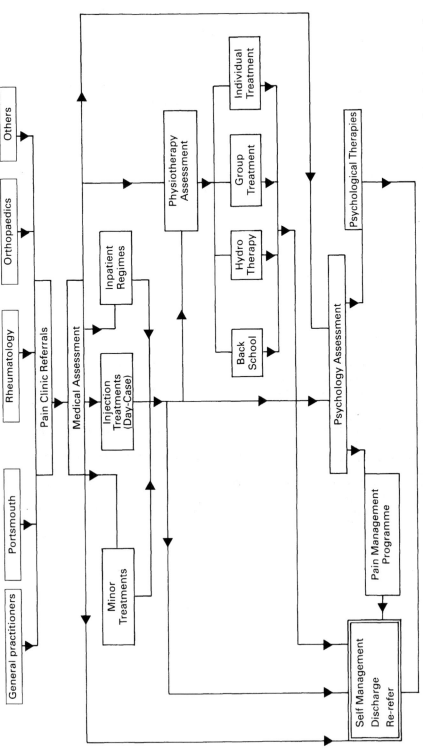

**Figure 1.1** Algorithm of possible routes through the pain clinic at St Richard's Hospital, Chichester. Decisions need to be made at a number of points about the most appropriate next step.

## Pain organizations

Many regional pain organizations have regular meetings, and most countries now have their own pain societies which have annual meetings where all disciplines involved in pain management can exchange ideas. National pain societies frequently advise their government departments of health and various specialty governing bodies. The International Association for the Study of Pain (IASP) has become the international body to which all national pain societies are affiliated. The IASP promotes the field at an international level and is also involved in publishing consensus guidelines and terminology for pain conditions. There is a world meeting held under the auspices of IASP every 3 years.

The main international journal is *Pain*. There has recently been a proliferation of other journals in the field, including *Journal of Pain and Symptom Management*, *Journal of Palliative Care*, *Pain Clinics* and *Clinical Journal of Pain*. Some chronic pain literature is published in the anaesthetic journals and some important articles may be published in the mainstream medical literature, such as *The Lancet* or *New England Journal of Medicine*.

## References

1. Bonica JJ. Organization and function of a pain clinic. *Adv Neurol* **4**: 433–443, 1974
2. Fordyce WE. *Behavioural Methods for Chronic Pain and Illness*. St Louis: CV Mosby, 1976
3. Sternbach RA. *Pain Patients: Tracts and Treatments*. New York: Academic Press, 1974
4. Flor H, Fydich T, Turk DC. Efficacy of multidisciplinary pain treatment centers: a meta-analytic review. *Pain* **49**: 221–230, 1992
5. Rowlinson JC, Hamill RJ. Organization of a multidisciplinary pain center. *Mt Sinai J Med* **58**: 267–272, 1991
6. Hannenburg AA, McArthur JD. Establishing a pain clinic. *Int Anesthesiol Clin Boston* **21**: 1–10, 1983
7. Bullingham RES, McQuay HJ, Budd K. Pain control centres: problem of organization and operation in the UK. *Clin Anaesthesiol Lond* **3**: 211–221, 1985
8. International Association for the Study of Pain. *Desirable Characteristics for Pain Facilities*. Seattle: IASP, 1990
9. Mushin WW, Swerdlow M, Lipton S, Mehta MD. The pain centre. *Practitioner* **218**: 439, 1977

# The pain patient

S. J. Dolin

## Epidemiology of pain

Pain is a common experience and is costly for both the individual and for the health service. A number of epidemiological studies have examined the extent of the problem.

The *Nuprin Pain Report*[1] found that most people experienced pain, and reported on average three to four different kinds of pain experience per year. Back pain was experienced by 16% of all adults, headache by 15% and joint pain by 11%. In further studies 24% of families had one family member who experienced chronic pain, while 14% of individuals reported chronic pain, and 75% of these had sought medical attention for the pain within the last year.[2] When pain clinic patients were compared to a sample from a general population, pain clinic attenders had a higher self-assessment of physical, emotional and social distress. Those with serious psychosocial disturbance were more likely to attend pain clinics.[3]

In the Christchurch psychiatric epidemiology study 81.7% of the population reported pain in one or more sites. The majority reported more than one life-disrupting experience of pain. Pain was most common in the joints, back, head and abdomen. Women reported more pain than men. In general the prevalence of pain increased with age.[4]

The epidemiology of chronic pain in children and adolescents is relatively undocumented.

## Clinical presentation

Patients presenting to pain clinics are most likely to present with back pain, headache, joint pain or abdominal pain. They will ideally have been through an appropriate diagnostic work-up, and will arrive with either a positive diagnosis which has not responded to surgical or medical therapy or at least the exclusion of serious underlying pathology. A substantial percentage of patients presenting to pain clinics will have a discrepancy between the degree of pain, suffering and disability and the amount of objective evidence for the presence of pathology that could account for the clinical state. These patients may believe their pain is not accepted as being real by the medical profession or even by friends and family and there may be a need to have the pain legitimized. There may be a persistent desire for a diagnosis and a surgical solution, in spite of multiple investigations and even previous surgery. An important role of the pain clinic is to terminate the round of referrals that the patient may have been on, and to approach the problem from a symptom-control rather than a diagnostic perspective.

Patients with chronic pain will nearly always have tried a variety of medications. Most will have tried simple or compound analgesics (e.g. paracetamol and codeine). Benefit from these will be variable. Many patients will report that these medications offer little benefit and some patients will have stopped taking all medications. Patients may have been started on opioid analgesics by pressurizing their doctors into providing these, which are considered inappropriate in chronic benign pain. Patients with high intakes of opioids may need to be detoxified, and this represents a complex problem in the pain clinic. Benzodiazepines are widely used by patients presenting to pain clinics. There is little evidence that benzodiazepines offer any advantage in chronic pain states, but coming off these drugs may offer a challenge to the pain clinician. Patients may also have been prescribed tricyclic antidepressants or more recently selective serotonin reuptake inhibitors such as fluoxetine (Prozac). These drugs may be helpful with sleep disturbance and depression as well as chronic pain.

## Sociological profile

Enquiries into family dynamics have demonstrated that some patients with chronic pain may come from dysfunctional families. There may well be another member of the family who suffers from chronic pain or who is handicapped. A family history of alcoholism, abuse and depression is also more common in patients with chronic pain.[5] Patients from lower socioeconomic groups are more likely to ascribe pain to physical rather than psychosocial causes,[6] but it is unclear whether or not patients from lower socioeconomic groups are more likely to seek a pain clinic referral.

## Psychological profile

- The patient's role within the family and within society may be altered.
- There may be a decline in income with loss of employment.
- Independence can be threatened and the patient may assume a dependent role.
- Feelings of helplessness and meaninglessness are common.
- Sleep is commonly disturbed by pain.
- Chronic sleep deficit can lead to exhaustion and irritability.
- Activity levels may well be reduced, while some patients may alternate excessive activity with periods of relative inactivity. Some patients may spend many hours of the day resting.
- The patient may have a pronounced preoccupation with symptoms and pain can take the place of significant social interaction.
- Patients with chronic pain have an inability to enjoy social life, leisure and sexual activity.

- Depression is common in chronic pain states. However, the relationship between the two is complex. As the pain often predates the depression it may be that depression is secondary to pain. However, depression with painful somatic symptoms is also well-recognized. Depression associated with chronic pain has a lower incidence of suicidal ideation than depression with somatic manifestations.[5] It has been proposed that chronic pain is a variant of depression and that painful physical symptoms may protect against more painful mental aspects of depression.[7] However, this view is not universally accepted.
- Interpersonal conflict is commonly reported, with high divorce rates.

## Role of litigation and compensation

There is much evidence in the medical literature that patients who are receiving disability payments or who have litigation pending from an injury are less likely to respond to medical therapy than patients who do not.[8] One of the factors predicting successful outcome from multidisciplinary pain treatment was absence of financial compensation.[9] Settlement of claims was reported to have a positive effect on symptoms.[10] However the presence of ongoing litigation and disability benefits should not affect the decision to offer pain clinic therapies to the patient. It has been argued that those who are pursuing litigation or are on disability benefits may be more severely affected by an injury, or may have fewer employment opportunities due to lack of skills and so not benefit from the advantages of continued activity and employment.

## References

1. Taylor H, Curran MM. *The Nuprin Pain Report.* New York: Louis Harris, 1985
2. Crook J, Rideout E, Browne G. The prevalence of pain in a general population. *Pain* **18:** 299–314, 1984
3. Crook J, Tunks E. Defining the chronic pain syndrome: an epidemiological method. *Adv Pain Res Ther* **9:** 870–877, 1985
4. James FR, Large RG, Bushnell JA, Wells JE. Epidemiology of pain in New Zealand. *Pain* **44:** 279–283, 1991
5. Blumer D, Heilbronn M. Depression and chronic pain. In: Cameron O (ed.) *Presentations of Depression.* New York: John Wiley, 1987
6. Hollingshead AB, Redlich FC. *Social Class and Mental Illness.* New York: John Wiley, 1958
7. Engel G. Psychogenic pain and the pain prone patient. *Am J Med* **26:** 899–918, 1959
8. Sander RA, Meyers JE. The relationship of disability to compensation status in railroad workers. *Spine* **11:** 141–143, 1986
9. Guck TP, Meilman PW, Skultety FM *et al.* Prediction of long-term outcome of multidisciplinary pain treatment. *Arch Phys Med Rehabil* **67:** 293–296, 1986
10. Gotten N. Survey of 100 cases of whiplash injury after settlement of litigation. *JAMA* **162:** 865–867, 1956

# Measurement of pain

J. A. Pateman

Why do we need to measure pain? Both clinicians and managers within the health service have an interest in the measurement of pain. Clinicians need to compare single patients and groups of patients, and to monitor the progress of individuals, as well as to validate new treatments for research purposes. Managers are responsible for maximizing the return for their money, and many pain programmes are expensive, so they may demand objective proof of efficacy, as well as documentation of the level of need within their local population. Chronic pain problems cause a lot of lost potential within the community, both in terms of economic potential and personal suffering. However the impact on an individual can be subtle, and so measures such as mortality or gross morbidity will be of little use in assessing either an individual's progress or the level of disability within a patient group.

Many measures of pain are based on patient self-report. Arguably, self-report is subjective and so less reliable than objective measurements. However, since pain (as defined by the International Association for the Study of Pain[1]) is 'an unpleasant sensory and emotional experience associated with actual or potential tissue damage, or described in terms of such damage', it is clear that any attempts to measure pain will have to incorporate the effects of emotion and affect, and that observer-based reports of these experiences may in fact be more indirect and potentially unreliable than self-reports.

The simplest attempts to measure pain rely on a single dimension, such as pain intensity. Methods vary from descriptive terms to visual analogue scales. Pain has also been measured using objective assessment of activity, or pain-specific behaviours. However levels of activity do not necessarily correlate with pain intensity, as reported by Linton.[2] Attempts to encompass some of the other dimensions of the total pain experience and to quantify behavioural, emotional, economic and sociocultural factors have been developed. In many of these, the bias which might be introduced by an idiosyncratic response to a single question is reduced by using large numbers of questions. This increases complexity and can make a questionnaire beyond the reach of patients who are very unwell or have poor cognitive function.

## Single-dimension pain measures

Single pain measures can look at physical, functional or behavioural aspects.

- *Physical* pain can be measured by self-report in terms of intensity, location, physical symptoms or by external measures such as electro-myogram activity. To assess location and distribution of pain using a body map, the patient is asked to shade in the areas of pain and any radiations. Pain intensity (or any other aspect of pain) can be measured using several different types of scales. Measurements such as verbal descriptors, e.g. mild, moderate, severe and excruciating, or pictorial representation such as facial expressions are non-parametric, suffer from the limited number of possible responses and the tendency of patients to use the middle of the scale. This renders them less useful for research, but better in some clinical situations, where they are easily understood and quick to administer.

    More complex numerical rating scales such as 0–10 are still strictly non-parametric, but give a wider range of possible responses (Fig. 3.1a). Visual analogue scales with a 100 mm line and descriptive terms at each end are relatively simple to administer, can be adapted for patients who are too unwell to mark the line completely independently, and are in widespread use (Fig. 3.1b). However, older patients can find them difficult to understand, and reports of their reliability are conflicting. They are probably most useful in measuring changes in pain level in an individual patient.

- *Functional* measurement of pain assessed on single variables ranges from productivity, e.g. employment rate or recreational activity level, through physical abilities, e.g. distance walked, to up-time and down-time – time spent resting or mobilizing. These are objective measures so they have gained some popularity, and indeed self-reporting of some functional measures may be unreliable. However employment rate is a very blunt measure of function, reflecting more the age and work skills of the individual than any treatment effect.

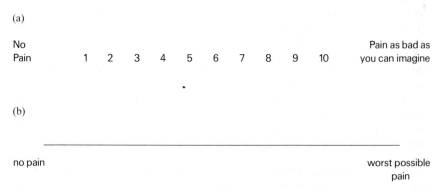

(a)

| No |  | | | | | | | | | | Pain as bad as |
|---|---|---|---|---|---|---|---|---|---|---|---|
| Pain |  | 1 | 2 | 3 | 4 | 5 | 6 | 7 | 8 | 9 | 10 | you can imagine |

(b)

no pain                                                                    worst possible
                                                                                    pain

Figure 3.1 (a) Numerical rating scale for pain; (b) linear analogue scale.

- *Behavioural:* Another way of measuring pain without relying on self-report is the use of *behavioural* scales. Patients with particular pain syndromes develop specific patterns of pain behaviours, such as grimacing, rubbing the affected part, guarding their movements or developing an abnormal gait. These behaviours can be scored according to their frequency; they are reliable and correlate with pain intensity, but are highly specific for individual pain conditions – the pain behaviour in a patient suffering for example pelvic pain or postherpetic neuralgia will be specific for each condition. The patient should be unaware that the behaviour is being recorded by an observer. Looking at self-reporting of pain behaviour, Ready et al.[3] found that use of medication was underreported by 50–60%.

## Multiple-dimension pain reporting

The simplest method of scoring pain on multiple dimensions is to use multiple visual analogue or number ranking scales. This is only a valid method if each response is not influenced by the previous ones, which in practice is unlikely.

- The *memorial pain assessment card* is one example of this type of assessment. It has linear analogue scales for pain intensity, analgesic effect and mood and also an eight-option set of verbal descriptors for pain intensity.
- *McGill pain questionnaire:* More complex assessments of pain take the form of questionnaires. One of the best known multidimensional scales is the *McGill pain questionnaire* (MGPQ). This was first described by Ronald Melzack in 1975.[4] He grouped together words commonly used to describe pain into several different sensory, affective and evaluative categories. Patients are asked to select the most appropriate word for their pain within each subcategory. For example, one group of words in the MGPQ are: hot, burning, scalding, searing.

This particular set describes heat, a sensory aspect. There are a total of 20 sets of descriptors (10 sensory, five affective, one evaluative and four miscellaneous), and patients are asked to choose the best word to describe their pain in each of the groups they feel is relevant to their pain. Thus not all groups are chosen by an individual patient. Within the groups, the words can be graded in order of increasing intensity and given a numerical value, so in the example given above, hot is a less intense adjective than scalding. Thus a total score or pain rating index (PRI) may be obtained based either on the total number of words chosen (NWC) or the rank order of chosen words. The PRI is given the suffix S if derived from sum or R from rank. Melzack assessed PRIs for various diseases and found that toothache or postherpetic neuralgia gave mean scores of less than 25, phantom limb, cancer and back pain scored slightly higher, while labour pain was in the low 30s.

This part of the MGPQ is combined with a present pain intensity (PPI) score, and a patient pain map where areas of the body affected by pain or radiation of pain can be shaded. The validity of scoring the MGPQ was confirmed by Turk *et al.*[5] The questionnaire takes about 20 min to complete, and its use may be limited by the patient's level of comprehension of the vocabulary. It is normally a written assessment, but can be administered orally by an independent observer. However, oral and written scores should not be subsequently compared with each other.

- The MGPQ can be used with the *Dartmouth pain questionnaire* (DPQ), which assesses general affect, time course and intensity of pain, and effect on behaviour. This has the potential benefit of highlighting the positive aspects of the patient's function rather than simply the impairment.
- Another briefer multidimensional pain scale is the 52-item *West Haven– Yale multidimensional pain inventory* (WHYMPI), based on cognitive-behavioural models of pain behaviour, and specifically developed for chronic pain patients.

  There are three parts to this scale. First it examines the impact of pain on the patient's life (interference with work and leisure, family support, pain severity, self-control, and negative mood); second the patients' perception of the response of others to their communication of pain and suffering (punishing, solicitous and distracting responses), and third the extent to which participate in activities of daily living (household chores, outdoor work, activities away from home and social activities). It is quicker to administer than the MGPQ and emphasizes the patients' subjective distress, their perception of self-control and ability to solve problems.
- The *Wisconsin brief pain inventory* (BPI) is another quickly completed scoring system, taking less than 15 min to complete. It scores worst, average and current pain on numeric scales, medication usage and efficacy, and quantifies the impact on quality of life. It was developed for use in oncology and arthritis patients. Its chief advantage is the very low number of patients who are unable to complete the questionnaire.
- Tursky and colleagues[6] developed a *pain perception profile* (PPP). This uses cross-modality matching, i.e. equating a quantifiable sensation with the one it is desired to measure, to assess sensation threshold, intensity, reaction and sedation. Again it is shorter than the MGPQ and potentially the data produced may be more valid when used to assess the variations of the pain experience in a patient over time.
- Many of the therapeutic interventions in chronic pain patients are designed to lead to an improved quality of life, rather than less pain. To assess the success of these interventions, a measure of impact on quality of life is appropriate. The *sickness impact profile* (SIP) was designed for this purpose, although not specifically for pain patients. Its aim was to get a fairly sensitive measure of health status, and use this to measure differences after time and between groups. Questions were designed to look at aspects of activities of daily life affected by chronic low-level sickness. The SIP looks at 12 areas of daily activity, assessing impact in three ways – overall, physical and psychosocial – and has a total of 136 statements. It can be completed either at interview or by the subject, and takes about 30 min. Its application to chronic pain patients has been validated.

## Personality and depression measures

- The *Minnesota multiphasic personality inventory* (MMPI) is a commonly used personality assessment in patients with chronic pain. It is a long questionnaire – 566 items – is time-consuming to complete, and some patients resent the psychological bias of the questions. There are 10 clinical scales, assessing hypochondriasis, depression, hysteria, psychopathic deviation, masculinity–femininity, paranoia, psychasthenia (anxiety, low self-esteem), schizophrenia, hypomania and social introversion. The subject is given a score for each scale, and values over 70 are considered abnormal. Patients with chronic pain tend to score highly on hypochondriasis, hysteria and depression scales. However interpretation requires training, and experience in the relevant patient population.
- Depression is more common in chronic pain patients, so measurement of depression rating is of obvious clinical relevance. One of the most commonly used measures is the *Beck depression inventory* (BDI). This is a self-reporting depression index and can be used to quantify changes in level of depression with treatment.

## Pain diaries

Some patients find it helpful to complete a pain diary. This is directed at charting the pain intensity using a numerical scoring scale, recording activities of daily living and medications. These need to be filled in at the time to avoid distortion, but provide an estimate of how the patient functions in his or her normal environment. The use of a pain diary varies between patients, and may become less reliable with time. Another disadvantage is that it focuses the patient's attention more on the pain, and the limitations on life that the pain imposes. This may interact with ongoing treatment. It also requires a level of comprehension and accuracy in record-keeping, so is unsuitable for elderly or infirm patients.

## Pain assessment in children

Pain assessment in children is complicated by the age and development of the child and his or her interaction with the parents. In infants with no verbal skills, this can be very difficult, with the assessor relying on such gross measures as crying or motor withdrawal. These are measures of general distress, so are non-specific at best. Toddlers begin to develop localizing and other signs which are more indicative of pain, such as rubbing, as well as more complex although less specific behaviours such as lip smacking, and aggressive behaviours. From the age of 3 children begin to be able to cope with simple rating measurements such as face scales, colour matching, and the Oucher scale. From about 5 years of age children can complete visual analogue and other simple scales. Multidimensional scales such as the MGPQ have been validated for patients older than 12.

# References

1. Merskey H, Albe-Fessard DG, Bonica JJ. Pain terms: a list with definitions and notes on usage. *Pain* **6**: 249, 1979
2. Linton SJ. The relationship between activity and chronic back pain. *Pain* **21**: 289–294, 1985
3. Ready LB, Sarkis E, Turner JA. Self-reported vs. actual use of medications in chronic pain patients. *Pain* **12**: 285, 1982
4. Melzack R. The McGill pain questionnaire: major properties and scoring methods. *Pain* **1**: 277–299, 1975
5. Turk DC, Rudy TE, Salovey P. The McGill pain questionnaire reconsidered: confirming factor structure and examining appropriate uses. *Pain* **21**: 385–397, 1985
6. Tursky B, Jammer LD, Friedman R. The pain perception profile: a psychological approach to the assessment of pain report. *Behav Ther* **13**: 376–394, 1982

# Further reading

Bergner M, Bobbitt RA, Carter WB, Gilson BS. The sickness impact profile: development and final revision of health status measure. *Med Care* **19**: 787–805, 1981

Chapman CR, Syrjala KL. Chapter 32. In: Bonica JJ (ed.) *The Management of Pain*, Lea and Febiger, 1990

Chapman CR. Chapter 74. In: Nimmo WS. Rowbotham DJ, Smith G (eds) *Anaesthesia*. Blackwell Scientific Publications, 1994

Daut RL, Cleeland CS, Flannery RC. Development of the Wisconsin brief pain questionnaire to assess pain in cancer and other diseases. *Pain* **17**: 197–210, 1983

Follick MJ, Smith TW, Ahern DK. The sickness impact profile: a global measure of disability in chronic low back pain. *Pain* **21**: 67–76, 1985

Keefe FJ, Block AR. Development of an observational method for assessing pain behaviour in chronic low back pain patients. *Behav Ther* **13**: 363–375, 1982

Kerns RD, Turk DC, Rudy TE. The West-Haven–Yale multidimensional pain inventory (WHYMPI). *Pain* **23**: 345–356, 1985

Melzack R *et al*. Labor is still painful after prepared childbirth training. *Can Med Assoc J* **125**: 357–363, 1981

Rollman GB. Measurement of pain in fibromyalgia in the clinic and laboratory. *J Rheumatol* **16**: 113–119, 1989

Williams R. Toward a set of reliable and valid measures for chronic pain assessment and outcome research. *Pain* **35**: 239–251, 1988

4

# Reflex sympathetic dystrophy – causalgia

J. H. Hughes

Reflex sympathetic dystrophy (RSD) and causalgia are chronic painful conditions predominantly involving the limbs and are characterized by burning pain, trophic and pseudomotor changes and loss of function. They involve a variety of conditions variously described as: causalgia,[1] Sudeck's atrophy,[2] posttraumatic pain syndromes,[3] minor causalgia[4] and RSD.[5] The French and orthopaedic literature frequently refer to algodystrophy. In 1953 Bonica suggested that these terms be included under the heading of reflex sympathetic dystrophy. Some suggest that causalgia remains a separate entity[6] or should be reserved for a similar syndrome involving trauma to a major nerve.[7]

The International Association for the Study of Pain (IASP) has defined RSD and causalgia under a heading of complex regional pain syndromes (CRPS).[8] These are subclassified into CRPS type I (RSD) and CRPS type II (causalgia). Causalgia is recognized to develop the signs of RSD but also to begin with a nerve injury.

Sympathetically maintained pain (SMP) is now defined as a pain that is maintained by sympathetic efferent innervation or by circulating catecholamines.[8] It may be a feature of several painful conditions including CRPS, postherpetic neuralgia and some cancer pains but is not an essential requirement for any individual condition. Pain relieved by sympathetic blockade may be described as SMP but does not imply a mechanism. Patients may have both SMP and sympathetically independent pain.

## Incidence and aetiology

The few prospective studies assessing the incidence of RSD are uncontrolled and the populations liable to bias. The incidence is probably higher than previously thought, the diagnosis made late with many cases going undiagnosed.[9] Most patients are adults but children may be involved.[10]

### Incidence

- Estimates of the incidence of RSD following trauma vary. It is possible that many patients have self-limiting episodes.[11]

- Colles' and other fractures traditionally have an incidence of under 2%;[12] more recent work suggests a rate of 30–37%.[13]
- Head-injured patients present with an incidence of 12%.[14]
- Peripheral nerve lesions have a reported incidence of 2–5%.[15]
- Presenting causes to the pain clinic are trauma 45–65%, postoperative 10–20%, inflammatory processes 2%, cardiac 3%, others 4% and no precipitating cause in 10–20%.[10,16]
- The female to male ratio is approximately 3 to 1 with a mean age of onset at 40–50 years.[10,16]

### Precipitating factors

The precipitating factors associated with RSD include:

- trauma (from inconsequential to major nerve damage)
- surgical trauma,[17] including immobilization in splints or plaster casts[18] and venepuncture[19]
- neurological disturbances[14] (central nervous system trauma, cerebro-vascular accident, parkinsonism, epilepsy)
- inflammatory diseases[5,20]
- neoplastic disease[21] (brain, lung, ovarian and breast most commonly)
- myocardial infarction[16]
- other factors include pregnancy,[22] familial[23] and iatrogenic[24] (isoniazid, ethambutol, cyclosporin)
- psychological states predisposing to RSD or its development remain controversial. Some consider the stress of organized sporting activity to precipitate or perpetuate RSD in children[9]
- there may be no apparent precipitating cause
- there are case reports of RSD involving small areas,[25] recurring at different sites with time,[27] being multifocal,[27] presenting as interstitial cystitis[28] or as a Münchausen's syndrome[29]

It should be noted that the severity of the injury may bear no relation to the severity of the RSD.

## Pathophysiology

In 1873 Létiévant postulated a mechanism where the peripheral nerve was the point of irritation, with transmission to the spinal centres causing abnormal neural activity and, if the impulses were strong enough, to higher centres. Since then there have been advances but the pathophysiology has not been fully elucidated. Traditional theories suggest an increase in sympathetic activity contributing to RSD: this is now being challenged.[30] Consensus exists for a history of trauma (accidental, surgical or patho-logical) that is not always identifiable and for sympathetic nervous system involvement. Current theories involve peripheral,[31] central[32] and mixed mechanisms.[33] Psychological mechanisms are also under review. The result is likely to involve several mechanisms that require integration before a final conclusion can be made.[34]

## Inflammatory mechanisms

Sudeck suggested an inflammatory process to explain RSD, in contrast to the generally accepted theory of sympathetic nervous system involvement. Current data support this theory.

- Immunoglobulins concentrating in the affected extremity confirm the idea of increased microvascular permeability.[29]
- Labelled phosphate nuclear magnetic resonance spectroscopy suggests impaired phosphate metabolism[35]
- Electromicroscopic studies show reduced muscle mitochondrial activity with other signs of oxidative stress.
- There is reduced oxygen extraction in the affected limb.[35]
- Veldman et al.[10] assessed their data in terms of increased regional inflammation and found it suitable for making the diagnosis of RSD.

## Peripheral end central neurological mechanisms

- Peripheral mechanisms involving the sympathetic system postulate involvement of $\alpha_1$-adrenoreceptor expression.[36] $\alpha_1$-Adrenoreceptor up-regulation on primary nociceptor afferents can occur in response to a barrage of stimulation. Nociceptive inputs to the spinal cord trigger sympathetic efferent activity that in turn stimulates the up-regulated receptors. Recent modifications suggest that non-nociceptive fibres are also susceptible to $\alpha_1$-adrenoreceptor up-regulation.[37] This accounts for allodynia and better explains the central alterations and self-perpetuation of SMP.
- Other mediators include the prostaglandins[38] and laboratory data suggest $\alpha_2$-adrenoreceptor involvement in peripheral up-regulation.[39]
- The motor manifestations may be explained by the effect of substance P release in the cord, producing prolonged dorsal horn cell depolarization.[40]
- In 1986 Roberts[41] reviewed the literature and proposed that 'SMP resulted from the tonic activity in myelinated mechanoreceptor afferents, that this activity is induced by sympathetic efferent actions on sensory receptors, and that this afferent input causes tonic firing in previously sensitized wide dynamic range or multireceptive neurons that are part of a central nociceptive pathway. A painful sensation results from this chain of actions.'
- Pain and disuse may cause a vicious cycle that reinforces and maintains the syndrome both peripherally and centrally.[42]

## Psychological mechanisms

- Psychological changes may be reactive to the development of RSD or may predispose some individuals to its development.[43]
- One hypothesis is based on clinical, psychological and pathophysiological data.[44] It assumes that at the time of physical trauma there is also a significant psychological stress, which may be related to the trauma or be coincidental. The patient's response is an inability to

cope and may involve premorbid factors. This pathopsychological condition provokes a psychophysiological cascade. This includes sympathetic overactivity, exaggerated illness behaviour, positive or negative reinforcement of that illness behaviour by social circumstances and continued symptomatology which promotes further psychological distress.

- In paediatric cases there is a suggestion that anxiety, life stress and depression play a role in the development of RSD.[43]

There remains a discrepancy between clinicians and basic scientists about the mechanism of RSD and how best to research it,[45,46] whilst others prefer the term sympathetically maintained pain.[41,47] The current taxonomy from the IASP[8] separating RSD and SMP and tightening the definitions may help reduce the confusion.

## Classification

Bonica[48] classified RSD into three grades (Table 4.1) based on the severity of pain and autonomic disturbance. A further classification[49] into acute, dystrophic and atrophic has also been made and each type could be subclassified by Bonica's classification. The classification is beneficial for teaching purposes but tends not to be used clinically.

**Table 4.1** Bonica's classification

*Grade 1 (severe)*
- Pain that is burning, knife-like or lancing, not relieved with rest and may be exacerbated by minimal stimulus (physical or emotional)
- Hyperaesthesia may be so severe that patients protect the area, often covering it with wet bandages[54]
- Frequently the sudomotor and vasomotor elements are severe

*Grade 2 (moderate) and grade 3 (mild)*
- Less severe and more common
- Pain is dull, throbbing, aching or diffusely burning
- The clinical picture may be so mild that the diagnosis goes unnoticed until it becomes irreversible

## Diagnosis

- The diagnosis is clinical with investigations or successful sympathetic blockade reinforcing clinical suspicion. Few patients show all the signs and symptoms, making diagnosis difficult in some. No single test confirms the diagnosis but objective testing helps in equivocal cases.
- A careful history is essential and must start with the first symptoms. Information about the patient's personality and social environment should be obtained.
- Patients may have more than one chronic pain and it is the clinician's responsibility to assess what processes are active and which are causing

the primary problem. The patient needs to be aware of this and know what degree of relief may be expected from the treatment given. It is common to find patients with associated myofascial problems.[10]

- A scoring system using some objective tests has been suggested as an aid for standardizing diagnosis and for making comparisons between studies.[50] It is based on 10 criteria with a single point if positive, half a point if equivocal and nil if absent. The criteria are: allodynia or hyperpathia, burning pain, oedema, colour or hair growth changes, sweating changes, temperature changes, radiographic demineralization, quantitative measurement of vasomotor or sudomotor disturbance (e.g. thermography), bone scan consistent with RSD and the response to sympathetic block. Scores over 5 probably have RSD, from 3 to 4.5 are equivocal and under 3 are negative.
- A separate study proposes three criteria; all must be present to make the diagnosis.[47] They are diffuse pain, loss of function and objective evidence of autonomic dysfunction (including cutaneous, subcutaneous, vascular flow, temperature, sweating, hair or nail changes).
- The differential diagnoses that need to be considered:[51] bony lesions, unrecognized sprain or fracture, arthritis, aseptic necrosis, Paget's disease, osteomas, infections, tumours (benign or malignant), diabetic osteopathy, posttrauma vasospasm, bursitis, tenosynovitis, calcification of tendons or ligaments, Raynaud's, phantom pain, frostbite, phlebitis, scleroderma, connective tissue diseases and myofascial syndromes.

## Clinical findings and course

A spectrum of severity exists from the obvious to the bizarre and frequently one symptom or sign predominates almost to the exclusion of others. Patients are therefore at risk of misdiagnosis.

The clinical findings vary but some are common to all:

- Pain occurs in over 90% of cases, does not correspond to known peripheral or segmental distributions, may spread proximally to involve all the limb or beyond to the ipsilateral or contralateral side of the body.
- Trophic changes (skin, hair, nails) usually occur but tend to be late in the disease.
- The pain continues after the precipitating factor has recovered or gone.
- Exercise often exacerbates the symptoms and signs.
- Symptoms vary with time; occasionally successfully treated patients have a recurrence.[33]

## Progression of the syndrome

RSD is described as a progressive disease passing through three stages, each lasting for 3–6 months.[49,52] The actual length of each stage is variable, from weeks to years.[53] This classification is useful as a generalization of progression but no study has confirmed this division. Individual cases do not always fit into the schema and patients may have features from more than one stage.

## Acute stage (stage 1 or hyperaemic stage)

This may start immediately after injury,[54] more commonly, days, weeks or months later. Onset may be insidious or fulminant.

- Pain is greater than that normally associated with the injury. It is burning or aching in character and exacerbated with movement, dependence, physical contact or emotional stimuli. Pain is limited to the distal part of the limb, following the blood vessels or peripheral nerves, but may spread to involve the whole limb or a previously unaffected limb.[52]
- Allodynia, hyperalgesia, hyperaesthesia, hyperpathia and dysaesthesia are common. Hypoaesthesia may also occur (see Table 4.2 for definitions).
- Skin may be warm, dry and red due to vasodilatation, or cyanotic and cold due to vasoconstriction. About 90% of patients will show a colour and/or temperature difference.[10]
- Increased sweating may occur with either a hot or cold limb.
- There is localized oedema and tenderness.
- There is accelerated hair and nail growth in the affected area.
- Muscle spasm and tremors occur.
- There is limitation of movement.

## Dystrophic stage (stage 2 or ischaemic stage)

- Pain continues, burning, aching or throbbing. It may reduce in intensity but frequently remains the major problem.
- There is marked allodynia, hyperalgesia and hyperpathia.
- Skin becomes cool, grey and cyanotic with a glazed look.
- Oedema becomes indurated.
- Thickening of joints and muscle-wasting further limit movement and increase weakness.
- There is reduced or no hair growth with the nails becoming brittle, cracked and grooved.
- There is spotty or diffuse osteoporosis.

**Table 4.2** Definitions

| | |
|---|---|
| Allodynia | Pain to a non-nociceptive stimulus |
| Hyperalgesia | Increased response to nociceptive stimulus |
| Hyperaesthesia | Increased sensitivity to stimuli (not special senses) |
| Hyperpathia | Excessive response to stimulus or after-sensation |
| Dysaesthesia | Unpleasant sensation to an innocuous stimulus |
| Hypoaesthesia | Decreased sensitivity |

## Atrophic stage (stage 3 or late stage)

- Pain, allodynia and hyperpathia frequently become less severe but may radiate proximal or distal to the site of injury or spread to involve the whole limb.
- Psychological and emotional disturbances may predominate.
- Skin becomes smooth, glassy, drawn, pale or cyanotic and cold.
- There are marked irreversible atrophic changes in muscle and subcutaneous tissue leading to thin, pointed fingers with loss of pulp pads.
- There are flexor tendon contractures similar to Dupuytren's.
- Joints are weak with limited movement and develop ankylosis.
- There is diffuse bony atrophy to advanced osteoporosis.
- Nails are brittle and ridged.

## Other clinical findings

- Reduced movement, weakness and fatigability frequently occur. Muscle spasm, dystonia and tremor may also occur;[55] they may precede the pain and occur in a mirror distribution or occasionally without pain. These features can develop during the acute or dystrophic stages and are nearly always present in the atrophic stage when sympathetic blockade has a variable effect.[40] Tremor increases with movement, is an enhanced physiological tremor and does not correlate with other symptoms. Resolution occurs on full recovery.[55] Weakness and incoordination may progress to the stage where the patient is unable to move (pseudoparesis).[10]
- Dermatological manifestations occasionally occur and include cutaneous ulceration and reticulate hyperpigmentation.[56]
- The trophic changes seen in adults only seem to occur in the most severe paediatric cases and are reversible.[33]

## Psychological considerations

- Psychological components may be solely reactive to RSD or may predispose some individuals to its development.[43] The pain is greater than that expected on physical examination; some consider it to be psychogenic[53] whilst others feel there is a population at higher risk of developing RSD.[33] Whichever the case, psychological changes are well-documented and require attention if successful outcomes are to be achieved.
- Patients often appear anxious, withdrawn and emotionally unstable. Drug addiction and suicidal tendencies sometimes occur.[10]
- Those who have had unsuccessful treatments coupled with suggestion that the problem is psychogenic often have an exacerbation of their psychological disturbance. This anxiety increases sympathetic activity and exacerbates the pain.[44]
- In paediatric cases, anxiety, life stress and depression play a role in RSD.[43] These stresses range from academic difficulties to physical abuse and include family conflicts such as parental separation and life-threatening illness in a sibling.

- The cultural background of the patient must be considered as the expression of pain includes psychosocial and cultural factors.[57]

## Investigations

### Blood tests

No tests are pathognomonic of RSD but it is not unusual to find hyper-triglyceridaemia, hypercholesterolaemia[51] or diabetes mellitus.[58] The use of full blood count, erythrocyte sedimentation rate and antibody screens is to exclude other disease states.

### Radiology

Radiological changes are not pathognomonic but do aid diagnosis. A semi-quantitative scoring system has been devised for RSD.[59]

- Diffuse soft-tissue swelling occurs in up to 90% of patients.
- In the acute stage, X-rays help little.[51]
- Osteoporosis develops in the dystrophic stage and progresses from patchy to diffuse.[58] It occurs within the area of RSD and is often in the epiphysial regions of small bones in the hand or foot.
- Similar changes occur in conditions with high bone turnover, such as thyrotoxicosis or following immobilization.

### Nuclear medicines[60]

Technetium ($^{99m}$Tc) scanning is of benefit in diagnosing RSD.[51] Phase 1 angiograms and phase 2 blood pool images are positive in 45% and 52% of patients. Delayed phase 3 scans (obtained 3–4 h later) showing diffuse regional uptake have over 80% sensitivity and specificity for RSD.[61]

- Early cases require a delayed scan only, show areas of multiple periarticular uptake[62] and sometimes occur before the clinical syndrome is evident.[63]
- One study suggests an increase in blood flow and volume during the acute stage with a decrease in the atrophic stage.[64] This has important implications when considering vasoactive treatments, e.g. calcitonin (vasoconstrictive) or guanethidine (vasodilating).
- In children decreased blood flow is more common in the early phase scan with soft tissue rather than bone uptake in the late one.[33]

### Thermography

This technique aids diagnosis,[65] and allows the course of disease and the effect of treatment to be monitored.[51] The equipment is expensive and not universally available.

- Diffuse temperature changes (increased or decreased) occur between the affected and normal limb.[10] Differences of 1°C or more are considered significant.[66]
- Thermographic differences may occur before cutaneous changes are evident, allowing an early diagnosis to be made[66] and disappear with resolution of the syndrome.[67]

## Pressure pain thresholds[68]

Pain pressure thresholds can be measured using a dolorimeter. The ratio between the affected and unaffected side helps diagnose early RSD.

Several readings are used and the average taken to calculate the ratio. When coupled with the clinical findings, ratios below 0.77 are suggestive of RSD.

## Intravenous phentolamine test[36,69,70]

There are good correlations between phentolamine ($\alpha$-adrenergic antagonist) test analgesia and sympathetic ganglion block. Patient acceptability is high with few side-effects. It allows those with sympathetically independent pain and placebo responders to be identified. Pain involving more than one limb or non-peripheral sites can be assessed simultaneously. Any therapeutic use for the test has yet to be elucidated.

- The patient lies supine with non-invasive blood pressure and electrocardiographic monitoring.
- An intravenous infusion is started and pain scores (visual analogue scores both with and without stimulus) monitored until a stable baseline is achieved (some patients respond to the infusion alone).
- Fluid loading with 3–500 ml N/saline followed at 2 ml/kg per h and pretreatment with 2 mg intravenous propranolol counters the effect of the phentolamine.
- Following a stable baseline, 35 mg of phentolamine is infused over 20 min. The patient should be blinded to the phentolamine administration for the best results. Sensory testing continues at 5-min intervals for a minimum of 30 min after infusion.
- A fall in pain score of 50% or more is considered significant.

## Differential nerve blockade[53]

- Initially a sympathetic block is performed (e.g. stellate ganglion block for the upper limb).
- If this fails then an appropriate peripheral nerve block is performed (e.g. axillary plexus block).
- If pain persists despite adequate blockade then a diagnosis of a central pain can be made.
- This assists with management planning in difficult cases.

### Doppler flow monitoring[71]

This technique helps confirm the effectiveness of sympathetic blockade, particularly if the procedure is performed under sedation or general anaesthesia. Increases in blood flow are detected within minutes of the block.

## Management

RSD is a complex condition with both physical and psychological elements. Many treatments are available. They should be aimed at restoration of function, relief of pain and provide psychological support. Active patient participation[57] is important and a multiple modality team approach often provides the best management.[72]

Attempting to prevent the development of RSD is important[73] and requires early treatment at the site of injury (including debridement, removal of foreign material, stabilization of fractures, surgical correction where required and treatment of infection), adequate analgesia (nerve blocks may provide analgesia and sympathetic block, so increasing blood flow), early mobilization and psychological support. Alternatively early diagnosis and treatment are required to break the cycle and halt its centralization.[74]

The most successful treatments involve blocking the effects of the sympathetic nervous system coupled with improving mobility via physiotherapy. Objective measures of progress can be helpful. Correlations have been demonstrated between visual analogue pain scales and limb volumes, active range of motion assessment (AROM) and the McGill pain questionnaire with joint pain indices.[75]

### Physiotherapy

- Physiotherapy is important in the treatment of RSD,[76] aims to maximize mobility and may be effective on its own.[53]
- Pain should be minimal; neural blockade often helps by allowing pain-free therapy, improved mobility, reduced anxiety and increased patient confidence. Injecting associated myofascial trigger points is often beneficial.

**Table 4.3 Treatment planning**

| Acute | Dystrophic | Atrophic |
|-------|------------|----------|
|  | Physical therapy | Aggressive rehabilitation |
|  | Tricyclic antidepressants | Psychological support |
|  | Transcutaneous electrical nerve stimulation | Tricyclic antidepressants |
|  | Sympathetic block | ?Sympathetic block |
|  | Psychological support | Systemic drugs |
|  | Conduction blocks | Behaviour management |
|  | Systemic drugs |  |
|  | Occupational therapy | Neurostimulation |
|  |  | Spinal opioids |
|  | Neuroaugmentation | Tendon lengthening |

Modified from Stanton-Hicks et al.[105]

- An exercise programme is essential for the best results and should include home activities.[77]
- Modalities include stress-loading, active and passive movement, muscle stimulation and pool therapy. The simultaneous use of transcutaneous electrical nerve stimulation (TENS) may help the therapist restore function.[77]

## TENS

- TENS provides analgesia of varying duration. Coupled with physiotherapy it provides good relief, especially in children.[78]
- TENS is easily taught to patients, is non-invasive, inexpensive and allows improved compliance with home exercise programmes.
- Despite an unknown mechanism of action, the best results occur in patients with a vasodilatory element to their SMP;[77] occasionally the pain is exacerbated.[9]

### Psychological therapies

- Psychological and psychiatric factors may have a role in the causation or maintenance of RSD. Patients who fail standard treatment should be considered for evaluation and management. This may prevent unnecessary treatments and the potential negative effects they have.[43]
- Care is required when suggesting a psychological assessment as patients may consider this an accusation of psychiatric disease.
- Similarly, caution is required when confronting patients to inform them that they have psychological problems. They often require an 'honourable exit' to avoid feeling trapped and having to admit to a psychological disturbance.[57]
- Reassuring patients and maintaining their motivation plays a significant role when treating many conditions. Anxiety exacerbates RSD and measures to reduce it are important in management.[51]
- If patients require admission to hospital it is important that they have a structured programme to minimize reinforcement of the 'sick role'. This includes the wearing of normal street clothes and a schedule of activities to encourage normal living.[9] This is often best achieved if the same ward and staff are used.
- Other family members may require counselling.
- Biofeedback has been used successfully[79] but not in large-scale studies. Patient improvements also occur when biofeedback is coupled to other treatment modalities,[77] including relaxation training.[80]
- Secondary gain may influence the response to treatment.[72]

### Sympathetic blockade

- Sympathetic blockade provides analgesia of varying duration and repeat blocks or a course are often necessary. How many constitute a course is undetermined; some suggest up to 15 whilst others limit the number to three or four.[76]

- This modality is beneficial after a short trial of non-invasive management has objectively been shown to fail.
- Reports suggest complete recovery in up to 80% treated with sympathetic blocks within 1 month of onset of symptoms and 75% if within 6 months.[81]
- Occasionally treatment failure is due to bilateral sympathetic innervation. It is then necessary to repeat the block on the contralateral side.[82]

### Regional sympathetic blocks (stellate for upper limb and lumbar for lower)[73]

- Characteristically the effect outlasts the duration of local anesthetic by hours or days. Ideally blocks are repeated as soon as possible after the effect wears off.
- The onset of the block is usually rapid, with warmth of the limb and reduction in pain. Reduced oedema follows hours later and function improves in days.
- Lumbar sympathetic blocks should be done with the aid of fluoroscopy.
- Sensory testing allows the most proximal level of sympathetic involvement to be assessed; this corresponds to the level of block required.[76]

### Intravenous regional blockade (IVRB); guanethidine, reserpine or bretyllum

IVRBs involve the administration of an active pharmacological agent with 0.5% prilocaine to reduce the pain of injection. The volumes used range from 40 to 60 ml depending on the extremity to be blocked and the patient characteristics. The tourniquet is kept inflated for 20 min after injection of the agent to minimize the risk of systemic effects. Some authors have noted a tourniquet effect and question the value of the pharmacological agents.[83]

The main advantages of IVRBs occur when disease prevents nerve blocks, in patients who refuse nerve blocks and when weaning patient from nerve blocks.[84]

Both qualitative and quantitative improvements occur,[85] with the duration of analgesia between treatments increasing.[86]

- Guanethidine: Intravenous block (guanethidine 20–30 mg, usually with 40–60 ml 0.5% prilocaine) produces skin temperature changes lasting approximately 3 days and pain relief of greater duration (days to weeks).[87] Side-effects may prevent or interrupt treatment; they increase with age and include orthostatic hypotension and thrombophlebitis.[88]
- Bretylium[89,90] in doses of 1.5 mg/kg in 0.5% prilocaine (40–60 ml) has provided significant analgesia for 20 days in patients who received less than a week's relief from stellate or lumbar sympathetic block. The mechanism of action is similar to guanethidine by inhibiting noradrenaline release from adrenergic nerve endings. Side-effects are initially hypertension and tachycardia (from noradrenaline release) followed by orthostatic hypotension. This can be minimized by fluid loading before tourniquet release and by maintaining a recumbent position for an hour afterwards.

- Reserpine[86] 1.25 mg with prilocaine has a similar effect to guanethidine. Side-effects include diarrhoea, syncope and depression.[90]
- Other drugs: Recent case reports show that IVRBs using 60 mg of ketorolac in a total volume of 40 ml provides analgesia of several days' duration. Repeat blocks may also extend the duration of analgesia.[91] Controlled trials have yet to be carried out. Methylprednisolone 80 mg with lignocaine produces a good immediate response which is maintained at long-term follow-up.[92]

## Drug treatment

- Antidepressants (amitriptyline, doxepin, desipramine) are of benefit to those who show signs of depression, poor mood, sleep disturbance or unremitting severe pain.[9] Dosage for adults is 10–100 mg at night and in children 0.1–1 mg/kg starting at low dose.
- Anticonvulsant drugs (carbamazepine, valproate, phenytoin) sometimes help chronic sufferers and are of benefit for shooting stabbing pain. Often helpful in treating postsympathectomy pain.
- Calcitonin is used to stop the osteoporosis of RSD.[93] Patients with vasodilatory disease treated with calcitonin show a significant decrease in flows towards normal on technetium scanning.[64] Intramuscular doses of 100 units combined with physiotherapy significantly improve patients' chances of returning to work.[94] The long-term effect of calcitonin is unknown.
- Steroids[62] – dose regimens vary. Some start with prednisolone 20–30 mg daily and taper over a period of weeks; others use a large initial dose (prednisolone 60–80 mg) for 2–3 days then taper by 20 mg/day to 5 mg for several weeks. Use in children has not shown clear benefits and steroids should therefore be avoided in this group.[9]
- Opioids are occasionally required in the acute stage or in managing acute exacerbations. Chronically they are of little benefit and the smallest effective dose should be used. Epidural or intrathecal use may have a role. Their use remains controversial.
- Non-steroidal anti-inflammatory drugs may help on their own or for their opioid-sparing effect.[26]
- $\alpha_1$-Blockers (phenoxybenzamine, prazosin) have been effective in some patients. Phenoxybenzamine in doses of 40–120 mg/day may provide prolonged analgesia[95] and prazosin may also be beneficial.[96]
- Nifedipine[97] may be effective in doses from 10 to 30 mg t.d.s.
- Propranolol has been used in doses up to 320 mg/day with some benefit.[6] One double-blind cross-over trial showed no benefit.[98]
- Transdermal clonidine[36] causes local analgesia under the patch. This may be a useful treatment for small areas of RSD.
- Transdermal nitroglycerine applied over the primary arterial supply may improve RSD of a vasoconstrictive nature.[25]
- Topical capsaicin has provided temporary analgesia to areas of RSD and probably works by reducing or preventing an increase in substance P in the peripheral sensory nerves.[99]

## Neuroaugmentation

### Infusion techniques

- These prolong the period of analgesia, allow intensive physiotherapy, permit desensitization of central pathways and minimize the number of injections.[9]
- Techniques include epidurals,[18] nerve plexus,[100] paravertebral, pleural[101] and continuous stellate.[102]
- Inpatient bupivacaine epidural infusions provide excellent analgesia and allow continuous passive motion of the affected limb which is swapped to an opioid epidural to allow increased patient mobility.[103] Low-dose local anaesthetic with or without opioid allows the patient to ambulate. If urinary retention occurs, the infusion can be stopped for a few hours several times a day to avoid the need for catheterization.[9]
- With outpatient infusions the patients, helpers and medical staff have to evaluate the benefits against the logistical difficulties such as infection control, filling and maintaining pumps.
- Implanted pumps become cost-effective at approximately 3 months; otherwise external pumps are cheaper.
- Tolerance may develop but can be overcome by having a drug holiday for 1–3 months, during which a different opioid can be used (e.g. sufentanyl for morphine).

### Dorsal column stimulation

This technique may help when conservative management fails to provide lasting results. Greatest benefit occurs if the pain is in an area of a major peripheral nerve. Implantation involves a two-stage surgical procedure; first a temporary wire is positioned and attached to an external generating box. If this provides satisfactory clinical relief the second stage is to implant a permanent electrode and tunnel it to a subcutaneous generator.

One centre noted that the first stage may be poorly tolerated and some patients require a second electrode. Patients commented on good control for allodynia and hyperaesthesia but only minor improvement with persistent pain. Others have demonstrated significant improvements in pain.[104] The commonest complications were electrode movement, haematoma, temporary nerve palsies and scar formation around the electrodes.[105]

## Neuroablative procedures

Consensus suggests that neuroablative techniques should be reserved for situations where more conservative therapy has failed to maintain control. There must be a history of successful sympathetic blockade with local anaesthetic.[6]

Some suggest considering patients for neuroablative procedures if four blocks have provided some reduction in pain but not a cure.[76] Patients need to be well-motivated and to continue with the other modalities after the procedure. One study suggests that a small minority of cases required this type of therapy.[9]

- Radiofrequency sympathectomies[106] can be performed on a day-case basis and avoid the complications of open surgery. It has been shown to be safe but has not gained in popularity.
- Neurolytic sympathectomy[107]: phenol 7–10% or alcohol 50–100% may be used, having first confirmed needle placement with contrast media. The current feeling is that phenol does not provide permanent relief; recurrence occurs in up to 30% of patients but is often less severe than the original pain. Postsympathectomy neuralgia occurs in 20–40% of cases, starts 10–14 days after the procedure and usually resolves spontaneously during the following weeks. The pain is localized to the area of denervation, is described as dull and boring but occasionally sharp. It occurs more commonly with lumbar sympathectomy[106] Permanent damage to adjacent structures can occur.
- Surgery should be reserved for that group of patients who have only temporary relief following a significant period of intensive conservative therapy (3–6 months). The clinician must be sure of the diagnosis as most failures are considered to be due to incorrect diagnosis or inadequate sympathectomy. In one series[108] following surgical sympathectomy, over 90% had their pain reduced by 50% or more. The best results were in those patients with less severe disease of shorter duration. The more extensive the sympathectomy, the better the results. Only 3 patients were able to return to their full-time activities.

    With the arrival of minimally invasive surgery a series of patients have now undergone thoracoscopic ganglionectomy with patient satisfaction rates of up to 62%.[109]

    Surgery is occasionally indicated to release long-standing irreversible contractures.[74]

    Surgical ablative procedures including dorsal root entry zone lesions, rhizotomy, chordotomy, thalamotomy and excision of cortical structures have not proved to be of long-term benefit.

    On very rare occasions with severe disease, limb amputation has been the only treatment available.[23] Amputation is neither standard treatment nor is it always successful in relieving the pain.

### Management of motor abnormalities

The majority of patients with motor disturbances and RSD obtain some relief with sympathetic blockade or sympathectomy. Spasms may be treated with benzodiazepines or baclofen in doses of 90–120 mg/day.[40] Limitation of shoulder movement frequently accompanies upper limb RSD[10] and may be treated by suprascapular nerve block. Other treatments for RSD appear to have little effect on the motor disturbances.

## Outcome

- The condition may be self-limiting but many cases persist for years.[54] Long-term studies suggest that 25–40% of patients still have features of RSD at 10-year follow-up.[110]

- The overall morbidity for pain clinic referrals suggests that 60% have residual symptoms and only 1 in 5 patients are able to resume prior activity at 18-month follow-up.[16] The morbidity for non-responders to treatment is significant.[108]
- No outcome figures are available for patient recovery in the general population. The incidence following tibial fracture was reported at 30% and most cases had resolved by 6-month follow-up.[13]
- In paediatric populations 94% reported their schoolwork had suffered and only 46% were symptom-free at follow-up (median 3 years).[9]

## Conclusions

- RSD causes a spectrum of disability from the self-limiting to the irreversible and permanently debilitating.
- RSD is not rare and is probably underdiagnosed in both adult and paediatric populations.
- Management requires early recognition with aggressive treatment, including analgesia, physiotherapy and measures to avoid pain behaviour patterns developing.
- No single treatment modality is effective. Many patients will respond to treatment; not all will be cured but efforts have to be made to palliate their distress.

## References

1. Mitchell SW, Morehouse GR, Keen WW. *Gunshot Wounds and Other Injuries of Nerves*. Philadelphia: JB Lippincott, 1864, p. 164
2. Sudeck P. Uber die akute enzundiche Knochenatrophie. *Arch Klin Chir* **62:** 147, 1900
3. Livingston WK. Post-traumatic pain syndromes. *West J Surg Obstet Gynecol* **46:** 341, 1938
4. Homans J. Minor causalgia. *N Engl J Med* **222:** 870–874, 1940
5. Evans JA. Reflex sympathetic dystrophy. *Surg Gynecol Obstet* **82:** 36–43, 1946
6. Payne R. Neuropathic pain syndromes, with special reference to causalgia and reflex sympathetic dystrophy. *Clin J Pain* **2:** 59–73, 1986
7. Moesker A, Boersma FP, Schijgrond HW, Cortvriendt W. Treatment of posttraumatic sympathetic dystrophy (Sudeck's atrophy) with guanethidine and ketanserin. *Pain Clinic* **1:** 171–176, 1985
8. Merskey H, Bogduk N (eds) Classification of Chronic Pain, 2nd edn. Seattle: IASP Press, 1994
9. Wilder RT, Berde CB, Wolohan M, Vieyra MA, Masek BJ, Micheli LJ. Reflex sympathetic dystrophy in children. Clinical characteristics and follow-up of 70 patients. *J Bone Joint Surg – Am Vol* **74:** 910–919, 1992
10. Veldman PHM, Reynen HM, Amtz IE, Goris RJA. Signs and symptoms of reflex sympathetic dystrophy: prospective study of 829 patients. *Lancet* **342:** 1012–1016, 1993
11. Atkins RM, Duckworth T, Kanis JA. Algodystrophy following Colies' fracture. *J Hand Surg – Br Vol* **14:** 161–164, 1989
12. Poole C. Colles' fracture: a prospective study of treatment. *J Bone Joint Surg – Br Vol* **55-B:** 540–544, 1973

13. Sarangi PP, Ward AJ, Smith EJ, Staddon GE, Atkins RM. Algodystrophy and osteo-porosis after tibial fractures. *J Bone Joint Surg – Br Vol* **75:** 450–452, 1993

14. Gellman H, Keenan MA, Stone L, Hardy SE, Waters RL, Stewart C. Reflex sympathetic dystrophy in brain-injured patients. *Pain* **51:** 307–311, 1992

15. Omer GC, Thomas MS. Treatment of causalgia. *Tex Med* **67:** 93–96, 1971

16. Subarrao J, Stillwell GK. Reflex sympathetic dystrophy syndrome of the upper extremity: analysis of total outcome of management of 125 cases. *Arch Phys Med Rehab* **62:** 549–554, 1981

17. Sachs BL, Zindrick MR, Beasley RD. Reflex sympathetic dystrophy after operative procedures on the lumbar spine. *J Bone Joint Surg – Am Vol* **75:** 721–725, 1993

18. Finsterbush A, Frankl U, Mann G, Lowe J. Reflex sympathetic dystrophy of the patello-femoral joint. *Orthop Rev* **20:** 877–885, 1991

19. Brock TR. Reflex sympathetic dystrophy linked to venipuncture: a case report. *J Oral Maxillofac Surg* **47:** 1333–1335, 1989

20. Foster O, Askaria A, Lanham J, Perry D. Algoneurodystrophy following herpes zoster. *Postgrad Med J* **65:** 478–480, 1989

21. Olson WL. Reflex sympathetic dystrophy associated with tumor infiltration of the stellate ganglion. *J R Soc Med* **86:** 482, 1993

22. Coughlan RJ, Hazleman BL, Crisp AJ, Jenner JR, Thomas DP. Algodystrophy in preg-nancy. Three case reports. *Br J Obstet Gynaecol* **95:** 935–937, 1988

23. Erdmann MW, Wynn-Jones CH. 'Familial' reflex sympathetic dystrophy syndrome and amputation. *Br J Accident Surg* **23:** 136–138, 1992

24. Munoz-Gomez J, Collado A, Gratacos J, *et al.* Reflex sympathetic dystrophy syndrome of the lower limbs in renal transplant patients treated with cyclosporin A. *Arthritis Rheum* **34:** 625–630, 1991

25. Chester MH. Segmental manifestation of reflex sympathetic dystrophy syndrome limited to one finger. *Anesthesiology* **73:** 558–561, 1990

26. Barrera P, van Riel PL, de Jong AJ, Boerbooms AM, Van de Putte LB. Recurrent and migratory reflex sympathetic dystrophy syndrome. *Clin Rheumatol* **11:** 416–421, 1992

27. Karras D, Karargiris G, Vassilopoulos D, Karatzetzos C. Reflex sympathetic dystrophy syndrome and osteogenesis imperfecta. A report and review of the literature. *J Rheumatol* **20:** 162–164, 1993

28. Galloway NT, Gabale DR, Irwin PP. Interstitial cystitis or redex sympathetic dystrophy of the bladder? *Semin Urol* **9:** 148–153, 1991

29. Roig-Escofet D, Rodriguez-Moreno J, Ruiz Martin JM. Concept and limits of the reflex sympathetic dystrophy. *Clin Rheumatol* **8**(suppl 2): 104–108, 1989

30. Drummond PD, Pinch PM, Smythe GA. Reflex sympathetic dystrophy: the significance of differing plasma catecholamine concentrations in affected and unaffected limbs. *Brain* **114:** 2025–2036, 1991

31. Hanna MH, Feat SJ. Ketanserin in reflex sympathetic dystrophy. A double-blind placebo controlled cross-over trial. *Pain* **38:** 145–150, 1989

32. Bej MD, Schwartzman RJ. Abnormalities of cutaneous blood flow regulation in patients with reflex sympathetic dystrophy as measured by laser Doppler fluxmetry. *Arch Neurol* **48:** 912–915, 1991

33. Silber TJ, Majd M. Reflex sympathetic dystrophy syndrome in children and adolescents. Report of 18 cases and review of the literature. *Am J Dis Child* **142:** 1325–1330, 1988

34. Janig W. Can reflex sympathetic dystrophy be reduced to an alpha-adrenoreceptor disease? *APS J* **1:** 1622, 1992

35. Heerschap A, den Hollander JA, Reynen H, Goris RJ. Metabolic changes in reflex sympathetic dystrophy: a $^{31}$P NMR spectroscopy study. *Muscle Nerve* **16:** 367–373, 1993

36. Campbell JN, Meyer RA, Raja SN. Is nociceptor activation by alpha-1 adrenoreceptors the culprit in sympathetically maintained pain? *APS J* **1:** 3–11, 1992

37. Roberts WJ, Kramis RC. Adrenergic mediation of SMP: via nociceptive or non-nociceptive afferents or both? *APS J* **1:** 12–15, 1992

38. Asenjo F, Blaise G. Sympathetic dystrophy: new name, new concepts, new treatment? *Anesth Analg* **75:** 633, 1992
39. Sato J, Perl ER. Adrenergic excitation of cutaneous pain receptors induced by peripheral nerve injury. *Science* **251:** 1608–1610, 1991
40. Schwartzman RJ, Kerrigan J. The movement disorder of reflex sympathetic dystrophy. *Neurology* **40:** 57–61, 1990
41. Roberts WJ. A hypothesis on the physiological basis for causalgia and related pains. *Pain* **24:** 297–311, 1986
42. Gracely RH, Lynch SA, Bennett GJ. Painful neuropathy: altered central processing maintained dynamically by peripheral input. [Published erratum appears in *Pain* **52:** 251–253, 1993.] *Pain* **51:** 175–194, 1992
43. Bruehl S, Carlson CR. Predisposing psychological factors in the development of reflex sympathetic dystrophy. A review of the empirical evidence. *Clin J Pain* **8:** 287–299, 1992
44. Van Houdenhove B, Vasquez G, Onghena P, *et al.* Etiopathogenesis of reflex sympathetic dystrophy: a review and biopsychosocial hypothesis. *Clin J Pain* **8:** 300–306, 1992
45. Ochoa JL. Reflex sympathetic dystrophy: a disease of medical understanding. *Clin J Pain* **8:** 363–366, 1992
46. Janig W. Comment on: Reflex sympathetic dystrophy: a disease of medical understanding. *Clin J Pain* **8:** 367–369, 1992
47. Amadio PC, Mackinnon SE, Merritt WH, Brody GS, Terzis JK. Reflex sympathetic dystrophy syndrome: consensus report of an ad hoc committee of the American Association for Hand Surgery on the definition of reflex sympathetic dystrophy syndrome. *Plast Reconstruct Surg* **87:** 371–375, 1991
48. Bonica JJ. Causalgia and other reflex sympathetic dystrophies. In: (Bonica JJ, Liebsekind JC, Able-Fessard DG, eds) *Advances in Pain Research and Therapy*, vol 3. New York: Raven Press, 1979, pp. 141–166.
49. Steinbrocker O. The shoulder–hand syndrome. Associated painful homolateral disability of the shoulder and hand with swelling and atrophy of the hand. *Am J Med* **3:** 402–407, 1947
50. Gibbons JJ, Wilson PR. RSD score: criteria for the diagnosis of reflex sympathetic dystrophy and causalgia. *Clin J Pain* **8:** 260–263, 1992
51. Rothschild B. Reflex sympathetic dystrophy. *Arthritis Care Res* **3:** 140–153, 1990
52. Steinbrocker O, Argyros TG. The shoulder hand syndrome: present status as a diagnostic and therapeutic entity. *Med Clin North Am* **42:** 1533–1553, 1958
53. Schwartzman RJ, McLellan TL. Reflex sympathetic dystrophy. A review. *Arch Neurol* **44:** 555–561, 1987
54. Mayfield FH. Causalgia. American lecture series No: 58. Springfield, Ill. Charles CT Thomas, 1951
55. Deuschl G, Blumberg H, Lucking CH. Tremor in reflex sympathetic dystrophy. *Arch Neurol* **48:** 1247–1252, 1991
56. Webster GF, Schwartzman RJ, Jacoby RA, Knobler RL, Uitto JJ. Reflex sympathetic dystrophy. Occurrence of inflammatory skin lesions in patients with stages II and III disease. *Arch Dermatol* **127:** 1541–1544, 1991
57. Amadio PC. Pain dysfunction syndromes. *J Bone Joint Surg – Am Vol* **70:** 944–949, 1988
58. Chard MD. Diagnosis and management of algodystrophy. *Ann Rheum Dis* **50:** 727–730, 1991
59. Bickerstaff DR, O'Doherty DP, Kanis JA. Radiographic changes in algodystrophy of the hand. *J Hand Surg – Br Vol* **16:** 47–52, 1991
60. Werner R, Davidoff G, Jackson MD, Cremer S, Ventocilla C, Wolf L. Factors affecting the sensitivity and specificity of the three-phase technetium bone scan in the diagnosis of reflex sympathetic dystrophy syndrome in the upper extremity. *J Hand Surg – Am Vol* **14:** 520–523, 1989
61. Holder LE, Cole LA, Myerson MS. Reflex sympathetic dystrophy in the foot: clinical and scintigraphic criteria. *Radiology* **184:** 531–535, 1992

62. Fano N, Helm C. Bone scintigraphy in post-traumatic reflex dystrophy. *Scand J Rheumatol* **17**: 455–458, 1988

63. Weiss L, Alfano A, Bardfeld P, Weiss J, Friedmann LW. Prognostic value of triple phase bone scanning for reflex sympathetic dystrophy in hemiplegia. *Arch Phys Med Rehab* **74**: 716–719, 1993

64. Blockx P, Driessens M. The use of $^{99}$Tcm-HSA dynamic vascular examination in the staging and therapy monitoring of reflex sympathetic dystrophy. *Nuclear Med Commun* **12**: 725–731, 1991

65. Cooke ED, Glick EN, Bowcock SA *et al*. Reflex sympathetic dystrophy (algoneurodystrophy): temperature studies in the upper limb. *Br J Rheumatol* **28**: 399–403, 1989

66. Pochaczevsky R. Thermography in posttraumatic pain. *Am J Sports Med* **15**: 243–250, 1987

67. Coughlan RJ, Hazleman BL, Thomas DP *et al*. Algodystrophy: a common unrecognized cause of chronic knee pain. *Br J Rheumatol* **26**: 270–274, 1987

68. Bryan AS, Klenerman L, Bowsher D. The diagnosis of reflex sympathetic dystrophy using an algometer. *J Bone Joint Surg – Br Vol* **73**: 644–646, 1991

69. Raja SN, Treede R-D, Davis KD, Campbell JN. Systemic alpha-adrenergic blockade with phentolamine: a diagnostic test for sympathetically maintained pain. *Anesthesiology* **74**: 691–698, 1991

70. Arner S. Intravenous phentolamine test: diagnostic and prognostic use in reflex sympathetic dystrophy. *Pain* **46**: 17–22, 1991

71. Irazuzta JE, Berde CB, Sethna NF. Laser Doppler measurements of skin blood flow before, during, and after lumbar sympathetic blockade in children and young adults with reflex sympathetic dystrophy syndrome. *J Clin Monit* **8**: 16–19, 1992

72. Lebovits AH, Yarmush J, Lefkowitz M. Reflex sympathetic dystrophy and posttraumatic stress disorder. Multidisciplinary evaluation and treatment. *Clin J Pain* **6**: 153–157, 1990

73. Bonica JJ. Causalgia and other reflex sympathetic dystrophies. In Bonica JJ (ed) *The Management of Pain*, vol 1. 2nd edn. Philadelphia: Lea & Febiger, 1990, pp. 220–243

74. Adebajo AO, Hazleman BL. Shoulder pain and reflex sympathetic dystrophy. *Curr Opin Rheumatol* **2**: 270–275, 1990

75. Davidoff G, Morey K, Amann M, Stamps J. Pain measurement in reflex sympathetic dystrophy syndrome. *Pain* **32**: 27–34, 1988

76. Schutzer SF, Gossling HR. Current concepts review. The treatment of reflex sympathetic dystrophy syndrome. *J Bone Joint Surg – Am Vol* **A-66**: 625–629, 1984

77. Headley B. Historical perspective of causalgia. Management of sympathetically maintained pain. *Phys Ther* **67**: 1370–1374, 1987

78. Kesler RW, Saulsbury FT, Miller LT, Rowlingson JC. Reflex sympathetic dystrophy in children: treatment with transcutaneous electric nerve stimulation. *Pediatrics* **82**: 728–732, 1988

79. Barowsky EI, Zweig JB, Moskowitz J. Thermal biofeedback in the treatment of symptoms associated with reflex sympathetic dystrophy. *J Child Neurol* **2**: 229–232, 1987

80. Grunert BK, Devine CA, Sanger JR, Matloub HS, Green D. Thermal self-regulation for pain control in reflex sympathetic dystrophy syndrome. *J Hand Surg – Am Vol* **15**: 615–618, 1990

81. Wang JK, Erickson RP, Ilstrup DM. Repeated stellate ganglion blocks for upper extremity reflex sympathetic dystrophy. *Reg. Anesth* **10**: 125, 1985

82. Munn JS, Baker WH. Recurrent sympathetic dystrophy: successful treatment by contralateral sympathectomy. *Surgery* **102**: 102–105, 1987

83. Blanchard J, Ramamurthy S, Walsh N, Hoffman J, Schoenfeld L. Intravenous regional sympatholysis: a double-blind comparison of guanethidine, reserpine, and normal saline. *J Pain Symptom Manage* **5**: 357–361, 1990

84. Ford SR, Johnston R. Intravenous guanethidine and reserpine in reflex sympathetic dystrophy. *Clin J Pain* **6**: 159, 1990

85. Field J, Monk C, Atkins RM. Objective improvements in algodystrophy following regional intravenous guanethidine. *J Hand Surg – Br Vol* **18:** 339–342, 1993

86. Rocco AG, Kaul AF, Reisman RM, Gallo JP, Lief PA. A comparison of regional intravenous guanethidine and reserpine in reflex sympathetic dystrophy. A controlled, randomized, double-blind crossover study. *Clin J Pain* **5:** 205–209, 1989

87. Hannington-Kiff JG. Pharmacological target blocks in hand surgery and rehabilitation. *J Hand Surg – Br Vol* **9:** 29–36, 1984

88. Eulry F, Lechevalier D, Fats B *et al.* Regional intravenous guanethidine blocks in algodystrophy. *Clin Rheumatol* **10:** 377–383, 1991

89. Hord AH, Rooks MD, Stephens BO, Rogers HG, Fleming LL. Intravenous regional bretylium and lidocaine for treatment of reflex sympathetic dystrophy: a randomized, double-blind study. *Anesth Analg* **74:** 818–821, 1992

90. Ford SR, Forrest WH, Eltherington L. The treatment of reflex sympathetic dystrophy with intravenous regional bretylium. *Anesthesiology* **68:** 137–140, 1988

91. Vanes DN, Ramamurthy S, Hoffman J. Intravenous regional block using ketorolac: preliminary results in the treatment of reflex sympathetic dystrophy. *Anesth Analg* **74:** 139–141, 1992

92. Tountas AA, Noguchi A. Treatment of posttraumatic reflex sympathetic dystrophy syndrome (RSDS) with intravenous blocks of a mixture of corticosteroid and lidocaine: a retrospective review of 17 consecutive cases. *J Orthop Trauma* **5:** 412–419, 1991

93. Lechevalier D, Crozes P, Thomachot B *et al.* Influence of calcitonin treatment on the osteocalcin concentration in the algodystrophy of bone. *Clin Rheumatol* **11:** 346–350, 1992

94. Gobelet C, Waldburger M, Meier JL. The effect of adding calcitonin to physical treatment on reflex sympathetic dystrophy. *Pain* **48:** 171–175, 1992

95. Ghostine SY, Comair YG, Turner DM *et al.* Phenoxybenzamine in the treatment of causalgia. *J Neurosurg* **60:** 1263–1268, 1984

96. Abram SE, Lightfoot RW. Treatment of long-standing causalgia with prazosin. *Reg Anesth* **6:** 79–81, 1981

97. Prough DS, McLeskey CH, Poehling GG *et al.* Efficacy of oral nifedipine in the treatment of reflex sympathetic dystrophy. *Anesthesiology* **62:** 796–799, 1985

98. Scadding JW, Wall PD, Parry CBW, Brook DM. Clinical trial of propranolol in post-traumatic neuralgia. *Pain* **14:** 283–292, 1982

99. Cheshire WP, Snyder CR. Treatment of reflex sympathetic dystrophy with topical capsaicin. *Pain* **42:** 307–311, 1990

100. Klein DS, Klein PW. Low-volume ulnar nerve block within the axillary sheath for the treatment of reflex sympathetic dystrophy. *Can J Anaesth* **38:** 764–766, 1991

101. Reiestad F, McIlvaine WB, Kvalheim L, Stokke T, Pettersen B. Interpleural analgesia in treatment of upper extremity reflex sympathetic dystrophy. *Anesth Analg* **69:** 671–673, 1989

102. Owen-Falkenberg A, Olsen KS. Continuous stellate ganglion blockade for reflex sympathetic dystrophy. *Anesth Analg* **75:** 1041–1042, 1992

103. Cooper DE, DeLee JC, Ramamurthy S. Reflex sympathetic dystrophy of the knee. Treatment using continuous epidural anesthesia. *J Bone Joint Surg – Am Vol* **71:** 365–369, 1989

104. Robaina FJ, Dominguez M, Diaz M, Rodriguez JL, de Vera JA. Spinal cord stimulation for relief of chronic pain in vasospastic disorders of the upper limbs. *Neurosurgery* **24:** 63–67, 1989

105. Stanton-Hicks M, Campbell JN, Hassenbusch SJ. Update on sympathetically mediated pain. American Pain Society 11th Annual Scientific Meeting. October 1992, San Diego

106. Wilkinson HA. Percutaneous radiofrequency upper thoracic sympathectomy: a new technique. *Neurosurgery* **15:** 811–814, 1984

107. Ogawa S. Sympathectomy with neurolytics. In: (Hyodo M, Oyama T, Swerdlow M, eds) *The Pain Clinic IV*. Utrecht: VSP Publishers, 1992, pp. 139–146

108. Olcott C 4th, Eltherington LG, Wilcosky BR, Shoor PM, Zimmerman JJ, Fogarty TJ. Reflex sympathetic dystrophy – the surgeon's role in management. *J Vase Surg* **14:** 488–492; discussion 492–495, 1991

109. Robertson DP, Simpson RK, Rose JE, Garza JS. Video-assisted endoscopic thoracic ganglionectomy. *J Neurosurg* **79:** 238–240, 1993

110. Field J, Warwick D, Bannister GC, Gibson AG. Long-term prognosis of displaced Colles' fracture: a 10-year prospective review. *Injury; Br J Accident Surg* **23:** 529–532, 1992

# 5

# Neuropathic pain

P. M. Jameson

## Aetiology and incidence

Neuropathic pain is due to injury to the nociceptive pathway. Injury may occur peripherally or centrally and may involve damage to the pain receptors, peripheral nerves, posterior roots, the spinal cord or central regions of the brain. This injury can involve numerous pathological conditions in isolation or in combination, such as infection/inflammation, trauma, ischaemia or degeneration (Table 5.1). The pathological process will cause an altered or reduced sensory state to the affected area with the majority of neuropathic pain states having a peripheral sensory element rather than a visceral element.[1] In short the painful condition is due to a malfunction of the nociceptive pathway, be that peripherally or centrally.

Painful conditions with a neuropathic component are often seen in the pain clinic setting (up to 25% of patients attending pain clinics). It is estimated that there are up to 550 000 patients suffering from neuropathic pain in the UK (incidence of 1% approximately). It appears to be a major problem in the ageing population with up to a third of patients over 60 years and half of those over 70 years attending pain clinics having a neuropathic element to their presenting condition.[2]

Table 5.1 Condition with a neuropathic element

Trigeminal neuralgia
Postherpetic neuralgia
Scar pain
Postsurgical neuroma
Postirradiation neuropathy
Phantom limb pain
Sympathetic pain
Neuropathies (diabetic, ischaemic)
Causalgia
Thalamic/central

## Clinical features

The neuropathic pain state may involve damage to the nociceptive pathway anywhere along its length from the periphery to central regions. The presentation of the pain can be varied but there are certain sensory symptoms that are characteristic of neuropathic pain.

- Allodynia is the sensation of pain caused by a stimulus that would normally not produce pain, for example the light touch of clothing or bedclothes producing a burning sensation.
- Hyperalgesia is the sensation of pain that is of inappropriate severity caused by a noxious stimuli.
- Continuous, spontaneous, paroxysmal pain: Continuous pain is always present, and may be felt as skin sensation such as burning, pricking, stabbing or a deeper musculoskeletal type pain such as a cramping or aching pain. The pain may have a periodic element or involve spontaneous, paroxysmal 'electric shock'-type sensations that may last a few seconds.
- Hyperpathia is the symptom of pain that may be delayed in onset and may only appear after repeated stimulation. The pain may have an increased spatial area and may also have an explosive onset. This may be caused by innocuous or noxious stimuli.
- Pain onset is difficult to predict, due to problems in knowing the precise nature of injury to the nociceptive pathway and to developing changes occurring in the peripheral and central nervous system. The onset of neuropathic pain may be immediate or delayed and the nature may change over time.

## Pathology

Neuropathic pain states are made up of many heterogeneous syndromes that make any one pathological process difficult to understand. But there is a growing understanding through various studies that both peripheral and central nervous tissue injury can lead to painful states with similar characteristics. It may be that a number of these neural tissue injuries may lead to further long-term changes in the nociceptive pathway at higher levels and that a number of interlinked pathological processes may occur in unison. This leads to a complicated picture of multiple pathological processes that may be interlinked in the periphery that may cause further central changes at a spinal or central level.

Before discussing these processes in more depth it should be stated that pain attributed to a neuropathic origin may well be a normal physiological response to nociceptor stimulation that is due to occult tissue damage or a progressive disease process. And therefore other more easily treatable causes of the painful condition must be excluded before a diagnosis of neuropathic pain is made.

It should also be noted that neuropathic pain is never predictable to a pathological condition. The same disease process or injury may cause many varied patterns of neuropathic pain in differing patients or it may leave the patient painfree.

## Peripheral mechanisms

- Abnormal nociceptor sensitization involves an abnormality in the return of normal C-fibre function such that they become sensitized, failing to respond normally, and they may exhibit spontaneous activity and have lower thresholds of activity or have thresholds for endogenous rhythmic firing (forming ectopic neural pacemaker nodules or sites). The C-fibres may become sensitized to respond in an excitatory manner to sympathetic stimulation[1,3] (this may be due to patches of demyelination along the axon),[4] and therefore they may respond to treatment strategies involving manipulation of sympathetic activity.
- Axon sprouts develop when primary afferent neurons are damaged, particularly in complete transection and in partial transection (diabetic neuropathy, die-back metabolic neuropathies, herpes zoster). Neurons sprout in their attempt to regenerate and reinnervate and may form neuromas in continuity. The sprouts or damaged afferents may become sensitive to low-threshold mechanoreceptors and therefore demonstrate abnormal sensitivity to mechanical, noradrenergic, thermal and ionic stimulation. They may also repetitively fire independent of any sensory apparatus, forming ectopic neural pacemaker nodules.[4] This can result in the symptom of allodynia.
- Ephapse formation involves the formation of abnormal electrical connections between adjacent axons, so allowing for a potential ephaptic crosstalk between axons.[5] This may allow mechanoreceptor axons to stimulate the nociceptive pathway.
- Crossed afterdischarge involves the depolaritzation of previously silent neurons by repetitive impulse activity from neighbouring neurons. The exact mechanism is uncertain but it is thought to involve mediation by potassium ions or neurotransmitters and, unlike ephaptic crosstalk, close apposition of adjacent neurons (with an absence of intervening glia) is not essential. It may be that crossed afterdischarge can under certain circumstances be involved in a positive feedback process whereby ever more potassium ions or neurotransmitters are released, leading to a larger number of neurons being stimulated.[4]
- Dorsal root ganglion involvement: The changes and pathological processes involved in peripheral nerves may also occur in the dorsal root ganglion. These may include sprout formation, ephaptic crosstalk and crossed afterdischarge. Also formation of ectopic pacemaker nodules in the injured cells may occur. Changes in the availability of nerve growth factor causing cell death may well be involved in the pathological process.[6]

## Central mechanisms

There are three possible mechanisms of central neuropathic pain that will be discussed. They may well occur in isolation or as a part of a larger process involving each other and some or all of the pathological processes thought to involve the peripheral nervous system.[7]

- Afferent impulses that cause central changes: Changes in the long-term excitability of dorsal horn cells are thought to be caused by changes in cell membranes which involve excitatory amino acid receptors. This has led to increasing interest in those receptors selective for $N$-methyl-D-aspartate (NMDA).[8] These changes may be caused by an initial massive afferent barrage by unmyelinated afferent on the dorsal horn. The changes may be irreversible following a single episode of afferent insult and once triggered they may be driven by a lower level of afferent input from injured peripheral nerves.[9] The afferent barrage may cause such synaptic excitation that dorsal horn cells may die due to amino acid excitotoxicity.[8] Excessive or prolonged exposure to excitatory amino acids may lead to irreversible changes in central nociceptive pathway structure.
- Chemical changes that cause central changes: Peripheral axon or cell damage may lead to changes in the neural transport substances and growth factors[10] involved in normal nervous system function. This may lead to death of dorsal root ganglia cells and so lead to a deafferentation of central cells. The loss of afferent input may lead to a loss of co-ordinated inhibitory processes, and spinal pathways may become hyper-excitable, expanding their receptor fields and exhibiting spontaneous excitation[11]. Central homeostatic mechanisms may come into play, detecting this loss of input, and raise the excitability of the central pathways to try and compensate for the decreased input. These changes involve transport mechanisms and are much slower in time scale (days to weeks) and so could be an explanation for the delayed onset of pain that is sometimes a characteristic of neuropathic pain.
- Changes in central control mechanisms: The nociceptive pathway has been shown to involve not just a simple one-way system of neural connections but also a number of interlinked and complex feedback systems that can alter by selecting and filtering information what flows through the pathway.[12] These feedback loops may have relevance to neuropathic pain as they are dynamic, being affected by not only the input of sensory pain fibres but also by the effect of higher central input. Depending on the effect of the central input the reaction to nociceptive input may be variable. The feedback loops are thought to have a limited operating range, outside of which they become unstable and so altering their feedback effects on the passage of nociceptive input. This sudden loss of stability may provide one explanation for the characteristic symptom of paroxysmal episodic pain seen in some neuropathic pain conditions.

## Treatment of neuropathic pain

Neuropathic pain has been inadequately treated in the past. The traditional treatment strategies such as simple analgesics, anti-inflammatory agents and opioid analgesics may be of little value. Also the conditions associated with neuropathic pain commonly occur in the elderly population,[2] so complicating any treatment strategies. This may be due to problems with compliance to prescribed drug regimes (30–60% relapse in treatment compliance)[13] or to the alterations in pharmacokinetics and pharmacodynamics that occur in the elderly population. There are a number of systemic diseases with an element of neuropathic pain, such as diabetic neuropathy or vitamin $B_{12}$ deficiency, where the treatment of the disease process may be the most effective treatment of the neuropathic pain rather than the use of neuropathic treatment strategies alone.

Other treatment strategies have developed, including adjuvant analgesics, anaesthetic procedures, neurostimulation and surgery. The mainstay of treatment for neuropathic pain conditions is drug therapy.

**Medical therapy**

- Tricyclic antidepressants are of use in the treatment of allodynia, burning or constant pain, and in postherpetic neuralgia, painful diabetic neuropathy, causalgia. Commonly used examples include amitriptyline,[14] doxepin, dothiepin, desipramine[15] and clomipramine. The mode of action is thought to involve an increase in the levels of serotonin (5-hydroxytryptamine) and noradrenaline in the brainstem by blocking neural reuptake. This is thought to cause an inhibitory effect on the nociceptive pathway via descending pathways on the dorsal horn region of the spinal cord. A further additional effect, seen when given in combination with morphine, may be due to an increase in free morphine due to altered protein binding. Serotonin has also been implicated in the activation of endogenous opioid mechanisms. Side-effects may include sedation, drowsiness, dry mouth, hypotension, urinary retention and constipation. These effects may be compounded by pre-existing autonomic neuropathy. These effects may prevent many patients from reaching therapeutic levels and gaining pain relief, or may lead to a lack of compliance to therapeutic regimes. It is of importance that treatment is prolonged to gain a therapeutic effect and patients are advised of treatment plans and possible side-effects. They may be reassured that the majority of adverse effects other than a dry mouth will settle with chronic treatment. Sedation may be of positive benefit in the correction of altered sleep patterns that are a further problem associated with neuropathic pain syndromes. The use of tricyclic antidepressant agents in this setting is not focused on their antidepressant action[14] – it is important to explain this to all patients to prevent misunderstanding and lack of compliance. Many patients have a depressive element to their overall clinical state due to the nature of chronic unrelieved pain. The choice of agent may be dependent on the severity of side-effects that the patients suffer.

  Amitriptyline: The starting dose should be small and commenced at night – 25 mg in the young, 10 mg in the elderly (side-effects should be monitored). The dose should then be gradually increased by 10–25 mg increments at 2-weekly intervals to 75 mg in the young (50 mg in the elderly) and should be held at this level for 4–6 weeks. If pain persists the dose may be increased with care (25 mg increments) to

150 mg (100 mg in the elderly) until relief occurs or side-effects supervene.[2] Doxepin or dothiepin may be a useful alternative as they may be less sedative and are less cardiotoxic. A similar regime of initial low dose followed by a gradual titration to response is recommended.

Desipramine: This agent is a selective inhibitor of the reuptake of noradrenaline and not serotonin reuptake. It has the least anti-cholinergic side-effects of the first-generation tricyclic antidepressants and causes relatively little sedation. It may be of use as a second- or third-line agent if other tricyclics are ineffective or not tolerated. A similar dosage regime of low initial dose slowly increased to 150 mg daily.[15]

- Anticonvulsants are used when shooting pain or 'pins and needles' are a major feature, in trigeminal neuralgia, or metatarsalgia (Morton's neuralgia). Examples include phenytoin, carbamazepine, sodium valproate and clonazepam. These agents block sodium channels and are able to suppress spontaneous discharge in A-$\delta$ and C-fibres. The sodium channel blocks are frequency- and voltage-dependent in their action, allowing the drugs to target spontaneously active nerves. Anticonvulsants block sodium channels such that they are effective against paroxysmal rather than intermittent firing neurons.

A positive therapeutic trial of carbamazepine for trigeminal neuralgia and glossopharyngeal neuralgia is diagnostic of these conditions (see Chapter 18 for treatment plans, doses and side-effects).

Sodium valproate: Starting dose of 200 mg at night, increasing to 200 mg twice daily after 1 week and to 200 mg three times daily (with food) by the third week. Optimal plasma levels for shooting pain are said to be at the lower levels of the therapeutic range of 278–694 $\mu$g/l. Side-effects include hepatotoxicity clinically (jaundice, vomiting, anorexia, weakness, rarely fatal hepatic failure) and subclinical serological changes in liver function. Regular liver function monitoring may be advisable. Other side-effects may include increased appetite, weight gain and transient hair loss.[2]

Clonazepam: Starting dose of 1 mg (500 $\mu$g in the elderly) at night for 4 nights, increasing slowly over 4 weeks to maintenance doses of 4–8 mg daily in divided doses. Side-effects may include fatigue, drowsiness, dizziness, muscle hypotonia and irritability and mental changes. Care should be taken with patients with renal or hepatic impairment; clonazepam should not be used in patients suffering from porphyria.

- Other sodium channel blockers: A relatively new therapeutic intervention for neuropathic pain involves the use of use-dependent sodium channel blockers such as lignocaine (intravenously) and mexiletine (oral). The mode of action is thought to be similar to that of carbamazepine in that neuropathic pain may be responsive to use-dependent sodium channel blockers. It has been found that lignocaine given intravenously 5 mg/kg body weight[16] may be effective as a diagnostic tool to identify if a patient's neuropathic pain is responsive to sodium channel blockade. If the lignocaine trial is effective then oral therapy with mexiletine (or carbamazepine) may be started. A dosage regimen starting with mexiletene 150 mg daily for 3 days increasing to 300 mg for a further 3 days, and then 10 mg/kg body weight daily is suitable to reduce the incidence of side-effects.[17] Care should be taken with both agents and treatment should only be commenced as an inpatient. There is a risk of cardiovascular side-effects such as bradycardia, hypotension and more general side-effects of nausea, hiccups, confusion, convulsions, tremor, nystagmus. Further work is required with this therapy to establish efficacy fully and to identify which conditions are most responsive to these drugs.[18]

- Opioids: The use of opioids in the treatment of neuropathic pain is the subject of debate. Some work suggests that neuropathic pain is unresponsive to opioids,[18] while other suggest that there is a spectrum of responsiveness from partial to complete relief.[19] The reasons for this variability may be due to the loss of postsynaptic receptor sites, be that by the degeneration of endorphinergic or encephalinergic inhibitory interneurons, or due to the formation of new central nervous pathways bypassing inhibitory interneurons. These changes may be variable ranging from partial to complete, therefore leading to a differing response from patient to patient. The problems of selecting which patient may be responsive to opioids coupled with the potential hazards of opioid use, particularly dependence, have led to avoidance of the use of opioids when they may be of major therapeutic value. This problem can be overcome by titration dosing of opioid therapy using a patient-controlled analgesic system[20] to assess opioid sensitivity rapidly without the risk of dependence. There is also increasing interest in the use of epidural and intrathecal implantable systems for the long-term administration of opioids to try to gain better pain control without the side-effects of large amounts of systemic opioid therapy.[21]

- Capsaicin cream has initially been used to treat pain with symptoms similar to those produced by capsaicin – burning paraesthesia, dysaesthesia and allodynia. Therefore it has been used for postherpetic neuralgia, diabetic neuropathy, stump pain, trigeminal neuralgia and scar pain. It has also been used to include cluster headaches, psoriasis, osteoarthritis, postmastectomy pain, apocrine chlorhidrosis, vulvar vestibulitis and pruritus associated with dialysis.[22,23] Capsaicin causes the release of substance P from nerve terminals. This neuropeptide is involved in the transmission of nociceptive information and therefore the initial use of capsaicin may result in pain. With continuing application the nerve terminal becomes depleted of substance P and so this leads to the loss of pain caused by substance P release.[24] There also appears to be a more central effect on neurons in which substance P acts as a neurotransmitter. This may be due to systemic absorption or active neuronal transport.

Capsaicin 0.025–0.075% is applied topically to the painful area at least four times a day and if effective this is continued indefinitely. Patients should be informed that the effect may take several days to occur and that the discomfort of initial treatment should subside, though this is not always the case. The treated area may initially be very painful (herpes zoster) and the patient may not persist with treatment. If the initial treatment is especially painful Emla cream (topical local anaesthetic) may be applied pretreatment to increase compliance. To date reports are of small numbers of patients and there is little objective evidence of its effectiveness, but it does appear safe and there do not appear to be any long-term side-effects with either dermal or oral preparations.

- Topical aspirin in chloroform has been used in postherpetic neuralgia. The mode of action is not fully understood but work to date suggests that aspirin may have a direct effect on the cutaneous, free-nerve endings of pain receptors. Crushed aspirin dissolved in chloroform (4%) applied topically to the painful area will lead to a reduction in pain after 20–40 min that can last for up to 2–4 h.[25] When used in the acute herpetic neuralgic state it may lead to a reduction in the severity of the post-herpetic neuralgia.[26] The treatment is well-tolerated with no adverse effects recorded to date.
- Ketamine has been used in phantom limb pain,[27] allodynia and hyper-algesic symptoms.[28] Ketamine is thought to produce its effect due to its action as a non-competitive antagonist at the NMDA receptor site. Initial studies have involved the use of low-dose intravenous techniques (250 $\mu$g/kg over 5 min) or subcutaneous infusion techniques. Care is required in its use, as in larger doses it is used as a general anaesthetic agent. Side-effects include sedation, confusion, delirium, hallucinations and dreams (nightmares).
- Clonidine has been used in chronic sympathetically maintained pain syndromes (see Chapter 4). Clonidine is an $\alpha_2$-adrenergic agonist, and is thought to relieve pain by inhibition of neurotransmission in the spinal cord dorsal horn (pre- and postsynaptic mechanisms). Administration is via the epidural route and side-effects may include decreased blood pressure, heart rate and sedation.[29]

### Neurostimulation

These therapies include transcutaneous electrical nerve stimulation (TENS), acupuncture, percutaneous electrical nerve stimulation, dorsal column stimulation and deep brain stimulation.

TENS has been used in postherpetic neuralgia, phantom limb pain and central poststroke pain.[30] Part of the effect of TENS is thought to be due to an alteration in the activity of non-opioidergic interneurons in the spinal dorsal horn, through A-$\beta$ cutaneous fibre stimulation.[2] This may be due either to high-frequency stimulation working by 'gating' in the spinal cord or by an acupuncture-like effect.[31] The effectiveness of this therapy is dependent on careful electrode placement, particularly if there are areas of sensory deficit, and therapy may be ineffective in conditions involving profound sensory deficit. Optimal frequencies of stimulation are thought to be of the order of 20–80 Hz.[32] The major advantages of this therapy are the absence of side-effects and that it is well-tolerated; unfortunately response rates are known to decrease (70% to less than 30% over a 1-year period).[31]

## Conclusions

The understanding of neuropathic pain and its pathophysiology is increasing. Specific treatment strategies have developed for particular characteristics of certain neuropathic pain states. Drug therapy is the mainstay of any treatment plan. Tricyclic antidepressants are the initial treatment of choice, but sodium channel blockers may be more appropriate for paroxysmal pain. The use of opioids should not be dismissed as a number of patients may gain benefit from their use but treatment plans involving assessment of opioid responsiveness are of particular use. The development of topical therapies (capsaicin and aspirin) may allow for improved pain control in specific neuropathic conditions with few problems due to their topical rather than systemic route. The development of new specific NMDA receptor antagonists may also be a major advance in neuropathic pain control.

Neuropathic pain remains difficult to control, with no 'quick fix' available and so it is vital that patient understanding and acceptance of this fact should be an integral part of all treatment strategies and so allow for a stepwise approach to long-term treatment.

## References

1. Bennet GF. Neuropathic pain. In: (Wall PD, Melzack R, eds) *Textbook of Pain*, 3rd edn. Churchill Livingstone, 1994, pp. 201–220
2. Bowsher D. Neuropathic pain syndromes and their management. *Br Med Bull* **47**: 644–666, 1991
3. Roberts WJ. A hypothesis on the physiological basis for causalgia and related pain. *Pain* **24**: 297–311, 1986
4. Devor M. Neuropathic pain and injured nerve: peripheral mechanisms. *Br Med Bull* **47**: 619–630, 1991
5. Janig W. Pathophysiology of nerve following mechanical injury in man. In: (Dubner R, Gebhart GF, Bond MR, eds) *Pain Research and Clinical Management*, vol 3. Amsterdam: Elsevier, 1988, pp. 89–108
6. Wilcox GL. Excitatory neurotransmitters and pain. In: (Bond M, Charlton E, Woolf CJ, eds) *Proceedings of the 6th World Congress on Pain*. Amsterdam: Elsevier Science, 1991, pp. 97–112
7. Wall PD. Neuropathic pain and injured nerve: central mechanisms. *Br Med Bull* **47**: 631–643, 1991
8. Woolf CJ. The pathophysiology of peripheral neuropathic pain – abnormal peripheral input and abnormal central processing. *Acta Neurochir* **58** (suppl): 125–130, 1993
9. Gracely RH, Lynch SA, Bennett GJ. Painful neuropathy: altered central processing maintained dynamically by peripheral input. *Pain* **51**, 175–194, 1992
10. Fitzgerald M, Wall PD, Goedert M, Emson PC. Nerve growth factor counteracts the neurophysiological and neurochemical effects of chronic sciatic nerve injury. *Brain Res* **332**: 131–141, 1985
11. Alexander J, Black A. Pain mechanisms and the management of neuropathic pain. *Curr Opin Neurol Neurosurg* **5**: 228–234, 1992
12. McMahon SB, Wall PD. The significance of plastic changes in lamina 1 systems. In: (Cervero F, Bennett GJ, Headley P, eds) *Processing of Sensory Information in the Superficial Dorsal Horn of the Spinal Cord*. New York: Plenum Press, 1989, pp. 249–272
13. Turk DC, Rudy TE. Neglected topics in the treatment of chronic pain patients in relapse, noncompliance and adherence enhancement. *Pain* **44**: 5–28, 1991
14. Max MB, Culnane M, Schafer SC *et al*. Amitriptyline relieves diabetic neuropathic pain in patients with normal or depressed mood. *Neurology* **37**: 589–596, 1987
15. Max MB, Kishore-Kumar R, Schafer SC *et al*. Efficacy of desipramine in painful diabetic neuropathy: placebo-controlled trial. *Pain* **45**: 3–9, 1991

16. Kastrup J, Petersen P, Dejgard A, Angelo HR, Hilsted J. Intravenous lidocaine infusion – a new treatment of chronic painful diabetic neuropathy? *Pain* **28:** 69–75, 1987

17. Dejgard A, Petersen P, Kastrup J. Mexiletine for treatment of chronic painful diabetic neuropathy. *Lancet* **1:** 9–11, 1988

18. Tanelian DL, Brose WG. Neuropathic pain can be relieved by drugs that are use-dependent. Sodium channel blockers: lidocaine, carbamazepine, and mexiletine. *Anesthesiology* **74:** 949–951, 1991

19. Arner S, Meyerson BA. Lack of analgesic effect of opioids on neuropathic pain and idiopathic forms of pain. *Pain* **33:** 11–23, 1988

20. Portenoy RK, Foley KM, Inturrisi CE. The nature of opioid responsiveness and its implications for neuropathic pain: new hypothesis derived from studies of opioid infusions. *Pain* **43:** 273–286, 1990

21. McQuay HJ, Jada AR, Carrol D *et al.* Opioid sensitivity of chronic pain: a patient-controlled analgesic model. *Anaesthesia* **47:** 757–767, 1992

22. Murphy TM, Hinds S, Cherry D. Intraspinal narcotics: non-malignant pain. *Acta Anaesthesiol Scand* **31** (suppl): 75–76, 1987

23. Clarke IMC. Peppering pain. *Lancet* **342:** 1130, 1993

24. Dubner R. Topical capsaicin therapy for neuropathic pain. *Pain* **47:** 247–248, 1991

25. La Motte RH, Lundberg LE, Torebjork HE. Pain, hyperalgesia and activity in nociceptive C-units in humans after intradermal injection of capsaicin. *J Physiol Lond* **448:** 749–764, 1992

26. King RB. Topical aspirin in chloroform and the relief of pain due to herpes zoster and post-herpetic neuralgia. *Arch Neurol* **50:** 1046–1053, 1993

27. De Benedittis G, Besana F, Lorenzetti A. A new topical treatment for acute herpetic neuralgia and post-herpetic neuralgia: the aspirin diethyl ether mixture. An open-label study plus a double-blind controlled clinical trial. *Pain* **48:** 383–390, 1992

28. Stannard CF, Porter GE. Ketamine hydrochloride in the treatment of phantom limb pain. *Pain* **54:** 227–230, 1993

29. Backonja M, Arndt G, Gombar KA, Check B, Zimmermann M. Response of chronic neuropathic pain syndromes to ketamine: a preliminary study. *Pain* **56:** 51–57, 1994

30. Rauck RL, Eisenach JC, Jackson K, Young LD, Souhern J. Epidural clonidine treatment for refractory reflex sympathetic dystrophy. *Anesthesiology* **79:** 1163–1169, 1993

31. Leijon G, Boivie J. Central post-stroke pain. The effect of high and low frequency TENS. *Pain* **38:** 187–192, 1989

32. Richards EG. Interventional therapy, transcutaneous electrical nerve stimulation and acupuncture. *Curr Opin Anaesthesiol* **3:** 786–790, 1990

33. Johnson MI, Ashton CH, Bousfield DR, Thompson JW. Analgesic effects of different frequencies of transcutaneous electrical nerve stimulation on cold-induced pain in normal subjects. *Pain* **39:** 231–236, 1989

# 6

# Muscle/soft-tissue pain

R. C. Bacon and S. J. Dolin

## Fibromyalgia

Fibromyalgia syndrome is a chronic pain disorder that is characterized by diffuse musculoskeletal pain, stiffness, tenderness, fatigue and sleep disturbance.

Fibromyalgia is not a new syndrome. Indeed, biblical references to Job's suffering of disturbed sleep, deep pain and exhaustion could be the earliest description of the syndrome. In the past it has been known under a number of different and sometimes misleading names. Fibromyalgia comes from the term fibrositis, first used by William Gowers in 1904 to describe muscular rheumatism of the back.[1] Later fibrositis was used to describe both regional myofascial pain syndrome and fibromyalgia, despite lack of inflammatory aetiology. More recently the term fibromyalgia was introduced[2a] and this has largely replaced other terminology including myofibrositis, myofasciitis, tension, muscular and psychogenic rheumatism and rheumatic pain modulation disorder.[2b]

The most recent diagnostic criteria for the classification of fibromyalgia by Wolfe et al.[3] are simple and have high specificity and sensitivity (Table 6.1).

### Aetiology

The aetiology of fibromyalgia is unknown. Infection, trauma, immunological disturbances and localized myofascial abnormalities are proposed aetiological factors, but there is little evidence for these.[4]

### Diagnosis and clinical features

#### History and examination

The prevalence of fibromyalgia is estimated at between 2 and 20%. The majority of patients are female aged 34–57 years at presentation.[5] The syndrome can occur in children and in the elderly and can accompany osteoarthritis.

**Table 6.1** Classification and definition of fibromyalgia*

*History of widespread pain*
Definition: Pain is considered widespread when all of the following are present: pain in the left side of the body, pain in the right side of the body, pain above the waist and pain below the waist. In addition, axial skeletal pain (cervical spine pain or anterior chest or thoracic spine/low back) must be present. In this definition shoulder and buttock pain are considered as pain for each involved side. 'Low back' pain is considered lower segment pain

*Pain in 11 of 18 tender point sites on digital palpation*
Definition: Pain, on digital palpation, must be present in at least 11 of the following 18 tender point sites. Digital palpation should be performed with an approximate force of 4 kg. For a tender point to be considered positive the subject must state that the palpation was painful. 'Tender' is not to be considered 'painful':

- *occiput:* bilateral, at the suboccipital muscle insertions
- *low cervical:* bilateral, at the anterior aspects of the intertransverse spaces at C5–7
- *trapezius:* bilateral, at the midpoint of the upper border
- *supraspinatus:* bilateral, at origins, above the scapula spine near the medial border
- *second rib:* bilateral, at the second costochondral junction, just lateral to the junctions on upper surfaces
- *lateral epicondyle:* bilateral, 2 cm distal to the epicondyles
- *gluteal:* bilateral, in upper outer quadrants of buttocks in anterior fold of muscle
- *greater trochanter:* bilateral, posterior to the trochanteric prominence
- *knees:* bilateral, at the medial fat pad proximal to the joint line

\* For classification purposes patients will be said to have fibromyalgia if both criteria are satisfied. widespread pain must have been present for at least 3 months. The presence of a second disorder does not exclude the diagnosis of fibromyalgia. From Wolfe et al.[3]

The patient with fibromyalgia can present with the following symptoms and signs,[4–6] although the degree to which they are present may vary with individual patients (Table 6.2).

- Pain is probably the most important feature of fibromyalgia. It is generally bilateral, affecting multiple areas, although pain in the neck, trapezius, arms, hips and lower back is the most frequently reported. Compared with rheumatoid arthritis, fibromyalgia patients complain of more intense pain over a larger body area.
- Exercise intolerance and muscle fatigue occur after small amounts of static work and few dynamic muscle contractions, which may be felt to be more disabling than pain. As a result there can be diminished work capacity.

**Table 6.2** Clinical features of fibromyalgia

Core features of fibromyalgia – generalized pain and widespread tenderness – are present in all patients

Characteristic features of the syndrome are present in more than 75% of patients – fatigue, non-refreshed or disturbed sleep, morning stiffness

Common features occur often (>25%) but are not essential to the syndrome. These include irritable bowel syndrome, Raynaud's phenomenon, headache, subjective swelling, paraesthesia, psychological abnormality and functional disability

Coexisting rheumatic conditions, e.g. arthritis, low back and cervical disorders and tendinitis, have symptoms which overlap with those of fibromyalgia

From Wolfe[5]

- Stiffness is generalized and does not diminish with activity, unlike rheumatoid arthritis.
- Subjective swelling and paraesthesia are more common in fibromyalgia than healthy controls. The mechanisms are unknown but there is a strong correlation between these symptoms and pain.
- Sleep disturbance is reported in 60–90% of fibromyalgia patients, which seems to correlate with fatigue.
- Psychological symptoms, including self-assessed anxiety, depression and mental stress are more common in fibromyalgia.
- Tender points are areas where slight to moderate pressure can produce painful sensations. Tenderness is measured either by direct digital palpation or pressure algometry. They are the most important physical findings in fibromyalgia if found in all four body quadrants. The location of tender points may vary between individuals and at certain times, but should be reproducible over a number of weeks.
- Cutaneous hyperaemia and reticular skin patterns have been reported in fibromyalgia. They are objective and do not rely on patient interpretation.
- Exacerbating factors may include cold, damp weather, physical exertion, anxiety and stress.
- A number of functional disorders are associated with fibromyalgia including tension headaches, irritable bowel syndrome, irritable bladder syndrome, primary dysmenorrhoea, premenstrual syndrome and mitral valve prolapse.[6] Hypersensitivity to cold, including Raynaud's phenomenon, can also be present.

### Investigations

All routine laboratory and radiological tests are normal in fibromyalgia.

### Differential diagnosis[7]

- myofascial pain syndrome
- temporomandibular joint dysfunction syndrome
- polymyalgia rheumatica/giant cell arteritis
- polymyositis/dermatomyositis
- endocrine myopathies
- alcoholic myopathy
- metastatic carcinoma
- chronic fatigue syndrome
- Parkinsonism

### Pathophysiology

The exact pathophysiological mechanisms are unknown in fibromyalgia. However there are some underlying pathological abnormalities described.[4,8,9]

- Muscle abnormalities: muscle biopsy in fibromyalgia has shown non-specific changes with light and electron microscopy. Histochemical staining for oxidative enzymes reveals red ragged fibres within muscle where there is a proliferation of mitochondria. These fibres are found where oxidative metabolism is compromised. Adenosine triphosphate and phosphocreatine are reduced in the trapezius muscles of fibromyalgia patients, possibly due to local hypoxia. Other findings in fibromyalgia patients which could suggest an abnormal microcirculation are abnormal oxygen tensions and reduced relaxation rates.[10] Patients with fibromyalgia have low aerobic fitness with reduced muscle blood flow and it is possible that fatigue can lead to unfit muscles which are more susceptible to microtrauma and pain.[11]

- Sleep disturbances: $\alpha$-Electroencephalogram (EEG) non-rapid eye movement (REM) sleep disturbances are present in fibromyalgia.[12] Sleep EEG recordings show $\alpha$ waves (7.5–11 Hz, normally seen in the awake state), intruding into $\delta$ waves (0.5–2 Hz, deep sleep), which may result in the non-restorative sleep disturbances that can affect pain perception. In healthy volunteers undergoing $\alpha$ intrusion on non-REM sleep it is possible to replicate muscle fatigue and tenderness over fibromyalgia tender points. It is unknown whether this sleep anomaly can cause fibromyalgia but it can contribute to a vicious circle of pain and disturbed sleep.
- Serotonin (5-HT) is an important central nervous system neurotransmitter. Low brain concentrations are associated with sleep disturbances, depression and increased pain perception. Serum levels of tryptophan, the precursor of 5-HT, have been reported to be reduced in patients with fibromyalgia.
- Substance P is a neurotransmitter involved with pain transmission. Substance P is significantly elevated in cerebrospinal fluid of fibromyalgia patients.
- Catecholamines may also be implicated in fibromyalgia. Patients have been reported to have elevated urinary noradrenaline concentrations which correlated with anxiety and tender point scores.
- Endorphins have been reported to be reduced in patients with chronic pain and could be involved with fibromyalgia. Evidence for this is indirect. Exercise activates endorphins and while it is impossible to induce fibromyalgic tender points in marathon runners, cardiovascular fitness training can result in improved symptoms in fibromyalgia patients.
- Immune system involvement is thought to account for the skin discoloration by altered neurovascular function. There is increased immunological deposition at the dermal–epidermal junction, probably reflecting increased vascular permeability in some patients.
- Psychological factors may also play a role. Despite a marked tendency to depression in fibromyalgia patients, there is no definite evidence that fibromyalgia is caused by psychological or psychiatric factors. Psychosocial problems are generally concomitant or a consequence of the syndrome.

## Relationship to chronic fatigue syndrome

Chronic fatigue syndrome is a disorder which shares many of the clinical features present in fibromyalgia. In both disorders the majority of patients are women of similar age, presenting with non-specific symptoms: fatigue, easy exhaustion, sleep disturbance, headache and muscular weakness, and a lack of reproducible or reliable laboratory findings. It has been proposed that these syndromes may share a common aetiology such as viral or other infectious agent.[13]

## Treatment

As little is known about the aetiology or pathogenesis of fibromyalgia, the management[14] is based on hypotheses. In addition there are few objective clinical features with which to measure outcome.

### Medical treatment[15]

- Tricyclic antidepressants in low doses have a useful role in the treatment of fibromyalgia, showing an improvement in tender point readings, pain scores and pain thresholds. They have both central and peripheral actions. Amitriptyline and cyclobenzaprine are the most widely studied, but imipramine and dothiepin have also been tried. Amitriptyline has a direct effect on sleep by causing REM suppression and prolonging stage 3 and 4 non-REM sleep. This is probably mediated by blocking 5-HT reuptake in the central nervous system. Tricyclics have analgesic properties, potentiating endogenous and exogenous opioids. They also act on the periphery by relieving muscle spasm and have an anti-inflammatory action. Low-dose antidepressants taken at night are well-tolerated and beneficial, the greatest effect being over the first 2–4 weeks, with follow-up over longer periods showing little further improvement. Doses should be kept to a minimum, starting with 5–10 mg of amitriptyline and slowly increasing to a maximum of 50 mg. Adverse effects of tricyclics include drowsiness, dry mouth and constipation.
- Benzodiazepines and phenothiazines have been tried but their use is limited by habituating or unpleasant side-effects. More recently there has been interest in fluoxetine, a selective 5-HT reuptake inhibitor, and S-adenosyl-methionine (SAMe), a chemical involved in brain methylation reactions.
- Non-steroidal anti-inflammatory drugs and prednisolone have been commonly used in fibromyalgia, although there is little evidence of their effectiveness.
- Tender point injections with local anaesthetics with or without steroids can provide some relief of tender points. As fibromyalgia patients may have multiple tender points, choosing which to inject may be a problem. Up to four tender points may be injected at a time and pain relief can last for months.
- Improved muscle blood flow by stellate ganglion blocks or regional intravenous blocks can reduce the number of tender points and improve pain scores.

### Non-medical treatment[16]

- Patient education and reassurance can be most beneficial. Establishing a diagnosis and explaining the known mechanism and contributing factors as well as explaining that this is a benign condition with a good functional prognosis in spite of continuing pain can reduce stress and anxiety.
- Psychological and behavioural therapy, such as biofeedback and cognitive-behavioural therapy, may be helpful. Behavioural management involves working with the patient to accept some degree of chronic pain, while accepting small benefits and performing within reasonable limits.
- Avoidance of precipitating and aggravating factors. Poor muscle fitness, obesity and poor posture should be corrected. Exposure to cold damp weather and inactivity are known aggravating factors that can be avoided.
- Aerobic training regularly over many weeks decreases pain and tender points. Its mechanism of action is unknown but theories include activation of endogenous opioids and stress-induced analgesia.
- Promotion of restorative sleep patterns by avoidance of alcohol, caffeine and nicotine can also be helpful.
- Other techniques have also been described, including heat, massage, transcutaneous electrical nerve stimulation (TENS), acupuncture, but none of these are of proven benefit.

## Prognosis

There is limited information on the prognosis, course or outcome of fibromyalgia. Patient's symptoms are usually stable with 60% continuing to have moderate to severe pain and fatigue and only a small percentage having complete remission.

## Myofascial pain syndromes

Myofascial pain syndrome is a regional muscle pain disorder characterized by a local area of deep muscle tenderness called a trigger point, and a reference zone of pain, which is worsened by palpation of the trigger point.[18] Active trigger points cause pain associated with myofascial pain syndromes while latent trigger points are generally without symptoms but may restrict movement and weaken the muscle. Latent trigger points can evolve into active trigger points.

Similarly to fibromyalgia, different terminology has been used to describe myofascial pain syndromes, often encompassing both disorders. Recent diagnostic criteria for myofascial pain syndromes have been defined[19] (Table 6.3).

### Aetiology and pathophysiology

Factors implicated in the aetiology of myofascial pain syndromes are numerous.[20] Formation of trigger points has been attributed to acute or

**Table 6.3** Diagnostic criteria for myofascial pain syndrome

*Major criteria*
Regional pain complaint

Pain complaint or altered sensations in the expected distribution of referred pain from a myofascial trigger point

Taut palpable band in an accessible muscle

Exquisite spot tenderness at one point along the length of the taut band

Some degree of restricted range of motion when measurable

*Minor criteria*
Reproduction of clinical pain complaint or altered sensations by pressure on the tender spot

Elicitation of a local twitch response by transverse snapping palpation at the tender spot or by needle insertion into the tender spot in the taut band

Pain alleviated by elongating (stretching) the muscle or by injecting the tender spot

From Simons[19]

chronic overloading of muscles, trauma, chronic infection, poor posture, emotional stress, nutritional, metabolic and endocrine abnormalities, e.g. vitamin and mineral deficiencies and hypometabolism. Regular exercises may have a protective effect against the development of myofascial pain syndromes. Latent trigger points can be activated by additional injury, intense heat or cold and damp weather.

- Histopathological studies focus on fibrositic or fibromyalgia tender points rather than myofascial trigger points and there has been confusion due to similar nomenclature previously applied to both syndromes. However, there is evidence that findings in myofascial pain syndromes and fibromyalgia are similar.[21]
- Electromyographic studies show that at rest the trigger point is inactive. Snapping palpation of the trigger point produces high-amplitude prolonged discharge, thought to be comparable to the twitch response, and higher motor unit activity when compared to normal muscle.[22]
- Endogenous opioids could be involved, as treatment with the opioid antagonist naloxone negates the effect of trigger point injections with local anaesthetic.[23]

The pathogenesis of myofascial pain is unknown but it has been proposed that there is an initiating event which leads to local muscle injury.[20] The muscle may develop abnormalities, possibly in the contractile elements, that may be potentiated by local ischaemia or damage to the metabolic pathways of the muscle cell. As all muscles are exposed to insults, those that proceed to develop trigger points may differ from normal muscle in structure, conditioning, physiology or in the development of a reflex arc involving spinal cord or other central mechanisms.

A number of abnormal spinal cord reflex circuits controlling outflow may be set up and through these circuits pain could be referred to distant sites.[24]

## Diagnosis

### Clinical features

There is limited information on age and sex distribution of myofascial pain syndromes. Trigger points are common and 54% of women and 45% of men have been shown to have areas of muscle tenderness.[25] The majority of patients however seem to be female (which may reflect an increased tendency to seek medical help) aged 30–60 years at presentation.[26,27]

Patients with myofascial pain can present with the following symptoms and signs:

- Pain is usually dull, well-differentiated, of variable intensity, continuous or intermittent and may be present at rest or only on movement. It is not usually localized in the trigger point itself but in its reference zone. The reference zones do not follow clear dermatomal, neurological, anatomical or myotomal patterns.
- Taut bands are palpable abnormalities in or around the muscle containing trigger points.
- Jump response is a behavioural response elicited from the patient who may cry out, jump, wince or suddenly move the limb segment activated by the affected muscle group when the trigger point is palpated.
- Twitch response: rapid snapping palpation of the taut band (fingertips put at right angles to the muscle fibre direction and suddenly pressed down while pulling the finger back, rolling the fibres against themselves) frequently produces sudden contraction of that area which may be felt or seen.
- Decreased muscle stretch: both active and passive stretch of the affected muscle is limited by pain locally or in the reference zone.
- Autonomic disturbances such as vasoconstriction, pilomotor activation, cutaneous erythema and temperature changes are sometimes seen in the trigger point or reference zone.
- Anxiety, depression, sleep disturbance, poor posture and reduced joint mobility are other features associated with myofascial pain syndromes.

### Investigations

All routine laboratory and radiological investigations are normal in myofascial pain syndromes.

### Differential diagnosis[10]

- polymyositis/dermatomyositis
- inflammatory arthritis
- tendinitis/bursitis/tenosynovitis
- multiple sclerosis
- neuralgias
- Ménière's disease
- torticollis
- thoracic outlet syndrome
- polyneuropathies
- infection

**Treatment**

There are few clinical studies on the treatment of myofascial pain. Management relies on avoidance of perpetuating factors and inactivation of the trigger points through counterstimulation and muscle rehabilitation.[24,28]

- Avoidance of perpetuating factors such as abnormal stresses including chronic overloading, chronic contraction or repetitive muscle use should be avoided. Patients' occupation and leisure activities may need to be assessed and advice given on posture, general fitness and physical conditioning. It may be necessary to correct mechanical abnormalities such as scoliosis.
- Counterstimulation involves inactivating trigger points through repetitive action. Spray and stretch and trigger point injections are the most commonly used but other methods include massage, acupuncture, ultrasound, icepacks, heat and TENS.
- Spray and stretch involves the application of a vapour coolant spray in a particular direction over the trigger point with simultaneous passive stretching of the muscle to interrupt and modify the trigger point. The stretching element is most important with the spray, facilitating muscle relaxation. The spray is directed parallel to the direction of the muscle fibres at a rate of 10 cm/s. Passive stretch is applied until the patient feels discomfort. The procedure can be repeated up to four times provided the skin is allowed to rewarm between stretches. It is best to avoid excessive sweeps or skin frosting as this can lower underlying muscle temperature and aggravate the trigger point. Examples of the technique are shown in Figure 6.1.
- Trigger point injection with local anaesthetic with or without steroids reduces pain and increases range of movement and exercise tolerance. It is primarily the mechanical disturbance of the trigger point by the needle which is thought to be important, rather than the drug injected, as dry needling and saline injections are also effective[23a] (but not as comfortable). The patient is positioned comfortably and the trigger point located accurately prior to injection. An aseptic technique is advised. A fine-gauge needle (25 or 27 G) is introduced quickly through the skin to avoid discomfort and the trigger point located with the tip. A twitch response or increased pain over the muscle or reference zone indicates correct position prior to injection of local anaesthetic. Passive stretching of the muscle for 1–2 min will restore the muscle to its normal length and help locate other trigger points. There may be an increase in pain for several hours after the procedure before the onset of pain relief. A series of injections may be necessary.
- Muscle rehabilitation with exercises involving posture, strengthening and active and passive stretching can be taught to the patient. This will increase muscle conditioning and reduce remaining trigger points and may prevent reactivation of the condition.

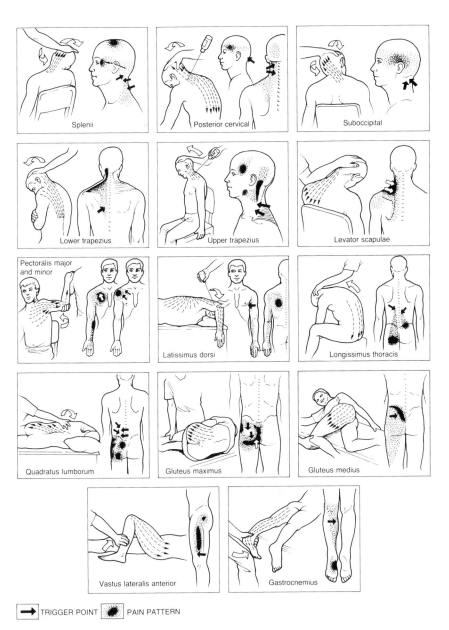

**Figure 6.1** Myofascial pain patterns: Location of trigger points and pain patterns, stretch positions and spray patterns for muscle groups commonly causing pain patterns seen in pain clinics. The curved white arrows identify the direction of pressure applied to stretch the muscle. The dashed arrows trace the impact of the stream of vapocoolant spray applied to release the muscular tension during stretch.

## Fibromyalgia versus myofascial pain syndromes

There is often confusion between fibromyalgia and myofascial pain syndrome.[29] It has been suggested that they are the same disorder with differing manifestations. Both syndromes present with one or more sensitive muscle points, affect women to a greater extent than men, have a similar age of presentation and are associated with sleep disorder and psychological factors. However, the two syndromes are defined separately, each having a set of diagnostic criteria. Critical differences do exist (Table 6.4).[28,30,31]

**Table 6.4** Comparison between fibromyalgia and myofascial pain syndrome

| Fibromyalgia | Myofascial pain syndrome |
| --- | --- |
| Generalized musculoskeletal pain syndrome (may be regional forms) | Local/regional syndrome of muscular pain and/or dysfunction |
| Aetiology unknown | Mechanical aetiology |
| Substance P-mediated? | Endorphin-mediated? |
| Chronic duration | Acute or chronic duration |
| Tender point area in muscle which is tender to palpation, usually in well-defined areas | Trigger point area in muscle associated with a taut band, reference zone, muscle twitch and jump response |
| Lower generalized pain thresholds more responsive to pain | |
| Prognosis guarded | Prognosis good with early treatment and elimination of perpetuating factors |

## Repetitive strain injury

Repetitive strain injury (RSI) is a painful condition mostly affecting hands and arms, which arises from repeated muscle activity, usually as a consequence of the patient's occupation. Other terms that have been used to describe RSI are shown in Table 6.5.

RSI is controversial, as recent compensation cases have demonstrated, and lack of physical signs, clear aetiology, pathological processes and clinical studies has led clinicians to question its existence.[32,33] Cost to both employer and employee can be substantial, as shown by experience of RSI in Australia. The 'Australian epidemic' started in the early 1980s, peaked in the mid 1980s, and declined in the late 1980s. Its rise was attributed to RSI becoming a socially acceptable disease potentiated by the medical profession, reinforced by ergonomists, supported by trade unions and with easy access to compensation. Its fall was attributed to a change in working practices, media derision and the rediscovery of mental factors in the syndrome.[34]

RSI is not a new syndrome that evolved with keyboard technology. The first report of a condition resembling RSI was given by Bernardino Ramazzini in 1713 when he described pain and fatigue in writers. Throughout the

**Table 6.5** Alternative names for repetitive strain injury

Chronic upper limb disorder
Cumulative trauma disorder
Muscle overuse syndrome
Occupational arm syndrome
Occupational cervicobrachial disorder
Occupational cramp
Occupational overuse syndrome
Occupational stress syndrome
Pain dysfunction syndrome
Refractory cervicobrachial pain
Regional pain disorder
Repetitive stress syndrome
Repetitive trauma disorder
Reversible strain injury
Static stress syndrome
Work-related upper limb disorder

19th century clinicians attempted to classify and define the pathological basis of writer's cramp and scrivener's palsy.[35]

### Aetiology and pathophysiology

The aetiology of RSI is multifactorial and no direct cause and effect has been found.[36] However a number of contributing factors have been recognized.

- biomechanical factors, including poor posture, frequent repetitive movements, joint position and muscle tension and stress
- faulty work organization, including duration of work, bonus and overtime incentives and poor supervision
- incompetent personnel training
- delayed reporting, incorrect and delayed diagnosis and inappropriate management

The exact pathophysiology of RSI is unknown. It has variously been interpreted as an overuse injury, a state of neural irritability, a psychogenic disorder, and a functional disorder of muscles and the central nervous system.

Some possible theories of pathogenesis are outlined below:[36,37]

- Excessive use of muscle causes pain and injury. Muscle exercise produces hypertrophy and hyperplasia with changes in metabolites, enzymes, fibre contractile characteristics and capillary density. If submaximal loads are applied too frequently or increased too rapidly this can result in tissue damage with release of myoglobin into the circulation. Repetitive microtrauma initiates a repair response. Rest alleviates the pain but return to work causes retraumatization.
- Sensory input leads to an increased-output, reflex arc within the spinal cord. Evidence for this is the neural quality of the pain associated

with hyperalgesia, hyperaesthesia and spread to adjacent areas. Increased sympathetic output is occasionally seen in RSI with sweating, colour and temperature changes.

- The brain can influence the development and perception of pain. Patients' personality may predispose to RSI with frustration, anger and disturbed sleep potentiating pain.

## Clinical features

The majority of RSI patients are women aged 20–50 years at presentation. Keyboard workers, machine operators, process workers, packers and musicians are particularly at risk. The onset is usually insidious, after months and years, rather than weeks of repetitive work.

### Symptoms[37]

- Pain is usually deep, burning or with an electrical quality. It is usually localized at first to hands and lower arms but extension to the upper limbs, shoulder, neck and back is common. The dominant limb is most frequently affected. Pain is relieved by rest and exacerbated by work, cold weather, damp and stress.
- Pins and needles may affect both hands.
- Fatigue may be the predominant feature and interfere with work to a greater extent than pain and cramp.
- There may be cramp.
- Other symptoms include a subjective feeling of swelling, disturbed sleep, headache, irritability and mood disturbances.

### Physical signs

Objective physical signs are generally absent in RSI. There may be lack of spontaneous movement, difficulty with fine movements, rapid fatigue, spasm and tenderness over nerves or muscle groups. Joints may feel stiff but there is a full range of movement. Crepitus can be found in a few acute cases[38] but in the majority there is a lack of physical signs.

### Investigations

Routine laboratory investigations and radiological tests, muscle biopsies and nerve conduction studies are normal in RSI.

### Differential diagnosis

- tennis elbow
- tenosynovitis
- carpal tunnel syndrome

## Management[37,38]

### Prevention

Ergonomics has been involved with prevention of RSI. Biomechanical factors that can be improved include poor posture, frequent repetitive movements, abnormal joint positions, badly designed equipment and stress. The employer should ensure adequate rest periods, suitable training and supervision, variety, opportunity, physical comfort, mental challenge and involvement in the workplace. The employee should be encouraged to report muscle discomfort before RSI develops.

### Treatment

There are few clinical studies on the treatment of RSI and most recommendations are based on anecdotal experience.

- Rest from the task precipitating RSI is the primary treatment and the only method that can guarantee pain relief. However, as with fibromyalgia, gradual increase in aerobic and muscle-building exercise can both relieve pain and prevent recurrence.
- Early return to work is recommended as this may become more difficult with time. With severe cases a change of occupation may be necessary.
- Counselling and cognitive-behavioural therapy include goal-setting, correcting false beliefs, relaxation training, accepting that depression and anxiety can sustain pain, and learning skills for coping with pain.
- Sleep disturbance can occur and treatment with low-dose tricyclic therapy can be useful.
- Physiotherapy can also be helpful. Application of local heat by convection, conduction or ultrasound can increase metabolic rate, arterial dilatation and soft-tissue flexibility and provide analgesia. Cooling therapies affect vasoconstriction, capillary flow, produce analgesia and may be helpful in reducing oedema. Other methods used include mobilizations, exercise programmes, relaxation techniques, muscle stretching and adverse mechanical tension techniques, acupuncture and TENS.
- Splints are often helpful in patients, particularly in the acute phase. They may provide protection from reinjury and allow joints, tendons and nerves to rest in the correct biomechanical position. Dynamic splinting will increase the range of movement. A disadvantage of splinting is immobilization which can be an additional problem if used for long periods of time.

### Prognosis

RSI generally improves with time and rest. Advanced injury can lead to permanent incapacity for repetitive work.

## Tendinitis

Tendinitis or inflammation of the tendon is a common overuse injury among athletes and in certain occupations. Overuse occurs when repetitive micro-trauma overcomes the tissues' ability to adapt. The overall incidence of tendinitis is rising as a result of increased health consciousness, with more people taking up recreational sport.

There is confusion over correct terminology for tendon disease. As tendons are composed of fibrous connective tissue with little vascularity, any inflammation usually occurs in surrounding peritendinous tissue. There-fore it has been suggested that the term peritendinitis is a better term and the term tendinosis should be used to describe degenerative lesions in the tendon itself.

### Impingement syndrome and rotator cuff tendinitis

The shoulder is the most used joint in the body and has the greatest range of movement. It is therefore not surprising that it is the commonest site for tendinopathies. Occupations and sports such as tennis and basketball that require repeated overhead movements often produce a painful shoulder. Impingement syndrome occurs when the smooth gliding of the supra-spinatous tendon in the subacromial space is impaired, usually caused by anatomical or pathological changes leading to a decrease of the space. In young people tendinitis with microtears and oedema is usually respon-sible, although other causes include calcium deposits, incomplete tears, osteophytes and anatomical variations.[39] Classically there is night pain with weakness and pain on abduction and external rotation. Treatment is initially conservative, including rest, non-steroidal anti-inflammatory drugs (NSAIDs) and physiotherapy, although surgical intervention is some-times necessary.[40]

### Bicipital tendinitis

Bicipital tendinitis is less common than impingement syndrome or rotator cuff tendinitis. Some 95% of bicipital tendinitis is secondary to impingement syndrome, although primary tendinitis may be caused by inflammation or trauma. Patients complain of pain over the anterior aspect of the shoulder radiating to the muscle belly. It is exacerbated by overhead movements and relieved by rest. As with other painful shoulder conditions the pain may be worse at night. On examination there is a tenderness in the biceps groove with the arm in 10° of internal rotation. Treatment is conservative initially with surgery reserved for patients who fail to respond.[41]

### Elbow tendinitis

Elbow tendinitis or tennis elbow can affect lateral, medial and posterior regions of the elbow. The tendons involved are primarily the extensor carpi radialis brevis in lateral tennis elbow; pronator teres and flexor carpi radialis in medial tennis elbow; and triceps in posterior tennis elbow.

Patients are usually over 35 years with a high level of sporting or occupational activity and those involved with racket or throwing sports are particularly at risk. Pain over the anatomical area and weakness may be present. A total of 20% of radiographs show calcification or exostosis at the epicondyle or tendon. The tendon shows degenerative changes secondary to overuse and there may be minimal inflammatory reaction. The term angiofibroblastic tendinosis describes the microscopic changes in the tendon that include fibroblastic infiltration and vascular atypical granulation tissue.[42]

Treatment is initially conservative, with rest, ice compression and NSAIDs. Promotion of healing is achieved with rehabilitation exercises, including aerobic and general conditioning. Patients should be encouraged to improve their sports technique and control the intensity and duration of activity. Surgery is indicated in patients with chronic symptoms lasting longer than 1 year.

### DeQuervain's tenosynovitis

The tendons of the wrist and fingers pass through retinacular tunnels at the wrist which prevent subluxation and act as pulleys. The synovial linings between the retinaculum and the tendons frequently become inflamed from overuse. DeQuervain's is the most common tenosynovitis and affects the first dorsal compartment containing the abductor pollicis longus and extensor pollicis brevis. DeQuervain was credited with giving the first description of this disorder in 1895 but a similar condition was described in Gray's *Anatomy* in 1883. Middle-aged women are most commonly affected and its frequency in the working population and athletes is increasing, with fishermen, golfers and those involved with racket sports particularly at risk. There is an association with rheumatoid arthritis, hypothyroidism, diabetes, osteoarthritis, gout, calcium deposition, Dupuytren's disease and collagen vascular disease. There is pain and swelling over the radial styloid process. Pain may radiate proximally and distally and can be exacerbated by wrist ulnar deviation and thumb flexion or adduction. Crepitus thickening of the extensor sheath, erythema, increased skin temperature and radial deviation may also be present.[43] Finkelstein's test, where the patient clenches the fist over the flexed thumb while the examiner pushes the base of the thumb towards the ulnar side, will produce pain at the ulnar radial process.

Treatment is initially conservative with rest and immobilization, thumb spicas and NSAIDs. Corticosteroid injection into the first dorsal compartment has proved to be particularly effective, with cure rates of 80–90%.[44,45] Surgery may be necessary in resistant cases.

### Patellar tendinitis

Patellar tendinitis, also known as jumper's knee or quadriceps tendinitis, affects athletes involved in repetitive activities such as jumping, climbing, kicking or running. Basketball, volleyball and tennis players, divers, high and long jumpers, mountain climbers, footballers and skaters are particularly at risk. Pain in the suprapatellar or infrapatellar regions is present and patients may report swelling and a feeling of giving way but there is no locking. Initially the pain may appear only at the beginning or end of activity but later may become persistent. There may be tenderness on palpation of the inferior or superior pole of the patella and cystic fluctuation or patella snapping may be present. Radiographs are usually normal but occasionally abnormal ossification centres, stress fractures, calcification of the tendon, and irregularity of the affected pole may be found. In young athletes patellar tendinitis is usually related to rapid growth spurts. Associated abnormalities include patellar hypermobility, patellar chondromalacia and Osgood–Schlatter's disease.[46]

Treatment remains controversial[47]. Ice, massage, NSAIDs, heat therapies, rest, immobilization and knee supports are recommended initially, but surgery is an option for chronic patients.

### Achilles tendinitis

With the increasing popularity of running for conditioning purposes, Achilles tendinitis has become a common overuse injury in recreational athletes.[48,49] The exact cause is unknown but predisposing factors include poor body mechanics, training errors or inadequate training conditions, age-related changes, inappropriate footwear and malalignment of the hip, knee and foot. Ballet dancers are particularly at risk because of the amount of force they exert on the tendon. Pain is present anywhere in the region of the Achilles tendon and initially follows strenuous activity. Later pain accompanies activity and limits participation. Pain may initially be worse at the beginning of a run and improve due to breakdown of adhesions. Stiffness can occur. There is usually tenderness 3–6 cm above the tendon insertion. This is intensified by squeezing the tendon medial to laterally. Decreased ankle dorsiflexion and hamstring tenderness are common. Tender nodular swellings are found in tendinosis and can accompany chronic symptoms. Rarely radiographs may show diffuse calcification of the soft tissue or tendon. Magnetic resonance imaging can distinguish between peritendinitis and tendinosis.

Initially there is thought to be inflammation in the surrounding tissue with thickening and oedema. This can impair the gliding function of the tendon. Histochemical studies have shown increased collagen breakdown and anaerobic enzyme activity.[50] If the stimulus is not removed, degenerative changes within the tendon may occur. Achilles tendinitis predisposes to rupture.

Treatment is usually conservative. Modifying exercise programmes, heel wedges, NSAIDs and cooling may help initially. Stretching and strengthening is probably the most important aspect of the treatment. Steroid injection into the tendon sheath relieves symptoms but care must be taken as intratendinous injection can cause rupture. Surgery is only necessary in refractory cases.

# References

1. Golders WR. A lecture on lumbago: its lessons and analogues. *Br Med J* **1:** 117–121, 1904
2a. Hench PK. Nonarticular rheumatism. Twenty-second rheumatism review: review of the American and English literature for the years 1973 and 1974. *Arthritis Rheum* **19** *No. 6 (suppl):* 1081–1088, 1976
2b. Smythe H. Fibrositis syndrome: a historical perspective. *J Rheumatol* (suppl 19): **16:** 2–6, 1989
3. Wolfe F, Smythe HA, Yunus MB *et al.* The American College of Rheumatology 1990 criteria for the classification of fibromyalgia: report of the Multicenter Criteria committee. *Arthritis Rheum* **33:** 160–172, 1990
4. Henriksson KG, Bengtsson A. Fibromyalgia – a clinical entity? *Can J Physiol Pharmacol* **69:** 672–677, 1991
5. Wolfe F. Fibromyalgia: the clinical syndrome. *Rheum Dis Clin North Am* **15:** 1–29, 1989
6. Yunus MB, Masi AT, Aldag JC. A controlled study of primary fibromyalgia syndrome: clinical features and association with other function syndromes. *J Rheumatol* (suppl 19) **16:** 62–71, 1989
7. Hench PK. Evaluation and differential diagnosis of fibromyalgia: approach to diagnosis and management. *Rheum Dis Clin North Am* **15:** 19–29, 1989
8. Boissevain MD, McGain GA. Towards an integrated understanding of fibromyalgia syndrome. I. Medical and pathophysiological aspects. *Pain* **45:** 227–238, 1991
9. Boissevain MD, McGain GA. Towards an integrated understanding of fibromyalgia syndrome. II. Psychological and phenomenological aspects. *Pain* **45:** 239–248, 1991
10. Bengtsson A, Henriksson KG. The muscle in fibromyalgia – a review of Swedish studies. *J Rheutmatol* (suppl 19) **16:** 144–149, 1989
11. Bennett RM, Clarke SR, Goldberg L *et al.* Aerobic fitness in patient with fibrositis. A controlled study of respiratory gas exchange and xenon[133] clearance from exercising muscle. *Arthritis Rheum* **32:** 454–460, 1989
12. Moldofsky H, Scarisbrick P, England R, Smythe H. Musculoskeletal symptoms and non-REM sleep disturbance in patients with 'fibrositis syndrome' and healthy subjects. *Psychosom Med* **37:** 341–351, 1975
13. Goldenberg DL. Fibromyalgia and its relation to chronic fatigue syndrome, viral illness and immune abnormalities. *J Rheumatol* (suppl 19) **16:** 91–93, 1989
14. Masi AT, Yunus MB. Fibromyalgia – which is the best treatment? A personalized, comprehensive, ambulatory, patient-involved management programme. *Baillieres Clin Rheumatol* **4:** 333–370, 1991
15. Goldenberg DL. Treatment of fibromyalgia syndrome. *Rheum Dis Clin North Am* **15:** 61–71, 1989
16. McCain GA. Nonmedicinal treatments in primary fibromyalgia. *Rheum Dis Clin North Am* **15:** 73–90, 1989
17. Felson DT, Goldenberg DL. The natural history of fibromyalgia. *Arthritis Rheum* **29:** 1522–1526, 1986
18. Simons DG. Muscle pain syndromes (I and II). *Am J Phys Med* **54:** 289–311, 1975; **55:** 1542, 1976
19. Simons DG. Muscular pain syndromes. In: (Fricton JR, Awad EA, eds) *Advances in Pain Research and Therapy*, vol 17. New York: Raven Press, 1990, pp. 1–41
20. Travell JG, Simons DG. Myofascial pain and dysfunction. *The Trigger Point Manual*. Baltimore: 1983, Williams & Wilkins
21. Bennett RM. Myofascial pain syndromes and fibromyalgia pain syndrome: a comparative analysis. In: (Fricton JR, Awad EA, eds) *Advances in Pain Research and Therapy*, vol 17. New York: Raven Press, 1990 pp. 43–65
22. Fricton JR, Auvinen MD, Dysktra D *et al.* Myofascial pain syndrome: electromyographic changes associated with local twitch response. *Arch Phys Med Rehab* **66:** (314–317) 1985

23. Fine PG, Milano R, Hare BD. The effects of myofascial trigger point injections are naloxone reversible. *Pain* **32:** 15–20, 1988
23a. Jaeger B, Shootsky SA. Double blind, controlled study of different myofascial trigger point injection techniques. *Pain* **31:** S292, 1987
24. Fricton JR. Myofascial pain syndrome. *Neurol Clin* **7:** 413–427, 1989
25. Sola AE, Rodenberger ML, Gettys BB. Incidence of hypersensitive areas in posterior shoulder muscles. *Am J Phys Med* **34:** 585, 1955
26. Cooper BC, Alleva M, Cooper DL *et al*. Myofascial pain dysfunction: analysis of 476 patients. *Laryngoscope* **96:** 1099, 1986
27. Fricton JR, Kroening R, Haley D *et al*. Myofascial pain syndromes of the head and neck: a review of the clinical characteristics of 164 patients. *Oral Surg Oral Med Pathol* **60:** 615, 1985
28. Goldman LB, Rosenberg NL. Myofascial pain syndrome and fibromyalgia. *Semin Neurol* **11:** 274–280, 1991
29. Simons DG. Fibrositis/fibromyalgia: a form of myofascial trigger points? *Am J Med* **81** (suppl 3A): 93–98, 1986
30. Scudds RA, Trachsel LCE, Luckhurst BJ, Percy JS. A comparative study of pain, sleep quality and pain responsiveness in fibrositis and myofascial pain syndrome. *J Rheumatol* (suppl 19) **16:** 120–126, 1989
31. Wolfe F. Fibromyalgia. Epidemiology of rheumatic disease. *Rheum Dis Clin North Am* **16:** 681–698, 1990
32. Campbell Semple J. Tenosynovitis, repetitive strain injury, cumulative trauma disorder and overuse syndrome, et cetera. *J Bone Joint Surg* **73-B:** 536–538, 1991
33. Hadler NM. Cumulative trauma disorder. An iatrogenic concept. *J Occup Med* **32:** 38–41, 1990
34. Ferguson DA. 'RSI': putting the epidemic to rest. *Med J Aust* **147:** 213–214, 1987
35. Quinter J. The RSI syndrome in historical perspective. *Int Disabil Studies* **13:** 99–104, 1991
36. Browne CD, Nolan BM, Faithfull DK. Occupational repetition strain injuries. Guidelines for diagnosis and management. *Med J Aust* **140:** 329–332, 1984
37. Huskinsson EC. Repetitive strain injury – the keyboard disease. Charterhouse Conference and Communications Ltd. 1992
38. Stone WE. Repetitive strain injuries. *Med J Aust* **2:** 616–618, 1983
39. Uhthoff HK, Sarkar K. Classification and definition of tendinopathies. *Clin Sports Med* **10:** 707–720, 1991
40. Bonutti PM, Hawkins RJ. Rotator cuff disorders. *Baillieres Clin Rheumatol* **3:** 535–550, 1989
41. Curtis AS, Snyder SJ. Evaluation and treatment of biceps tendon pathology. *Orthoped Clin North Am* **24:** 1993, pp. 33-43
42. Nirschl RP. Elbow tendinosis/tennis elbow. *Clin Sports Med* **11:** 851–870, 1992
43. Thorson E, Szabo RM. Common tendinitis problems in the hand and forearm. *Orthop Clin North Am* **23:** 65–74, 1992
44. Neustadt DH. Local corticosteroid injection therapy in soft tissue rheumatic conditions of the hand and wrist. *Arthritis Rheum* **34:** 923–926, 1991
45. Harvey FJ, Harvey PM, Horsley MW. DeQuervain's disease: surgical or non-surgical treatment. *J Hand Surg* **15A:** 83–87, 1990
46. Blazina ME, Kerlan RK, Jobe FW, Carter VS, Carlson GJ. Jumper's knee. *Orthop Clin North Am* **4:** 1973, pp. 665–678
47. Colosimo AJ, Bassett FH. Jumper's knee. Diagnosis and treatment. *Orthop Rev* **19:** 139–149, 1990
48. Leach RE, Dilorio E, Harney RA. Pathological hindfoot conditions in the athlete. *Clin Orthop* **177:** 116–121, 1983
49. Galloway MT, Jokl P, Dayton OW. Achilles tendon overuse injuries. *Clin. Sports Med* **11:** 771–782, 1992
50. Kvist MH, Lehto MUK, Jorza L *et al*. Chronic Achilles paratendonitis. *Am J Sports Med* **16:** 616–623, 1988

7

# Headache

**N. L. Padfield**

All of us have experienced headache at one time or another. In the majority of cases it resolves quickly and predictably with simple analgesics. Nevertheless it accounts for a huge amount of absenteeism and lost production at considerable cost to society. A large number of patients seek advice in pain clinics and pose a somewhat daunting problem to the tryo. A knowledge of the relevant anatomy, pathophysiology and careful and detailed evaluation of the patient's symptoms and signs in order to classify the condition correctly will aid the success in management of these difficult cases.

## Anatomy

### Blood supply to the head

The arterial blood supply to the head arrives from the common carotid artery which divides into internal and external branches and from the vertebral arteries arising from the subclavian arteries (Figure 7.1). The external carotid artery provides cervical, lingual, facial, maxillary, mandibular, pharyngeal, occipital, posterior auricular, and superficial temporal branches (these last three provide the majority of the arterial circulation to the scalp).

The vertebral arteries enter the foramen magnum to unite to become the basilar artery, which gives branches to the cerebellum, medulla, pons and midbrain and join the circle of Willis as communicating arteries to join the cerebral arteries, branches of the internal carotid artery whose branches supply the rest of the brain and meninges.

Venous blood is organized into superior and inferior sagittal venous sinuses at the superior and inferior borders of the falx cerebri which collect posteriorly into the transverse sinus along with the occipital sinus which then exit the skull either through the jugular veins or join the vertebral venous plexus. Anteriorly the ophthalmic veins join the facial veins and pterygoid venous plexuses to join the cavernous sinus which then exits the cranium via the petrosal sinuses to join the vertebral venous plexus. There are also small emissary vessels which perforate the skull to join the vascular supply to the surface structures.

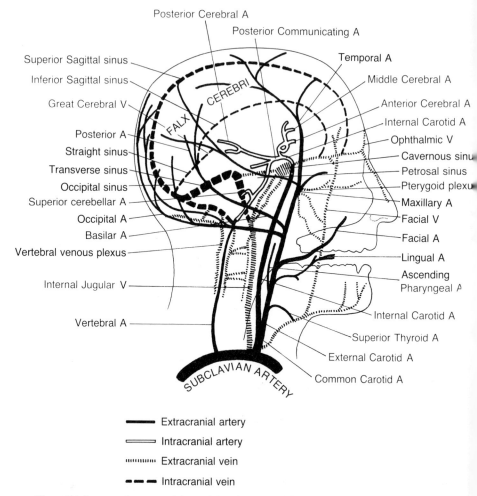

Posterior Cerebral A
Posterior Communicating A
Temporal A
Superior Sagittal sinus
Inferior Sagittal sinus
Great Cerebral V
Middle Cerebral A
Anterior Cerebral A
Internal Carotid A
CEREBRI
FALX
Posterior A
Ophthalmic V
Straight sinus
Cavernous sinu
Transverse sinus
Petrosal sinus
Occipital sinus
Pterygoid plexu
Superior cerebellar A
Maxillary A
Occipital A
Facial V
Basilar A
Facial A
Vertebral venous plexus
Lingual A
Internal Jugular V
Ascending
Pharyngeal A
Vertebral A
Internal Carotid A
Superior Thyroid A
External Carotid A
SUBCLAVIAN ARTERY
Common Carotid A

——— Extracranial artery
⊏⊐ Intracranial artery
⋯⋯⋯ Extracranial vein
– – – Intracranial vein

**Figure 7.1** Intra- and extracranial arterial and venous blood supply.

### Innervation of the head

The sensory nerve supply (excluding the special senses) travels with the blood vessels (Figure 7.2). The cranium has a sparse sensory innervation, mainly from unmyelinated nerve fibres with large receptive fields. The dura is the most sensitive structure supplied by adventitial plexus of sensory nerve fibres containing vasodilator neuropeptides. These include substance P, neurolinin A, calcitonin gene-related peptide, neuropeptide Y and vasoactive intestinal peptide,[1] which are stored in vesicles in the naked nerve endings.

The three branches of the trigeminal nerve supply the majority of the face, oral and nasal cavities and forehead, with the rest being supplied by the first three cervical nerves. Trigeminal fibres from the ganglion cells of the first

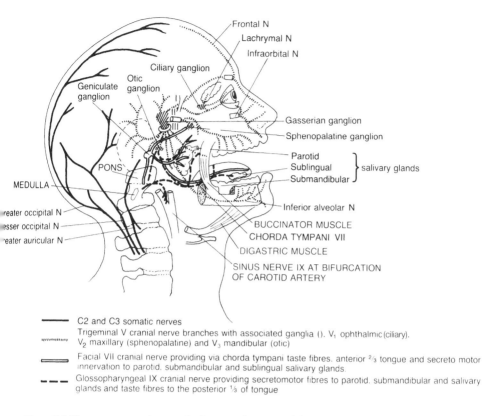

Figure7.2 The sensory supply to major intra- and extracranial structures.

division distribute themselves to the anterior, middle posterior cerebral arteries, anterior and posterior communicators on the same side. Hence the unilateral nature and the diffuse quality of pain and the difficulty in distinguishing between pain patterns produced by each of these three vessels. Some fibres also project into midlines structure such as the anterior cerebral artery, while others innervative the middle meningeal (dual, somatic) and middle cerebral (pial, visceral) arteries, which might explain the difficulty in separating pain from dural or pial origin. The rostral basilar artery along with the anterior cerebellar artery are supplied by axonal projections from the trigeminal ganglion, whereas the more caudal basilar and the vertebral arteries are supplied by the upper cervical dorsal root ganglion.

Afferent impulses from these two sources (trigeminal and cervical) converge on the second cervical segment of the spinal cord. The first-order synapse of central pathways is under the control of the endogenous pain system regulated by serotoninergic fibres from the nucleus raphe magnus and noradrenergic fibres from the locus coeruleus. The glossopharyngeal nerve and the vagus nerve supply the sensory innervation to the internal structures of the pharynx and larynx.

### Pain-sensitive structures of the head

- skin, subcutaneous tissue, muscle and its arteries, and the periosteum of the skull
- structures of the eye, ear, teeth and nasal cavity
- intracranial venous sinuses and their tributaries
- parts of the dura at the base of the skull
- dural arteries within the dura mater (anterior and middle meningeal)
- large arteries at the base of the brain
- V, IX, X cranial nerves
- first three cervical nerves

Note that the brain itself, its ependymal linings and much of its meningeal coverings are insensitive to pain.

## Classification

The International Headache Society has devised an international classification for headache and facial pain (Table 7.1).

**Table 7.1** International classification for headache and facial pain

1  Migraine
2  Tension-type headache
3  Cluster headache and chronic paroxysmal hemicrania
4  Miscellaneous headaches unassociated with structural lesions
5  Headache associated with head trauma
6  Headache associated with vascular disorders
7  Headache associated with non-vascular disorders
8  Headache associated with substances or their withdrawal
9  Headache associated with non-cephalic infection
10  Headache associated with metabolic disorders
11  Headache or facial pain associated with disorders of the cranium, neck, eyes, ears, nose, sinuses, teeth, mouth or other facial or cranial structures
12  Cranial neuralgias, nerve trunk pain and deafferentation pain
13  Headache not classified

For the purposes of this chapter categories 1, 2, 3 and part of 11 will be dealt with. Categories 4 and part of 11 will be dealt with in other chapters, whilst the remaining categories will not be touched upon since they are usually dealt with by other specialists outside the pain clinic.

## Evaluation and clinical presentation

Since headache can herald severe and life-threatening systemic disease, a careful history must be taken to determine the nature of the complaint.

At this stage it is important to emphasize that suspicion of any systemic disease must be referred to the relevant medical or surgical specialist for evaluation and appropriate treatment.

The corollary of this is that patients should only ideally be referred to the pain clinic when they have been fully evaluated and disease requiring specific medical or surgical treatment has been eliminated.

In the evaluation of symptoms one must determine:

- chronicity
- age of onset
- duration, frequency and variability of intensity
- onset to peak pain level time
- site
- character and severity of pain
- premonitory symptoms and aura
- associated symptoms
- precipitating factors

In addition to these, it is necessary to enquire into family history, medical and surgical history, past treatment, including substances of abuse and the results and nature of any previous diagnostic testing.

Warning bells should sound in the pain specialist's ears with the following factors:

- new headache of recent onset
- new headache of unusual intensity
- sudden change in a previously stable headache pattern
- nocturnal headache
- a short interval between pain onset and maximum intensity
- focal headache
- associated neurological dysfunction
- association with systemic illness, i.e. infection
- association with physical exertion
- headache associated with Valsalva manoeuvre

## The examination

The physical examination of the patient should focus on his or her general appearance, particularly taking note of the affect in terms of depression and anxiety. Various stereotypes have been suggested for different conditions. There is a female predominance amongst migraine sufferers who tend to be neat and trim, meticulous in details of condition and medication. In contrast there is a male predominance amongst cluster headache sufferers who tend to be plethoric with a square jaw and thick chin. The skin may reveal multiple telangiectasia and peau d'orange change over the malar surfaces and during an attack miosis, ptosis, lacrimation and facial flushing may be present. A tension headache sufferer may be of either sex and is often angry and aggressive, rubbing the temples or neck during the interview.

The patient with trigeminal neuralgia may find it difficult to talk, be dehydrated and have poor oral hygiene. The non-neuralgic atypical face pain may present in a similar fashion to the tension-type headache patient but may also show signs of abnormal grinding of the teeth.

### The head

Surgical scars, temporal arteries, sinuses, occipital nerves, trigger points, ocular anterior chamber, dental and periodontal tissues, oral cavity and salivary glands, temporomandibular joints and the external and middle ears must all be examined.

### The neck

Examination must look for decreased or faulty range of movement of the cervical spine, trigger points, signs of occult infection and malignancy, radicular or myelopathic signs in the extremities.

### Cranial nerves

Anosmia may suggest tumour involving the cribriform plate. Careful fundoscopy may reveal hypertensive or diabetic changes; palsies of the extrinsic ocular muscles may suggest intracranial pathology. Unilateral deafness may indicate acoustic neuroma. Serious intracranial lesions will arise from tumour, pus or blood (i.e. berry aneurysm, giant aneurysm, arteriovenous malformation).

## Investigation

Investigation is aimed to rule out systemic disease where headache is a prominent feature. A normal full blood count will rule out anaemia in association with collagen vascular disease. Abnormal results predicate an opinion from another medical specialty, i.e. rheumatology.

Positive findings at radiological examination of the cervical spine, skull and sinuses will generally reveal abnormalities requiring treatment by other specialties – ear, nose and throat, faciomaxillary or neurosurgery.

Further investigation, such as computed tomographic scan, magnetic resonance imaging scan, cerebral arteriography and digital subtraction, if indicated by a history suggestive of an intracranial mass lesion, predicates referral to another medical or surgical specialist.

Lastly, acute-onset headache or facial pain may be infective in origin and warrant a lumbar puncture. If you think a lumbar puncture is indicated, then make an urgent referral to an appropriate specialist.

When headache is a symptom of various general medical disease or specific disease to be found in the structures of the intra- and extracranial compartments, it is called organic headache. However, when it is not a symptom of such conditions it is called primary headache.

# Specific primary headache syndromes

### Vascular

- migraine
- cluster
- paroxysmal hemicrania

### Non-vascular

- cervicogenic
- tension-type
- myofascial

# Migraine

### Clinical features

- This is a periodic unilateral headache that appears most frequently by the third decade but can occur in childhood. The frequency of attacks varies from every few days to once every 5 or 6 months. The pain is usually throbbing and often settles behind one eye. There are often systemic symptoms such as nausea and vomiting, diarrhoea and associated photophobia. There may be alterations in mood, loss of libido and occasionally focal neurological deficits which can confuse the diagnosis. The headache usually lasts for at least 4 h and may continue for longer than 24 h. There is a female preponderance of 70%, with a prevalence of 6% for men and 15% for women,[1,2] and often there is a strong family history.
- Personalities are often described as obsessive and compulsive, but on performing the Minnesota multiphasic personality inventory on a large group of sufferers this was not confirmed, as patients revealed essentially normal personality profiles.
- There are often triggering factors such as tyramine-containing foods, alcohol, monosodium glutamate, nitrates, hormones and oral contraceptives, strong odours (like perfume) and strong sunlight.
- Migraine can occur: without aura; with aura, where the patient experiences pre-headache neurological disturbance commonly involving the visual cortex but also the sense of smell, motor function and feeling; and with prolonged aura, where the neurological disturbance persists beyond the immediate headache period.

### Pathophysiology

- Vascular changes associated with migraine can be simulated in the laboratory by activation of brainstem structures. Stimulation of the locus coeruleus causes reduction in regional cerebral blood flow, particularly in the visual cortex, but reflexly increases extracranial blood flow. Stimulation of the dorsal raphe nucleus and the trigeminal complex increases both cerebral and extracranial blood flow via a pathway leaving the brainstem in the parasympathetic part of the facial nerve, the greater petrosal nerve.

- Strong afferent stimuli like cold (icecream headache) are known to cause headache commonly in the habitual site in migraine sufferers. Patients who have had indwelling electrodes placed in the periaqueductal grey matter for the relief of intractable pain get migraine-like headaches. Both these facts support the theory of a central origin for migraine.

- Migraine sufferers have chronically low plasma 5-hydroxytryptamine (5-HT) levels[3] but these have been shown to double to control levels during a migraine attack.[4] While platelets release 5-HT during an attack, it is now thought that there is an increased turnover of 5-HT in plasma during interictal periods which results in low levels between attacks. During an attack the 5-HT turnover is reduced, thus 'normalizing' plasma levels, probably by a transient fall in enzyme degradation. The rise in plasma 5-HT may be seen as a defence mechanism; this could explain the ability of parenterally administered 5-HT agonists to abort migraine attacks.

- Increased glutamate and aspartate release and their consequent effect on the $N$-methyl-D-aspartate (NMDA) receptors are pivotal in spreading electrical depression implicated in the pathophysiology of migraine aura. By analogy with erythrocyte glutamate/aspartate active cellular uptake mechanism defects, it has been postulated that these are also responsible at the neuronal/glial cell level for the production of the migraine aura. While NMDA activity is attenuated by high magnesium levels, low levels, which are often found in migraine sufferers, potentiate NMDA activity.

- Migraine sufferers have low plasma and high platelet levels of methionine-enkephalin, which increase considerably during attacks.

- Calcitonin gene-related peptide (CGRP) has been found to rise during an attack but levels can be normalized with parenterally administered sumatriptan.

- Released neuropeptides activate endothelial cells, mast cells and platelets, to increase extracellular levels of amines, arachidonic acid metabolites, peptides and ions. Hyperalgesia and prolongation of pain levels result from activated cells and injured tissue. There is an early expression of the nuclear proteins c-*fos* with postsynaptic brainstem neurons of the trigeminal nucleus caudalis.[5]

- Migraine is thought to be a result of extracerebral cranial dilatation of the meningeal and dural arteries and arteriovenous shunts. Sumatriptan alleviates the effects by causing vasoconstriction of these vessels.[6] But this may not be the whole story, and neurogenic plasma extravasation which leads to sensitization of sensory nerve endings within the trigeminovascular system may also play a part in the genesis of pain.[7]

## Management

This will depend on the severity and frequency of attacks. It must take into account the impact on lifestyle of the headaches and the results of previous treatments. There may also be systemic diseases present that preclude certain treatments.

If the attacks are only every few months then abortive therapy should suffice. If however the attacks are frequent, severely compromise the patient's lifestyle or the patient suffers from the prolonged aura variant (which untreated has led to permanent neurological deficit), then treatment should be aimed at prophylaxis.

### Abortive therapies

- The 5-HT analogue sumatriptan is probably the most effective and reliable drug to abort an attack.[8,9] It can be given parenterally and will abort the headache at any stage.
- If the pain is not too severe, non-steroidal anti-inflammatory drugs (NSAIDs) and antiemetics may suffice, along with biofeedback training in suitable patients.
- Ergotamine has been successfully used in the past as it is an effective vasoconstrictor, but its use is contraindicated in any patient with coronary, cerebral or peripheral occlusive vascular disease. It is also contraindicated in any patient with a history of drug abuse, as its misuse or abuse can result in severe complications. However, in a highly select group of reliable patients its use can be extremely effective, but there are reservations about its continued prescription.[10]
- Various interventions, such as sphenopalatine block, injection of tender extracranial trigger areas, acupuncture and even intravenous infusions of lignocaine, have been found to be helpful in the acute situation.

### Prophylactive treatment

- Pizotifen, a 5-HT and histamine antagonist, has proven effective in migraine prophylaxis.
- β-Blockers have also proven effective, propranolol being the first choice, but nadolol or metoprolol may be substituted if somnolence or loss of libido is a problem. These drugs are of course contraindicated in the presence of cardiac failure, asthma or poorly controlled diabetes.
- Calcium channel blockers like verapamil have been effective in some patients who have not derived benefit from β-blockers. However there are more side-effects with these drugs.
- Antidepressants have been tried but the results are inconsistent and effectiveness will depend on careful patient appraisal.
- Clonidine, the $\alpha_2$-blocker, at low dosage has been helpful, especially in patients who have headaches triggered by tyramine. But it can often cause troublesome orthostatic hypotension. The various drug regimes have been reviewed by Solomon.[11]
- Serial sphenopalatine ganglion blocks performed daily for a week may be worth a trial in patients poorly controlled by β-blockers or antidepressants.

## Cluster headache

### Clinical features

Patients are predominantly male and affected on average in their fourth decade – 10 years later than migraine sufferers. There is usually no family history. The headaches occur in clusters after the seasonal change in the length of the day. The peak period is 90 min after the onset of sleep. The patient will experience on average 2–3 headaches per day, lasting 45–60 min. The cluster period usually lasts 8–10 weeks with remission usually shorter than 2 years. In some patients the attacks are 10 times more frequent and periods of remission are very reduced – a condition called chronic cluster headache. The pain is agonizing, retro-orbital, unilateral and temporal of a deep burning quality. It is associated with Horner's syndrome and lacrimation, facial flushing and conjunctival injection. Ocular and skin changes (peau d'orange, telangiectasia and furrowing of the forehead) may become permanent. The pain is so bad during an attack that it is quite common for patients to rock forwards and backwards in a chair and suicides have been reported. Attacks can, like migraine, be provoked by alcohol, nitrates, histamine, other vasoactive substances and high altitude.

### Pathophysiology

Cluster headaches are also an abnormality of brain blood how associated with discharge along the parasympathetic pathway, the greater petrosal nerve, and are associated with facial flushing, lacrimation and rhinorrhoea. An ocular Horner's syndrome is often observed, probably because post-ganglionic sympathetic neurons are compromised in the pericarotid plexus by oedema of the wall of the carotid syphon. Like migraine, therapy is directed at causing vasoconstriction of the extracerebral blood vessels.

### Management

Because the pain is so severe it should be treated as an emergency and abortive therapy instigated immediately.

- Oxygen inhalation remains the safest and most effective method of aborting the attack.[12] A close-fitting mask with a flow of 10 l/min will usually abort an attack within 10 min.
- Sphenopalatine blocks performed daily may also be used in combination with oxygen therapy to abort acute cluster headache.
- A short, rapidly reducing course of steroids has also been found to be effective, starting at 80 mg prednisolone, reducing daily by 10 mg.

## Chronic cluster headache

### Clinical features

The diagnosis of this rare form requires at least two attacks per week over a period of more than a year. The pattern may arise beginning with regular attacks of more than two a week or a chronic pattern may supersede an ordinary intermittent cluster headache pattern.

### Management

Lithium carbonate is the treatment of choice. However the therapeutic ratio is low and careful monitoring of plasma levels should be routine. The dose to start with is 300 mg for 2 days, then 300 mg b.d. thereafter. Thirst, polyuria, rash, fatigue and nausea may be the first symptoms of toxicity.

As a last resort, in chronic cluster headache some form of trigeminal ganglion destruction may be considered. This should obviously be performed by a clinician familiar with the technique and complications.

## Chronic paroxysmal hemicrania

### Clinical features

This is a rare variant of cluster headache where 80–90% of sufferers are women. The pain is principally ocular, frontal and temporal, associated with lacrimation and nasal stuffiness. It is usually completely relieved by indomethacin.

Daily attacks occur at a maximum of 15–30/24 h. While patients characteristically have attacks every day, their intensity and frequency vary. Each attack lasts 5–45 min with a usual duration of 30 min. Nausea and vomiting are rarely associated. Attacks can be provoked by bending or rotating the head. The symptoms disappear during pregnancy, only to reappear in the postpartum period. A review of the literature and a review of 3 cases emphasizes the importance of differentiation from cluster headaches.[13]

### Management

Treatment with indomethacin will give complete relief for as long as it is taken.

## Cervicogenic headache

### Clinical features

- The clinical features are unilateral headache with symptoms and signs of neck involvement,[14] where pain is provoked by pressure on the ipsilateral upper posterior neck region. The pain is associated with ipsilateral neck and arm pain and there is a reduced range of movement in the cervical spine. The pain is characteristically moderate, non-clustering, non-throbbing and of varying duration that starts in the neck and spreads forward.
- There is a female predominance and often there is a history of neck trauma. It must be differentiated from migraine without aura

and tension-type headache. In a recent study comparing patients with cervicogenic headache and migraine without aura, a clearcut difference was found between the two groups where onset of frontotemporal pain was virtually pathognomonic of migraine without aura.[18]

## Pathophysiology

Forehead pain may be caused by stimuli being transferred from the posterior part of the head/neck via C1–3 nerves. In the brainstem nerve fibres have a close relationship to the caudal part of the trigeminal nucleus. Cortical interpretation of the impulses may therefore be misinterpreted as coming from the ophthalmic division of the trigeminal nerve. The facet joints C2–3 and the cervical nerves C1–3 have been blocked with success and this leads to the diagnosis.[16]

## Management

Treatment involves blockade of the greater occipital nerve, the cervical zygapophyseal joints at C2–3 level and the supraorbital nerve with bupivacaine 0.5%. If this is successful, then more permanent relief may be afforded by cryotherapy to these nerves.

# Tension-type

### Clinical features

- This is the commonest form of non-vascular headache. It was in the recent past referred to as muscle contraction headache. However, it is often not associated with any muscle contraction at all.
- It is usually bilateral, though it can be unilateral, often involving the frontal, temporal and occipital regions. There is often associated neck symptomatology. It is often described as a band-like non-pulsatile ache or tightness. Its onset is gradual and lasts over a period of hours to days.
- There is usually considerable sleep disturbance with this kind of headache, with sufferers complaining of headaches at 4–8 a.m. and also in the afternoon at 4 p.m. While there is no strict family history, children learn to mimic their parents.
- There may well be unresolved conflicts in the emotional, marriage or psychosexual sphere with resultant latent depression and somatization in the form of abnormal muscle contraction. Stress, whether physical or emotional, is the common trigger.[17]
- Acute cervical spine injury, like whiplash, will exacerbate pre-existing tension-type headache, as will worsening pre-existing degenerative cervical spine conditions like spondylosis.

## Pathophysiology

The electromyogram (EMG) evidence of chronic muscle tension is often only found in patients who have migraine as well as tension-type headache. Whilst in one study, headache sufferers showed significantly higher temporal EMG activity compared with controls, the EMG data *per se* were of little value in assigning patients to specific diagnostic groups.[18] There is evidence that tension headache sufferers have very low platelet met-encephalin compared with sufferers from migraine without aura.[19]

## Management

- This can be abortive or prophylactic. The choice of treatment approach will depend on frequency and severity of attacks and the impact on the patient's lifestyle. The results of any previous diagnostic testing and therapy along with any history of drug abuse must be taken into consideration when deciding on a therapeutic course of action appropriate to each individual patient.
- If the patient only suffers every few months, then education in reduction or avoidance of physical or psychological stress in combination with simple analgesics and non-steroidals may suffice.
- But most patients will have been referred because of the intractable nature (apparently) of their headache, so that prophylactic approaches are more appropriate. Treatment with antidepressant compounds has been found to be very efficacious because not only are they analgesic; they can also restore normal ordered sleep patterns and treat underlying depression. Simple analgesics and non-steroidal compounds can be used simultaneously to treat exacerbations. Amitryptiline 25 mg is a good initial choice where the physician must titrate the dose against the side-effects of dry mouth, blurred vision, constipation and somnolence. If the last is a problem then a 5-HT reuptake inhibitor like fluoxitene 20 mg may be better tolerated. Care must be exercised in the presence of cardiac disease or advanced age.
- In young well-motivated non-depressed patients, monitored relaxation techniques combined with education in coping strategies and stress reduction can be very beneficial. Any skills learned in biofeedback, though, must be used regularly at home and work to sustain the beneficial effect.
- Cervical epidural steroids have their advocates in the treatment of chronic severe tension headaches. They may be particularly of use early on in the management of chronic tension-type headache in the more elderly depressed patient while waiting for antidepressant medical therapy to work.
- Occasionally it will be necessary to admit patients as the headache is the somatization end-point of a serious underlying psychiatric disorder such as major depression or uncontrolled anxiety states. This may be superimposed on drug abuse/dependence, where the patient may need to be detoxified or weaned from drugs. The help of a psychiatric colleague can be invaluable in these circumstances.

# Myofascial pain

### Clinical features

There are trigger or hyperirritable foci which can be identified by digital pressure that cause pain, which may then be referred within the muscle to the principal site of pain – active trigger point – or it may just be evoked locally by digital pressure – latent trigger point. In one study the muscles most commonly tender to digital pressure were found to be: lateral pterygoid (51%), the trapezius (52%) and the sternomastoid (51%). There was a female preponderance and the young age group was more tender than the old age group.[20] The pain is described as dull and aching, provoked by stress and repetitive movement under strain (as in ironing).

### Pathophysiology

The pathophysiology is unknown but it is thought that this may represent some injury to muscle or ligamentous tissue.

### Management

Very often this will gradually resolve over a period of a few months. Physiotherapy with graded exercises forms the mainstay of treatment, with the avoidance of immobilization. Acupuncture can often be a very useful adjunct. Relaxation therapy and biofeedback have also been found to be effective. However, there are some premorbid personalities that preclude complete resolution and when litigation is pending symptoms may persist or even increase.

# Missed pathology

Lastly there may be a small group of patients referred inappropriately to the pain management clinic suffering from serious conditions that require urgent referral to another specialty for investigation and treatment. Symptoms and signs of such dangerous conditions have already been alluded to. When an intracranial mass lesion is suggested, this will be due to:

● tumour
● pus
● blood

All of these require urgent referral to a neurosurgical unit. There will also be other miscellaneous causes that require treatment by other physicians and these include:

● giant cell arteritis
● diseases of the skull (osteomyelitis, mastoiditis, Paget's disease)
● diseases of the eye (glaucoma, iritis etc.)

These organic headache conditions are outside the scope of this chapter and can best be found described in the relevant general medical or surgical textbooks.

## References

1. Udman R, Edvinsson L. Neuropeptides in the cerebral circulation. *Cerebrovasc Brain Metabolism Rev* **1**: 230–252, 1989
2. Rasmussen BK, Jensen R, Schroll M, Olesen J. Epidemiology of headache in a general population – a prevalence study. *J Clin Epidemiol* **44**: 1147–1157, 1991
3. Stewart WF, Lipton RB, Celentano DD, Reed ML. *JAMA* **267**: 64–69, 1992
4. Ferrari MD, Saxena PR. On serotonin and migraine: a clinical and pharmacological review. *Cephalgia* **13**: 151–165, 1993
5. Ferrari MD, Odink J, Taparelli C, Van Kempen GMJ, Pennings EJM, Bruyn GW. *Neurology* **39**: 1235–1242, 1989
6. Moskowitz MA. Neurogenic inflammation in the pathophysiology and treatment of migraine. *Neurology* **43** (suppl 3): S16–S20, 1993
7. Ferrari MD. Sumatriptan in the treatment of migraine. *Neurology* **43** (suppl 3): S43–S47, 1993
8. Macfarlane R. New concepts of vascular headache. *Ann R Coll Surg* **75**: 225–228, 1993
9. Tansey MJ, Pilgrim AJ, Lloyd K. *J Neurol Sci* **114**: 109–116, 1993
10. Moskowitz MA, Cutrer PM. Sumatriptan: a receptor targeted treatment for migraine. *Annu Rev Med* **44**: 145–154, 1993
11. Dahlof C. Placebo controlled clinical trials with ergotamine in the acute treatment of migraine. *Cephalgia* **13**: 166–171, 1993
12. Solomon GD. Therapeutic advances in migraine. *J Clin Pharmacol* **33**: 200–209, 1993
13. Sjaastad O, Fredriksen TA, Pfaffenrath V. *Headache* **30**: 725–726, 1990
14. Newman LC, Lipton RB, Solomon S. Episodic paroxysmal hemicrania: 3 new cases and a review of the literature. *Headache* **33**: 95–97, 1993
15. Di Sabato F, Fusco B, Pelaia P, Giacovazzo M. Hyperbaric oxygen therapy in cluster headache. *Pain* **52**: 243–245, 1993
16. Sjaastad O, Bovim G, Stovner LJ. Common migraine ('migraine without aura'); localization of the initial pain attack. *Funct Neurol* **8**: 27–32.
17. Bovim G, Sand T. Cervicogenic headache, migraine without aura and tension-type headache. Diagnostic blockade of greater occipital and supra-orbital nerves. *Pain* **51**: 43–48, 1992
18. Rasmussen BK. Migraine and tension-type headache in a general population: precipitating factors, female hormones, sleep pattern and relation to lifestyle. *Pain* **53**: 65–72, 1993
19. Hatch JP, Moore PJ, Cyr-Provost M, Boutros NN, Seleshi E, Borcherding S. The use of electromyography and muscle palpation in the diagnosis of tension-type headache with and without pericranial muscle involvement. *Pain* **49**: 175–178, 1992
20. Ferrari MD. *Pathol Biol* **40**: 287–292, 1992
21. Jensen R, Rasmussen BK, Pedersen B, Lous I, Olesen J. Cephalic muscle tenderness and pressure pain threshold in a general population. *Pain* **48**: 197–203, 1992

# 8

# Facial pain

**N. M. Girdler**

Facial pain may be a temporary inconvenience or a life sentence. It often has special emotional, biological and psychological meaning to the patient. Apart from headache, which may also involve structures in the mouth and face, acute facial pain arising from dental disease is probably the most common pain in the body.[1] It has been estimated that 'toothache' is suffered for over 5 million days per year in the UK. However, although acute dental pain is the most common cause of facial pain, it is also the most readily treated; there are over 26 000 dentists in the UK expert in its management.

In contrast, it is the chronic types of facial pain that usually present to the pain specialist. These can be a major source of dilemma in diagnosis and management.[2] Chronic facial pain is believed to account for 40% of all chronic pain problems, affecting over 20% of the population.[3] Many cases can be effectively treated using simple therapeutic regimes but others may require multidisciplinary pain therapy.[4] Such conditions include pain arising from disorders of the temporomandibular joints, masticatory muscles, nose, paranasal sinuses, eyes, ears and salivary glands. It also encompasses the facial neuralgias, migrainous syndromes, psychogenic and referred facial pain. These complex cases will frequently present for specialist pain management and are therefore the prime subject area of this chapter.

## Anatomy and physiology of facial pain

The face, underlying oral and nasal cavities and the associated structures are principally innervated with sensory nerve fibres from the fifth cranial nerve (the trigeminal nerve).[5] The trigeminal nerve has three major divisions, the ophthalmic, maxillary and mandibular, each of which has many important branches (Figure 8.1). Nociceptive fibres in the trigeminal ramifications are mainly small myelinated A-$\delta$ fibres but up to a tenth may be unmyelinated C-fibres. Certain sites such as the cornea and dental pulp are predominantly or exclusively innervated by nociceptive afferents.

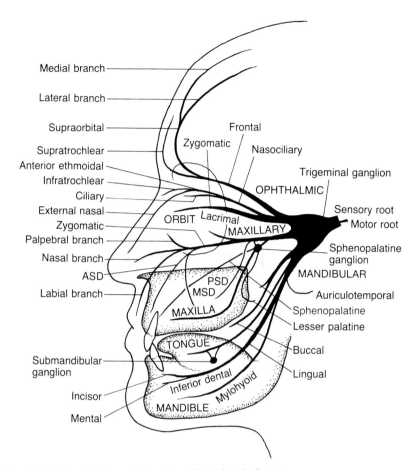

**Figure 8.1** Major divisions and branches of the trigeminal nerve.

The posterior third of the tongue and the faucial region is innervated by the glossopharyngeal nerve. The skin over the angle of the mandible is innervated by the second and third cervical segments (Figure 8.2). There is also some contribution to innervation of the face from the nervus intermedius of the facial nerve and the vagus nerve.

Impulses originating in the trigeminal field travel via the peripheral nerve branches to the trigeminal ganglion.[6] Cell bodies of first-order neurons form the trigeminal ganglion which lies in a depression in the petrous temporal bone, lateral to the internal carotid artery and at the posterior end of the cavernous sinus. The central processes of trigeminal and other first-order sensory nerves converge and enter the brainstem where they synapse in one of three separate nuclei which extend from the pons to the upper spinal cord. The specific modalities determined by each nucleus are as shown in Table 8.1.

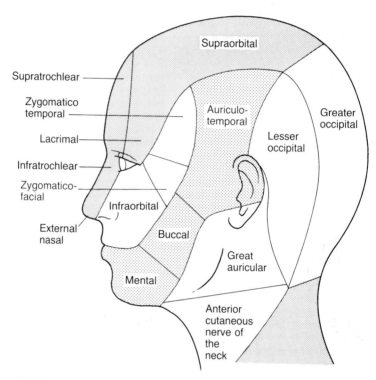

**Figure 8.2** Cutaneous nerve supply of the face and head.

The wide-ranging distribution of trigeminal neurons in the brainstem provides a system for referred pain in the trigeminal system[7] (Figure 8.3).

Second-order neurons transmit to the thalamus and are subsequently relayed bilaterally to the hypothalamus and to the sensory, temporal and frontal cortices. The autonomic response to pain occurs in the hypothalamus, while the sensory cortex is involved with analysis of the site and distribution of pain, the temporal cortex with memory and the frontal cortex determines the psychological reaction to pain. There is a disproportionately large representation of the orofacial region in the higher levels of the somatosensory system, which accounts for the exquisite sensibility of the orofacial tissues.

Peripheral cellular damage can be mediated by physical, chemical, inflammatory or immunological injury and is associated with increases in local concentrations of serotonin, histamine, kallidin, bradykinin and prostaglandins. These chemicals have the ability to depolarize nociceptors, produce action potentials and thereby initiate painful stimuli. Neuropeptides such as substance P, neurokinin A, calcitonin gene-related peptide, noradrenaline and $\gamma$-aminobutyric acid assume a role as neurotransmitters in the more central trigeminal nociceptive pathways. The endogenous opioid peptides, enkephalins and endorphins, have varying degrees of analgesic potential and are important in central pain control.

**Table 8.1** Modalities of the mesencephalic, sensory and spinal nuclei

| Nucleus | Modality | Source of afferents |
|---|---|---|
| Mesencephalic | Proprioception | Muscles of mastication<br>    facial expression<br>    tongue<br>    ocular movement<br>Periodontal ligament |
| Sensory | Touch<br>Pressure | Skin<br>Mucous membranes<br>Bone<br>Gingivae<br>Cornea |
| Spinal | Pain<br>Temperature | Skin<br>Mucous membranes<br>Bone<br>Dental pulp<br>Gingivae<br>Cornea |

## Classification of facial pain

Since facial pain has a multiplicity of causes it is helpful to being with a simple classification.[8] The most common causes of facial pain can be divided clinically into those arising from:

- local disease
- neurological disorders
- psychogenic conditions
- referred pain

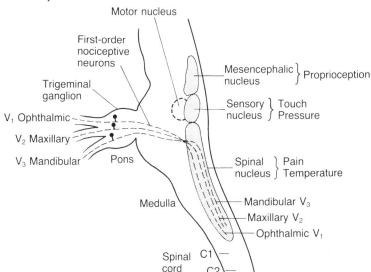

**Figure 8.3** The relations of the trigeminal ganglion and trigeminal nuclei in the brainstem. Nociceptor neurons converge in the spinal nucleus where they synapse.

## History

In order to maximize the value of the history, the following information about the nature of the pain must be determined.[9]

- site – area of maximum severity, trigger points, radiation
- quality – sharp, stabbing, throbbing, dull or burning
- periodicity – speed of onset, duration, frequency, diurnal or seasonal variation
- provoked by eating, yawning, talking, heat or cold
- relieved by heat, cold, analgesics, splints or collars
- associated symptoms – swelling, facial analgesia, nasal obstruction, jaw dysfunction, tooth grinding, also concurrent neck, back, chest, abdominal or pelvic pain

Then questions should be specifically directed towards obtaining details of the patient's:

- general health – medical history, review of systems
- social history – occupation, stress, smoking, alcohol
- family history – marital status, children, siblings, parents
- drugs and allergies – past, current

## Examination

Each patient must be examined in a systematic manner with particular emphasis on structures of the head, neck and face.[10]

### Visual inspection

Careful assessment of:

- swelling
- asymmetry
- skin/scalp lesions
- scars
- fundoscopy
- auroscopy
- nasal inspection

### Palpation

#### Lymph nodes

Evaluation of consistency – swollen, soft, firm, tender, mobile, fixed. Each group is examined in a logical sequence:

- deep cervical
- superficial cervical

- occipital
- preauricular
- submandibular
- sublingual

### Salivary glands

Assessment of swelling, tenderness or erythema. Appearance and patency of the salivary ducts.

- parotid
- submandibular

### Temporomandibular joint and masticatory muscles

- range of mandibular movement
- pain/noises in and around the temporomandibular joint during function
- test for muscle tenderness/spasm – temporalis and masseter, by direct palpation; lateral pterygoid, by pushing the jaw forwards against resistance or by palpating directly behind the maxillary tuberosity
- trigger zones

## Cranial nerve assessment

The function of each cranial nerve must be appraised. Any abnormality suggests organic disease and indicates the need for referral to the appropriate specialist for treatment.

## Intraoral examination

- teeth – percussion test: tapping teeth with a blunt instrument to assess periodontal pathology; ethyl chloride pulp test: small wad of soaked cotton wool applied to test pulp vitality; electric pulp test: low electric current used to determine pulp vitality
- gingivae
- buccal/labial oral mucosa
- hard/soft palate tongue
- tonsils
- fauces
- pharynx

## Diagnostic nerve blocks

Local anaesthetic nerve blocks can be diagnostic as well as palliative.[11]

### Mandible

- Inferior dental nerve block: The inferior dental nerve is anaesthetized where it enters the mandibular foramen just above the lingula. After palpation of the mandibular internal oblique ridge the needle is advanced along the medial aspect of the mandibular ramus for about 2 cm where the solution is then deposited. This will anaesthetize the ipsilateral mandibular teeth, the mandibular bone and the soft tissue of the lower lip (Figure 8.4).

- Lingual nerve block is performed by injecting the lingual tissues just behind the third molar teeth.
- Mental nerve block: The mental nerve can be anaesthetized where it emerges from the mental foramen between the root apices of the lower premolars.
- Long buccal nerve block: This nerve is blocked as it passes down the external oblique ridge of the posterior mandible.

### Maxilla

- Infraorbital nerve block: This will anaesthetize the ipsilateral anterior maxilla, upper incisor teeth and the soft tissues of the cheek, upper lip and lateral aspect of the nose. The infraorbital block is best performed via an indirect intraoral approach; the infraorbital margin is palpated and the globe protected with a finger while the needle is advanced through the upper labial mucosa and the solution deposited 1 cm below the midline of the infraorbital margin (Figure 8.5).
- Supraorbital nerve block: Performed directly by depositing local anaesthetic along the supraorbital margin.
- Palatal nerve blocks: The local anaesthetic solution is placed around the greater palatine or nasopalatine foramina.

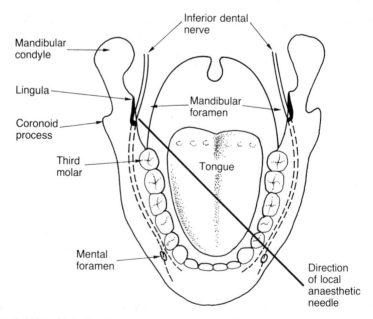

**Figure 8.4** Site of injections for an inferior dental nerve block.

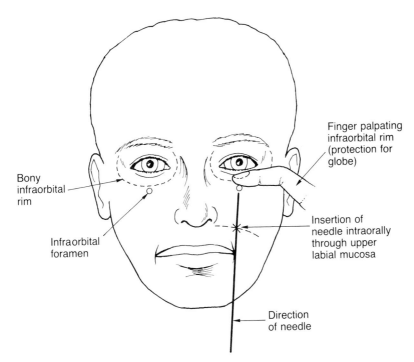

**Figure 8.5** Diagram of infraorbital nerve block.

### Temporomandibular joint and neck

Local anaesthetic deposited just anterior to the mid-tragus will block the auriculotemporal nerve and eliminate arthralgic temporomandibular joint pain. If cervical referral is suspected, nerve blocks can be performed on selective spinal nerves from C2 to C4.

### Muscles of mastication

Depositing a small amount of local anaesthetic around a muscle belly may be diagnostic by abolishing a trigger point or relieving muscle spasm.

## Investigations

### Radiography

The simplest and most useful initial investigation that can be performed in all units is radiography of the face. The most helpful screening radiographs are as follows:

- Orthopantomogram (OPG): This is a full-mouth radiograph which will show obvious dental disease, bony pathology in the mandible and disease in the inferior aspect of the temporomandibular joints. Detailed joint pathology can be seen more clearly if the radiograph is taken whilst the mouth is wide open. The OPG also shows the dental aspect of the maxillae and the floor of the maxillary antra. Alternative views where an OPG is not available are the left and right lateral obliques.

- Occipitomental radiographs: Pathology in the maxilla, paranasal sinuses and orbits is best visualized in occipitomental (OM) radiographs. Angulations of 45°, 30° and 10° will show all aspects of the middle part of the face. As an adjunct, lateral facial and base of skull radiographs may be helpful in excluding maxillary antral and nerve trunk pathology respectively.
- Computed tomograms (CT) and magnetic resonance image (MRI) scans: By far the most revolutionary recent development in the investigation of facial pain has been the introduction of CT and MRI scanning. The visualization of deep bony and soft-tissue structures has led to the diagnosis of previously hidden pathology, in particular the localization of tumours. Furthermore, in complex psychogenic types of facial pain, negative scans give essential confirmation that there is no organic disease present.

### Laboratory tests

Tests should be used to screen for underlying diseases such as those of infective or autoimmune origin:

- full blood picture
- erythrocyte sedimentation test
- autoantibody screen

### Specialized investigations

- sialography – to show calculi and salivary gland disease
- temporomandibular joint arthrography – indicates intra-articular pathology
- fine-needle aspiration biopsy – useful for swollen nodes
- open biopsy – for suspicious soft-tissue or bony lesions

## Clinicopathological features and management

### Dental and oral pain

It is unlikely that cases of toothache will present to the pain specialist. Most cases are straightforward to treat and come well within the remit of the dental, oral or maxillofacial surgeon. Nevertheless, toothache is the commonest cause of acute facial pain and it can be misinterpreted as other facial pain conditions. A basic understanding of some common forms of toothache is helpful to avoid missing the obvious in many cases of facial pain. Conditions that are classified as toothache include pulpitis, periodontitis, pericoronitis, stomatitis and osteitis.

- Pulpitis occurs when the dental pulp or dentine is exposed and presents as a severe, stabbing pain in response to hot, cold or sweet stimuli. If the pulp becomes inflamed the pain becomes intense and throbbing, giving a classical toothache. Dental caries, cracked cusps, lost restorations and split crowns all give rise to pulpal pain. Affected teeth will be acutely sensitive to cold; application of ethyl chloride will be excruciating to the patient!

  Treatment may involve placement of a sedative dressing, a new restoration, pulp extirpation with root canal therapy or extraction of the tooth. An unusual feature of pulpitis which may lead to pain specialist referral is that the pain is poorly localized and may radiate into the adjacent jaw and sometimes the ipsilateral jaw. Even when the toothache has been relieved, facial pain may persist. It is often difficult to distinguish pulpitic pain from symptomatic neuralgia and atypical facial pain.

- Periodontitis: Death and necrosis of the dental pulp can lead to inflammation at the apex of the root, which is termed apical periodontitis. This pain is dull, continuous, throbbing and well-localized but with considerable radiation and associated swelling and tenderness. The tooth is exquisitely tender to touch, so chewing is avoided. The adjacent mucosa will be red and tender. If untreated, suppuration occurs rapidly with the formation of a dentoalveolar abscess.

  Treatment involves drainage of the infected area via the root canal of the tooth or by extraction.

- Pericoronitis is caused by infection of the flap of gingiva that surrounds a partly erupted or impacted tooth. The condition is common amongst patients in their late teens and early 20s when the wisdom teeth (third molars) are erupting. Many third molars do not have enough room to erupt and thereby become impacted and susceptible to pericoronitis. Patients present with acute pain and swelling around the angle of the mandible and occasionally severe trismus (limitation of jaw opening). The submandibular and cervical lymph glands are often enlarged and tender.

  Radiographs will show the impacted tooth and treatment will eventually necessitate extraction once the acute infection has resolved with antibiotics.

  Pericoronitis can be misdiagnosed for other forms of facial pain, especially temporomandibular joint pain and spasm in the muscles of mastication. It is easy to attribute pain to impacted teeth just because they are there. In fact, impacted teeth that have no communication with the oral cavity are rarely the cause of pain.

- Stomatitis or oral ulceration can have a traumatic, infective, auto-immune, neoplastic or systemic aetiology. Ulcers of the oral mucosa give rise to a continuous pain and, depending on their severity, may considerably restrict dietary intake. Mucosal ulceration is usually easily identified as a cause of facial pain. Ironically, the more sinister ulcers, such as squamous cell carcinoma, are usually painless and may go undetected in remote corners of the oral cavity. It may be many months before painful malignant infiltration of the lingual nerve actually prompts the patient to seek advice.

Treatment involves identifying and treating the underlying cause of the stomatitis.

- Osteitis (or dry socket) is commonly due to a localized inflammation in a tooth socket following extraction. The pain is very severe, gnawing, throbbing and associated with a foul taste in the mouth.

  Treatment involves placing a sedative, oil of cloves dressing in the socket along with a prescription for analgesics and antibiotics. Sometimes there may be a piece of root or bony sequestrum retained in the socket so a radiograph should also be taken.

- Osteomyelitis and osseous malignancy: On rare occasions severe osteomyelitis or malignancy may initially present as a toothache or ill-defined facial pain. The symptoms from both conditions are a dull, persistent pain, tooth mobility and later altered sensory function of the fifth nerve. A screening radiograph will show the bony erosion or infiltration.

  Urgent specialist maxillofacial referral is of course essential.

### Temporomandibular joints and masticatory muscles

Myofascial pain arising from the temporomandibular joints and masticatory muscles is the most common cause of facial pain after toothache.[12] Temporomandibular joint dysfunction, also known as myofascial pain dysfunction or facial arthromyalgia, is a chronic disorder characterized by pain arising from the joints and masticatory muscles with joint noises and trismus.

Symptoms may vary from a clicking, uncomfortable jaw joint on chewing to a continuous dull ache with acute exacerbations, often described as earache. The pain radiates widely to the temporal, masseteric, occipital and mastoid areas or down into the neck (Figure 8.6). The patient may give a history of jaw clenching and nighttime tooth grinding (bruxism). It commonly occurs in association with headache, earache, back pain, abdominal cramp and dysmenorrhoea and has many features of a stress-induced syndrome. A high proportion of patients are young or middle-aged females with anxiety neuroses.

The pathophysiology of temporomandibular joint dysfunction is complex.[13] Essentially the pain appears to arise from a combination of traumatic arthrosis and painful muscle spasm. Thus, the synonymous terms myofascial pain-dysfunction and facial arthromyalgia may be more accurate descriptors for the condition. The problem is commonly initiated by emotional stress which leads to muscle hyperactivity, bruxism and joint overloading. Trauma to the mandible and alterations in the occlusion of the teeth can also contribute to the aetiology. Examination of the patient will usually reveal tenderness and clicking around the mandibular condyles, which should be palpated via the external auditory meatus. The masseter and temporalis muscles will be painful and there will be limitation of jaw opening. Intraoral palpation behind the maxillary tuberosities will often elicit exquisite tenderness from the lateral pterygoid muscles – the so-called pterygoid sign. Muscle palpation can also trigger acutely painful episodes in remote parts of the face and mouth. Inspection of the teeth may show considerable wear of the crown surfaces due to bruxism or a poorly balanced occlusion (bite) due to uneven tooth loss.

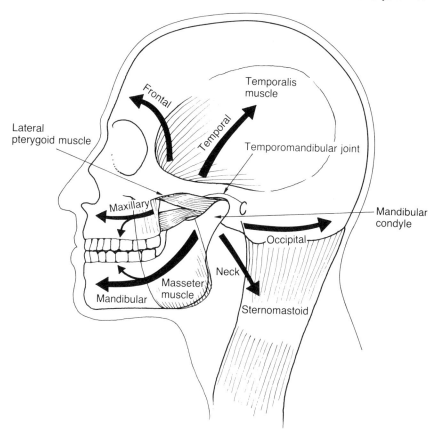

**Figure 8.6** Patterns of radiation of pain originating in the temporomandibular joint and muscles of mastication

Management of this condition requires an understanding of dentistry, pharmacology, neurology, rheumatology and psychiatry.[14] Investigations should include radiography of the jaw joints and serology to exclude the arthritides. An auriculotemporal nerve block or a local anaesthetic injection around a specific masticatory muscle may be diagnostic. Specialist arthrography or arthroscopy will indicate adhesions or damage to the intra-articular disc. In cases where pathological changes are detected or where a mechanical aetiology is suspected, patients should be referred for a specialist maxillofacial opinion. Although the need for surgical intervention is rare for temporomandibular joint dysfunction, there are some cases where open surgery is the only cure.

- Reassurance and simple analgesia: Most cases of temporomandibular dysfunction are classical myofascial arthromyalgias and are amenable to treatment using a number of standard regimes. First-line management includes an explanation of the condition and reassurance that there is no organic disease present, followed by recommendations to take a soft diet and to rest the jaw. Referral to a dentist for the replacement of lost teeth with dentures or for construction of a bite guard will help many patients by reducing joint loading. A combination of a non-steroidal anti-inflammatory analgesic such as piroxicam, 10 mg b.d., and a skeletal muscle relaxant like baclofen, 10 mg b.d., for a short period, will often break the cycle of pain and muscle spasm. Physiotherapy using short-wave and ultrasound can also be considered to relieve muscle spasm. Most patients will respond well to a combination of these simple protocols.

- Tricyclic antidepressants: There will always be some cases that fail to respond to standard treatment regimes. It is these chronic intractable cases that will present to the pain specialist. Often there will be a predominant psychological component which is exacerbating the underlying condition. The use of tricyclic antidepressant drugs has been shown to be of immense value in the treatment of chronic cases even in those who are not depressed." They are thought to control chronic pain by enhancing central pain suppressor activity as well as elevating mood. The precise site of action is unknown but the pharmacological properties appear to be related to the inhibition of synaptic uptake of serotonin and noradrenaline. Drugs with fewer sedative and anticholinergic side-effects such as dothiepin are preferred in contrast to amitriptyline. Dothiepin can be prescribed starting with a dose of 25 mg nocte, increasing to 75 mg over 3 weeks and then maintaining this regime as necessary. In some cases anxiolytics, such as temazepam 10 mg nocte, may be helpful in patients who are prone to nighttime tooth grinding.
- Local anaesthetics: Immediate symptomatic pain relief can be achieved by injecting long-acting local anaesthetics, such as mepivacaine, directly into the joint capsule or around muscle attachments. Such patients should be forewarned that transient facial palsy can occur following injections around the temporomandibular joint. Local anaesthetic solution (1 ml) is sufficient to inject into the joint itself, while 2 ml should be injected at muscle attachments. The masseter and temporalis muscles are very amenable to local anaesthetic injection to relieve spasm. The lateral pterygoid muscle is more inaccessible but it can be anaesthetized by submucosal infiltration injection at the back of the maxillary tuberosity. More prolonged pain relief can also be achieved by intraarticular steroid injections.
- Botulinum toxin: There has been recent experimental work which suggests that injections of botulinum toxin into the masseter muscle could, by producing selective and temporary paralysis, alleviate intractable muscle spasm. Such innovative treatment is best restricted to use by the maxillofacial specialist.
- Biofeedback/acupuncture: Biofeedback-assisted relaxation and acupuncture can both relieve pain symptoms and psychological distress as part of a stress management scheme.

In summary, there is a large armamentarium of therapies that can be used in the pain clinic to treat temporomandibular joint dysfunction. In most cases it is a matter of selecting a combination of treatment modalities that give the best relief for that individual.

## Nose and sinuses

- Sinusitis: Symptoms of acute sinusitis are severe, dull ache centred on the cheek and radiating to the ipsilateral orbit. In many cases sinusitis may present as and be mistaken for a toothache. The pain is worse on bending forwards and the antra are tender to pressure, as are the upper premolar and molar teeth. The patient usually has a nasal obstruction and discharge. OM radiographs will show an opaque sinus, often with a fluid level. Chronic sinusitis, in contrast, rarely gives rise to facial pain.

   Acute sinusitis most frequently affects the maxillary antrum. It usually follows an upper respiratory tract infection or a dental infection. Streptococci and staphylococci are the main pathogens.

   Treatment is antibiotic therapy and ephedrine nose drops to shrink the nasal mucosa.
- Tumours of the nose and sinuses, although normally painless, can present with pain if they cause obstruction or secondary infection. In any investigation of facial pain such lesions should always be excluded by careful examination of an OM radiograph.

## Ears and eyes

- Pain originating from aural disease is usually relatively well-localized and can be readily distinguished from other types of facial pain. It is normally associated with other signs of ear disease such as deafness, vertigo, tinnitus and discharge. In such cases specialist ear, nose and throat referral is appropriate. Sometimes a painful otitis externa can be a source of more generalized facial pain, but this should be easily detected during examination. The close proximity of the jaw joint to the ear means that patients often complain of earache as an initial symptom of temporomandibular joint dysfunction. The dental pain of pulpitis and pericoronitis can also be poorly localized and present as earache, as can malignant tumours of the tongue.
- Eye conditions such as corneal ulceration, iritis and acute glaucoma are all causes of facial pain. But these are all well-localized and are usually obvious on examination. One important point during eye examination is to remember to test the corneal reflex; although rare, the possibility of a cerebellopontine angle tumour as an underlying cause of facial pain may be detected by testing this reflex.

## Salivary glands

Disorders of the parotid and submandibular gland can present with facial pain. The common conditions are mumps, suppurative parotitis and salivary calculi.

- Mumps will result in bilateral painful swelling of the parotids and the patient will be febrile. Serology for the S and V antibodies of mumps will confirm the diagnosis and treatment is largely symptomatic. In suppurative parotitis the pain is usually dull, well-localized and provoked by eating. The affected gland is swollen, tender and pus may be expressed from the inflamed parotid duct. Antibiotic therapy is the treatment of choice.
- Salivary calculi are relatively common and present with obstruction of the affected gland, which becomes painfully swollen after eating. Plain radiographs may reveal a radiopaque calculus but sialography is usually indicated to exclude gland damage. The calculus can either be surgically removed or fragmented with a lithotriptor and allowed to flush out naturally.
- In rare cases salivary gland pain may be caused by a tumour. If none of the above diagnoses is applicable then a CT scan must be performed to exclude tumour growth.

### Lymph nodes

Facial pain may arise from infective cervical lymphadenitis. Severe pain is unusual, tenderness is more common and slight trismus may occur as movements of the jaw are painful. Diagnosis should be evident on examination and will usually lead to a primary infection in the drainage area.

### Autoimmune arteritis

Giant cell arteritis can give rise to severe facial pain in the elderly. The temporal arteries are normally affected but inflammatory foci may occur in any branch of the external carotid. If a superficial vessel is involved, such as the temporal artery or facial artery, the pain may be acute and well-localized. If the maxillary artery is affected the pain presents as intermittent claudication in the tongue and masticatory muscles during function. The erythrocyte sedimentation rate will be raised and arterial biopsy will confirm the diagnosis. Aggressive treatment with systemic steroids is imperative to prevent involvement of the ophthalmic artery and ultimate blindness. Therapy should commence with 60 mg prednisolone daily for 10 days, then reducing the doses as the condition comes under control.

### Neuralgias

The primary neuralgias, which affect the main trunks and branches of the trigeminal, glossopharyngeal and superior laryngeal nerves, are significant causes of facial pain (see Chapter 18). There are also secondary facial neuralgias, which are caused by external irritation of a nerve.[16] These can be classified as extracranial or intracranial, depending on the location of the external irritant.

- Mental nerve compression: One of the commonest types of extracranial neuralgia found in elderly patients is an intermittent, severe, paroxysmal pain affecting the lower jaw and lip. This is caused by bony compression of the mental branch of the mandibular nerve within a narrowing and ossifying thermal foramen. Occasionally it can be due to Paget's disease. Radiographs show evidence of a narrowed mental foramen.

Treatment involves surgical decompression of the nerve. A similar type of pain occurs in edentulous patients with old faithful lower dentures. With age the alveolar bone resorbs, the mental nerve becomes more superficial and is more susceptible to compression by the denture base. A sharp pain is initiated by eating and can be elicited by pressure over the site of the nerve. Treatment is to relieve the denture or surgically reposition the mental nerve.

- Causalgia in the facial region is a well-localized, persistent throbbing or burning pain which occurs at a site of previous surgery. Although it is rare, when it does occur it usually follows third molar extraction. Pain persists for months or years after tooth removal. It may be difficult to distinguish causalgia from atypical facial pain and often the patient will have tried multiple treatments, all unsuccessfully.

Permanent nerve blocks can be performed by surgical section, cryotherapy or alcohol injection. Cryotherapy is the preferred technique as this claims the advantage that touch and pressure sensation eventually return but the smaller nociceptive fibres fail to regenerate.

- Postherpetic neuralgia: Herpes zoster can affect the trigeminal ganglion and give rise to severe facial pain. Pain is often the initial symptom, followed by a vesicular eruption of the skin, restricted to a specific area supplied by the affected branch of the trigeminal nerve.

To aid rapid recovery, topical acyclovir is applied to the lesions five times daily. Postherpetic neuralgia is a rare complication caused by destruction of myelinated nerve fibres by the zoster virus. It causes episodes of localized facial pain. Strong analgesics may be required in treatment. This subject area is covered in more detail in Chapter 17.

- Intracranial neuralgias: A whole range of intracranial lesions may cause secondary neuralgias. The more frequent disorders to bear in mind for obscure facial pain patterns are disseminated sclerosis and space-occupying lesions. The former may present with bizarre groups of neurological disturbances, whilst the latter usually show good localizing signs in addition to facial pain. The acoustic neuroma will affect the trigeminal, facial and vestibulocochlear cranial nerves causing facial pain, sensory loss, deafness and ataxia. Middle cranial fossa tumours will encroach on the optic, ophthalmic, maxillary, oculomotor, trochlear and abducent nerves to produce facial pain, cutaneous analgesia and disturbances in vision and ocular movements. Suspicion of such lesions will require specialist referral and investigation.

- Migrainous syndromes: Syndromes of migraine and migrainous neuralgia (cluster headache) are described fully in Chapter 7.

## Psychogenic conditions, including atypical face pain

Pain of emotional origin is the third most frequent cause of facial pain, after toothache and jaw joint dysfunction.[17] Psychogenic pain may arise as a result of stress or it may be a feature of a neurosis, an abnormal personality trait or a psychosis. Psychogenic pain often presents with identical features to organic pain but clinical and radiographic investigation does not reveal an apparent cause. A detailed social, family and personal history may provide the clue to a possible psychogenic aetiology.

- Atypical facial pain presents as a continuous ache with intermittent excruciating episodes localized in the facial soft tissue or bones.[18] It may be unilateral or bilateral and persists for long periods. It is more common in women and most patients have suffered for months or years by the time they present to a pain clinic. Most patients with atypical facial pain have associated symptoms such as temporomandibular joint dysfunction or other psychogenic pains.

   Diagnosis of atypical facial pain is based on a detailed social, family and personal history with a careful examination and extensive investigations to exclude all organic disease. Radiographic investigation should include an OPG, temporomandibular joint, OM and base of skull views. A CT scan is also important in chronic cases. Serology should include haemoglobin estimation, erythrocyte sedimentation rate, blood film analysis as well as rheumatoid factor, serum iron, vitamin $B_{12}$ and folate estimations. A diagnosis is not made purely by the exclusion of physical disorder. A history of stress in the form of adverse life events or chronic problems must be identified and other psychogenic symptoms established.

   Patients who are suspected of having personality disorders or frank psychoses should be referred for specialist psychiatric treatment. The remainder of cases can be readily treated in the pain clinic. Patients should be reassured that their pain is real and not imaginary, arising in cramped muscles and dilated blood vessels as a response to stress. They must also be reassured that no serious physical disorder is present. The patients who do not respond to reassurance alone can then be treated with antidepressant medication in slowly increasing doses. A suggested treatment regime is to use the tricyclic antidepressant dothiepin 25 mg nocte, increasing to a maximum of 225 mg nocte over 12 weeks until pain control is achieved. If no response is achieved then a phenothiazine, trifluoperazine, 2-6 mg, can be added for a further 8 weeks. Medication should be continued for at least 3–6 months at a dosage that gives appropriate pain relief. Later the medication can be slowly withdrawn but any relapse of pain will indicate the need for reintroduction of medication. During treatment patients will need regular reinforcement and monitoring to detect untoward drug side-effects. This treatment regime has been shown to give good pain relief in the majority of patients with psychogenic facial pain.

   Other treatment modalities which can be effective in the management of atypical facial pain include transcutaneous nerve stimulation, acupuncture and topical drug therapy. Transcutaneous nerve stimulation is thought to work by using external electrical impulses to produce counterirritation and pain relief via the gate theory. Acupuncture is a widely ranging Chinese therapy, based on metaphysical concepts, which is of proven value in the treatment of numerous disease processes including atypical facial pain. Topical application of drugs such as capsaicin and clonidine has recently been proposed for the relief of neuropathic facial pain disorders.

- Atypical odontalgia (phantom tooth pain) is a variant of atypical facial pain characterized by a severe throbbing pain in a tooth or teeth which are hypersensitive to all stimuli without the evidence of major pathology.[19] Patients often undergo extensive dental restorative and endodontic treatment in an attempt to cure the pain. Multiple unnecessary extractions may be performed but these do not cure the pain which persists even in an edentulous jaw.

  Diagnosis and management follow the same protocol as for atypical facial pain. Cases of localized atypical odontaigia may be effectively managed in the short term by selective blocking of specific dental branches of the trigeminal nerve.

- Oral dysaesthesia is a burning pain in the tongue or gums with disturbance of taste, dry mouth, denture intolerance or an uncomfortable bite. It often occurs in combination with atypical facial pain. Patients may undergo exhaustive investigations of their salivary glands, teeth and dentures. Many are concerned that the symptoms are caused by the mercury content of amalgam fillings.

  The replacement of all amalgam fillings with synthetic white restorations may have a placebo effect but symptoms normally return after a short period. Pain is usually managed using antidepressant medication as for atypical facial pain.

## Referred pain

- Cervical spine and muscles: Cervical referral into the head and face often coexists with other forms of chronic facial pain. Spinal nerves C2 and C3 project into the facial region and have diffuse bilateral projections in the brainstem. Disorders affecting the sternocleidomastoid and trapezius muscles often give rise to cervicofacial referral. Missed diagnoses of cervico-occipital pathology are common in intractable facial pain. If the lesion is in the trigeminal tract the corneal sensation and reflex will be retained. Examination of the neck for muscle tenderness and trigger zones is critical if cervical referral is not to be missed. Cervical strain or a prolapsed intervertebral disc between the second and fourth cervical vertebrae may give rise to pain at the angle of the mandible and sensory neuropathy. Cervical spondylosis can present with pain radiating to the face which is exacerbated by movement. Radiographs will reveal loss of intervertebral spaces and osteophytes. High cervical epidurals are useful in the treatment of cervically referred facial pain.
- Heart: Ischaemic pain from the myocardium may radiate into the lower jaw, occasionally without concurrent chest pain, although there is usually simultaneous pain in the ipsilateral arm. The pain is precipitated by exercise, emotion and eating, and remits in several minutes. Pain due to malignant invasion of the superior mediastinum may present as bilateral facial pain but will also be associated with severe chest symptoms.

## Conclusions

The diagnosis and management of facial pain conditions are complex. The wide distribution of interconnecting nociceptive pathways in the trigeminal region can produce pain symptoms that are difficult to localize and evaluate. Ironically, it is these very cases that present to the pain clinic. Initial clinical assessment and investigation should exclude any significant pathology for which specialist dental or surgical referral is essential.

In general, the expertise of the pain specialist will focus on the chronic facial pain conditions arising from temporomandibular joint and myofascial pain-dysfunction, the neuralgias, migrainous syndromes and psychogenic pain syndromes. A large armamentarium of physical, pharmacological and psychological therapies is available for the management of these enigmatic conditions. A successful outcome will often require a combination of modalities as well as considerable time, patience and understanding on the part of the clinician.

## References

1. Mumford JM. *Orofacial Pain: Aetiology, Diagnosis and Treatment*. London: Churchill Livingstone, 1982
2. Hillman L, Burns MT, Chander A, Tai YM. The management of craniofacial pain in a pain relief unit. *Anesth Pain Control Dent* 1: 85–89, 1992
3. Fricton JR. Recent advances in temporomandibular disorders and orofacial pain. *J Am Dent Assoc* 122: 24–32, 1991
4. Peterson JK, Milgram P. *Pain Relief in the Orofacial Regions*. Copenhagen: Munksgaard, 1989
5. Dubner R, Sessle BJ, Storey AT. *The Neural Basis of Oral and Facial Function*. New York: Plenum, 1978
6. Sessle BJ. The neurobiology of facial and dental pain; present knowledge, future directions. *J Dent Res* 66: 962–981, 1987
7. Maciewicz R, Mason P, Strassman A, Potrebic S. Organisation of trigeminal nociceptive pathways. *Semin Neurol* 8: 255–263, 1988
8. Bell WE. *Orofacial Pains: Classification, Diagnosis, Management*. Chicago: Year Book, 1989
9. Fricton JR, Kroening RJ, Hathaway KM. *TMJ and Craniofacial Pain: Diagnosis and Management*. St Louis, MO: Ishiyku Euro America, 1988
10. Sharav Y. Orofacial pain. In: (Wall PD, Melzack R, eds) *Textbook of Pain*. Edinburgh: Churchill Livingstone, 1989, pp. 441–454
11. Lipton S. *Relief of Pain in Clinical Practice*. Oxford: Blackwell Scientific, 1979
12. Zarb GA, Carlson GE. *Temporomandibular Joint: Function and Dysfunction*. Copenhagen: Munksgaard, 1979
13. Mitchell RJ. Etiology of temporomandibular disorders. *Curr Opin Dent* 1: 471–475, 1991
14. Fricton J, Hathaway K, Bromaghim C. Interdisciplinary management of TMJ and craniofacial pain; characteristics and outcome. *J Cranio Dis Oral Facial Pain* 1: 1–16, 1988
15. Harris M. Medical versus surgical management of temporomandibular pain and dysfunction. *Br J Oral Maxillofac Surg* 25: 113–120, 1987
16. Kerr FWL. Craniofacial neuralgias. In: (Bonica JJ, Liebeskind JC, Albefessard D, eds) *Advances in Pain Research and Therapy*. New York: Raven Press, 1979, pp. 283–295
17. Feinmann C, Harris M. Psychogenic facial pain management and prognosis. *Br Dent J* 156: 205–208, 1984
18. Leeser JD. Tic douloureux and atypical facial pain. In: (Wall PD, Melzack R, eds) *Textbook of Pain*. Edinburgh: Churchill Livingstone, 1989, pp. 535–543
19. Schnurr RF, Brooke RI. Atypical odontalgia: update and comment on long-term follow-up. *Oral Surg, Oral Med, Oral Pathol* 73: 445–448, 1992

# 9

# Neck pain

## J. A. Pateman and S. J. Dolin

The head is supported by the neck in an upright posture but can perform a wide range of complex movements. In the bony skeleton of the neck there are nearly 40 separate small articulations and a complex network of ligamentous supports and muscle groups. In addition many vital structures pass from the head to the body through a comparatively narrow area in close proximity to the spine and to each other. This combination of structure and function renders the neck extremely vulnerable to trauma, degenerative conditions of the bones and joints, muscle problems, and damage to the nerves and vessels within the neck. Pain in the neck region is a common complaint, affecting over 10% of the adult population at any one time, and 35% of adults have had at least one episode of neck pain.[1] Radiological evidence of the most common degenerative problem of the neck, cervical spondylosis, is very common after the age of 30. However, severe disability and loss of function are less common than with lumbar pain.

Pain may arise from almost any of the structures within the neck (Table 9.1).

## Clinical examination

On initial assessment of the patient the history of the neck pain should include character, localisation, radiation, onset and duration, episodicity, a history of trauma, and exacerbating or relieving factors.

Examination begins with assessment of the posture, including the general posture, and any abnormal curvature of the thoracic or lumbar spine. Skin pallor or redness and shortening of ligaments are important. Palpation may reveal increased muscle tone, local or diffuse tenderness over bone or muscle, and the full range of active and passive movements should be assessed, including flexion, extension, lateral flexion and rotation. Specific manoeuvres to test the joints of the cervical spine include head compression, traction to distract the joints, and a Valsalva manoeuvre, which increases intrathecal pressure.

Investigations will include X-rays, anteroposterior and lateral views show the bony structure, including osteophyte formation and extraosseous calcification. Open-mouth views demonstrate the atlantoaxial joint, and

**Table 9.1** Sources of neck pain

| | |
|---|---|
| Bones and ligaments | Cervical spondylosis |
| | Rheumatoid arthritis |
| | Ankylosing spondylitis |
| | DISH (diffuse idiopathic skeletal hyperostosis) |
| | Ossification of the posterior longitudinal ligament |
| Nerves | Radiculopathy – entrapment, disc prolapse |
| | Myelopathy |
| | Brachial plexus – thoracic outlet syndrome, brachial plexus neuropathy |
| | Cervical neuralgia |
| Muscular | Whiplash |
| | Myofascial pain |
| | Cervical dystonia |
| Referred pain | Head (teeth, acromioclavicular joint, temporomandibular joint), lung, heart (angina), aorta, pharynx, abdomen (gallbladder, hiatus hernia), cervical nodes, central nervous system (headaches, tumour, meningism), shoulder |

oblique views may be useful in elucidating suspected nerve impingement. Computed tomographic (CT) scan and magnetic resonance imaging (MRI) are useful to show soft tissues, and a barium swallow will indirectly demonstrate the soft tissues in front of the vertebra, and confirm dysphagia caused by osteophyte formation.

## Specific syndromes

### Skeletal abnormalities

#### Cervical spondylosis

Radiographic evidence of cervical spondylosis is almost universal by middle age; however there is little correlation between severity of X-ray findings and symptomatology. Changes are more common in the lower cervical spine, and begin with the development of osteophytes in the vertebral bodies. The facet joints are progressively involved. Intervertebral disc degeneration may lead to loss of height. Progression of the disease may lead to compression of nerve roots causing a radiculopathy. There may rarely be involvement of sympathetic nerves, leading to dysphagia, vertigo and visual disturbances. This may also occur due to vertebrobasilar insufficiency.

Symptoms include:

- pain: initially diffuse, more localized if nerve roots are involved; may be referred to the face or to the anterior chest

- stiffness
- sensory loss: radicular in origin, usually the upper limb, but can affect the face, tongue and shoulder
- spinal cord compression: myelopathy
- sympathetic: dysphagia, vertigo, visual disturbance
- arterial – vertebrobasilar insufficiency: due to vascular compression or coincident atheroma
- headache: occipital is common in upper cervical disease

On examination findings include lower cervical tenderness and associated muscle spasm. Deep trigger points may be found if there is facet joint involvement, or superficial ones in myofascial disease (see Chapter 6). Limitation of active and passive movements occurs.

Investigations should include cervical X-rays, and if necessary oblique and open-mouth views. Diagnostic changes include increased subchondral bone density, osteophyte and pseudocyst formation and narrowing of the joint spaces.

Treatment: the natural history of the disease is episodic, with gradual progression over years. Primary treatment should be aimed at reducing inflammatory response with non-steroidal anti-inflammatory drugs (NSAIDs). Localized pain in involved facet joints or associated myofascial trigger points can be treated with injection of local anaesthetic with or without steroid in a dose of 2 ml 0.25% bupivacaine and 8–16 mg Depo-Medrone at each trigger point. Cervical epidural injection of local anaesthetic and steroid mixtures may be performed percutaneously with X-ray control. Once pain has been addressed, improvement of mobility with physiotherapy is important; this includes the use of techniques such as heat, massage, cervical traction and exercise. The onset of a radiculopathy or myelopathy requires urgent investigation and orthopaedic or neurosurgical consultation.

### Rheumatoid arthritis

Rheumatoid arthritis occurs in 5% of British women. In the neck, the upper cervical spine is the most commonly involved area, seen in up to 80% of patients' X-rays. Of particular vulnerability is the atlantoaxial joint, where subluxation of the odontoid peg may occur spontaneously or during manipulation of the neck. Lateral and vertical subluxation of the joint may also occur, and subluxation of the second or third cervical vertebrae.

Pain may be localized to the neck or referred to the face from the upper cervical nerve roots. It is exacerbated by movement. Myelopathy may occur at any level. Other features of rheumatoid arthritis should be sought in making the diagnosis, particularly peripheral joint involvement and rheumatoid nodules. Serial X-rays show soft-tissue swelling, periarticular osteoporosis, loss of joint space, erosions and deformity. The diagnosis may be suspected from the finding of a high erythrocyte sedimentation rate (ESR), and in 80% of cases a positive rheumatoid factor.

Treatment is of the underlying disease process, with NSAIDs in high doses during acute exacerbations, and opioids only if absolutely necessary. Physiotherapy may be useful after acute episodes. If there is subluxation of a joint a collar or surgical stabilization may be indicated.

### Ankylosing spondylitis

Ankylosing spondylitis is a disease which predominantly affects men. It has an incidence of 2 per 100 000 in Caucasians, and 95% have the human leukocyte antigen (HLA)-B27. Ankylosing spondylitis affects mainly the axial skeleton, particularly the sacroiliac joints, and also the neck. Onset is usually in early adult life. It is primarily an inflammatory process occurring at the margins of bone where tendons, ligaments and joint capsules adhere. Bony erosion occurs initially but healing leads to bone formation at the site and loss of flexibility.

Clinical features are of gradual onset of pain and morning stiffness improved by exercise, with diminished movements of the neck. This may initially be episodic, but rigidity eventually becomes marked. Limitation of range of movements affects the whole spine, with loss of the normal lumbar lordosis, and there is pain on springing of the sacroiliac joints. In established ankylosing spondylitis, complications arise such as iritis, aortic incompetence, amyloidosis, and a restrictive pulmonary abnormality due to involvement of the thoracic cage. Neurological damage may occur due to an increased vulnerability to spinal trauma.

Radiographic changes show loss of definition of joint margins, erosions and then sclerosis of the whole joint. Sacroiliac involvement is necessary to make the diagnosis. The ESR may be raised acutely, as may plasma viscosity. Although HLA-B27 is almost universal in ankylosing spondylitis patients, it should be remembered that only 1% of HLA-B27 carriers develop the condition, possibly due to an infective trigger.

Treatment is conservative, with NSAIDs and physiotherapy, aimed at maintaining an upright functional posture. Local trigger points may occur and should be treated with local anaesthetic or steroid mixtures as above.

### Diffuse idiopathic skeletal hyperostosis

Diffuse idiopathic skeletal hyperostosis (DISH), also known as Forestier's disease, occurs in middle-aged Caucasian men. It is a disease of ectopic calcification of the anterior and lateral spinous ligaments. Usually the thoracic region is most involved, but the neck may also be affected. Limitation of movement is more predominant than pain. With impingement on nerves, myelopathy or radiculopathy may arise. If anterior calcification is florid, dysphagia may occur.

Ossification of the posterior ligament predominates in a group of elderly male Asian patients. This may be a variant of DISH.

### Nerve entrapment

Nerve entrapments cause pain and motor or sensory loss and may occur from the spinal cord through nerve roots out to peripheral nerves, giving different clinical pictures.

### Myelopathy

Cervical myelopathy occurs due to cord compression, most commonly in the lower cervical spine because the spinal cord is slightly larger in this region. The clinical features are of a lower motor neuron lesion at the level of compression, with upper motor neuron signs below this. Sensory disturbances are common, but differ from those seen in a radiculopathy by being non-dermatomal in pattern.

There are two main presentations: first, acute cervical myelopathy, with a sudden onset, often in young patients due to cervical disc prolapse or to trauma. The less acute form has an onset over weeks rather than hours, and may present with clumsiness or gait disturbance. This is often due to cervical spondylosis, but can be caused by other degenerative diseases of the bones, tumour, haematoma and infection. Some elderly patients with narrowed cervical canals develop cord compression on flexion of the head.

The differential diagnosis of a compressive myelopathy is of one secondary to radiation, or primary disease of the spinal cord, classically syringomyelia. More marked positional symptoms may be due to an inflammatory myelopathy, such as multiple sclerosis.

If the onset of a myelopathy is suspected in a patient being treated for neck pain, urgent investigation including MRI scan is indicated. Anteroposterior X-ray views showing narrowing of the cervical canal diameter increase the likelihood of a diagnosis of cord compression, but if negative do not exclude large space-occupying lesions.

### Radiculopathy

Compression of nerve roots within the neck may occur secondary to many conditions affecting this area, but some particular patterns of involvement predominate:

- Acute radiculopathy is most commonly due to trauma or disc prolapse in young patients and may occur at any cervical level.
- Radiculopathy due to cervical spondylosis usually affects the middle or lower cervical nerve roots and occurs in an older population. The development of an acute radiculopathy in this group may be precipitated by minor trauma, if the intervertebral foramen is already narrowed with osteophytes.
- Chronic radiculopathy may arise insidiously or persist after an acute episode. It is usually due to degenerative diseases of the cervical skeleton. However, caution should be exercised when there is a suspicion of malignancy, as differentiation of involvement with tumour from coexisting degenerative disease can be difficult.

The clinical features are of a dermatomal distribution of pain and sensory disturbance in the neck, shoulder and arm (Figure 9.1). The pain is typically neuropathic in character, with a persistent burning and/or intermittent lancinating component. Tenderness may be noted at the site of pathology. Symptoms can be increased by stretching the root with any manoeuvre that depresses the shoulder on the affected side, such as carrying a heavy

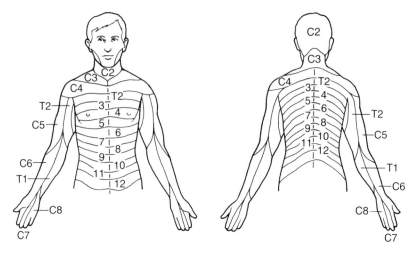

**Figure 9.1** Anterior and posterior distribution of cervical and thoracic dermatomes.

weight. They will also be increased by increasing intrathecal pressure, e.g. coughing, sneezing, the Valsalva manoeuvre and sometimes by lateral flexion to the affected side, rotation away from the involved side or compression of the spine from above, which all cause narrowing of the intervertebral foramen. Conversely, symptoms may be relieved by shoulder abduction, reducing tension on the nerve root. The diagnosis may be made by electromyogram (EMG) or evoked potentials. MRI scan may demonstrate impingement and differentiate between tumour recurrence and degenerative changes.

Treatment is of the underlying cause where appropriate, or by conservative measures such as NSAIDs, physiotherapy including cervical traction and soft collar support of the neck. Segmental epidural block with local anaesthetics may relieve severe pain. Neuralgic components can be treated with anticonvulsants. As in many conditions of the neck, severe pain may lead to secondary muscle spasm, and then trigger point injections may be appropriate.

### Thoracic outlet syndrome

The subclavian vessels and the lower trunk of the brachial plexus may be compressed as they leave the neck (Figure 9.2). The most common cause is a cervical rib, either a complete anatomical rib or a fibromuscular band. About 1 in 200 of the population have bilateral cervical ribs, but only 10% give rise to symptoms of thoracic outlet syndrome. This may be due in part to poor posture. Thoracic outlet syndrome may also be due to a fracture of the clavicle or first rib, or mechanical factors, including the habitual lifting of heavy weights on one shoulder, and body building leading to compression by hypertrophied muscle.

Symptoms include pain in the neck, shoulder or upper arm. Sensory disturbances occur in the lower dermatomes of the brachial plexus, typically C8 and T1. Weakness of the small muscles of the hand may occur, and in 10%

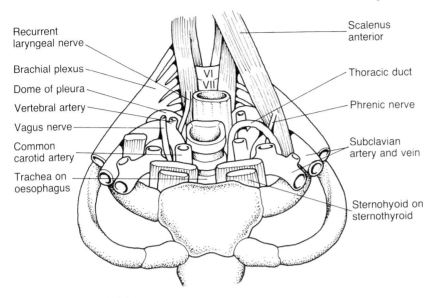

Recurrent
laryngeal nerve

Brachial plexus

Dome of pleura

Vertebral artery

Vagus nerve

Common
carotid artery

Trachea on
oesophagus

Scalenus
anterior

Thoracic duct

Phrenic nerve

Subclavian
artery and vein

Sternohyoid on
sternothyroid

**Figure 9.2** The thoracic inlet.

of cases there is vascular occlusion of the upper limb, which may present as Raynaud's phenomenon, venous thrombosis or swelling of the arm after exercise.

Investigations to confirm the diagnosis include X-rays of the cervical spine, EMG, somatosensory evoked potentials and MRI. Treatment is initially conservative with exercises to improve shoulder girdle posture. Surgery to divide the band or resect the cervical rib may be indicated if vascular symptoms predominate, but vasomotor symptoms may persist postoperatively, and then chemical or surgical sympathectomy is indicated.

### Neuropathies

Cervial neuralgia is rare than facial neuralgia (see Chapter 8). It may arise from the glossopharyngeal nerve or the dorsal rami of the upper cervical nerve roots (C2–4). The sensory distribution of each nerve root (and potential areas of referred pain) are shown in Table 9.2.

Glossopharyngeal neuralgia is a rare condition similar to trigeminal neuralgia but affecting the ninth cranial nerve. The pain is a severe paroxysmal

**Table  9.2** Sensory distribution of nerve roots

| Nerve root | Cutaneous supply |
|---|---|
| C1 | Suboccipital muscles, no cutaneous supply |
| C2 | Forms greater occipital nerve, skin over occiput |
| C3 | Branch to greater occipital nerve, third occipital nerve, skin near midline posteriorly below occipital protuberance |
| C4 | Skin immediately below third occipital nerve |

lancinating pain occurring in the throat, ear and upper neck. It occurs in elderly patients, and may be provoked by swallowing and speech.

The ventral roots of C5 to T1 form the brachial plexus. These may be involved in a brachial plexus neuropathy occurring in middle-aged patients, and may have a familial, viral or toxic aetiology. Pain in the shoulder girdle progresses over a few weeks, then resolves spontaneously, but is followed by rapidly progressive patchy sensory and motor loss in the upper limb, which may be bilateral. Recovery takes several months, with 90% complete recovery by 3 years, although the condition may recur.

## Muscular diseases of the neck

### Whiplash

Rapid changes of velocity from vehicular or sports injuries cause sudden violent extension and flexion of the neck. Whether the initial impulse is acceleration or deceleration, both movements occur. Severe extension of the neck can cause a tear of the anterior longitudinal ligament, anterior herniation of the intervertebral disc, and chip fractures of the body of the vertebra. Damage to soft tissues such as the oesophagus may occur. Tissues damaged by hyperflexion injuries include the posterior part of the inter-vertebral disc, the longitudinal spinous ligaments and the zygapophyseal joints. Muscle damage is partly caused by reflex contraction of the muscles in response to stretching, and varies in extent, ranging from microscopic bleeding to complete rupture. The small neck joints may be damaged, and may continue to sublux if not supported by ligaments which have also been overstretched. Sympathetic nerves in close approximation may also be damaged.

Severe whiplash is apparent immediately after the trauma. Severe pain occurs and is increased by movement, with associated spasm of the neck muscles and occipital headache. Dizziness and visual disturbances may also occur. Less severe trauma may cause acute neck sprain.[2] The upper cervical vertebrae are most vulnerable. Partial tearing of ligaments and muscles of the atlanto-occipital region occur. Symptoms may not arise until the following day. The predominant feature is pain in the upper neck and occiput. Associated sympathetic dysfunction leads to visual or vestibular disturbance. On examination, the spinous processes of the affected cervical vertebrae will be tender, and spasm of muscles is promi-nent. Active movements are reduced and traction on the neck increases pain. On X-ray, loss of the normal lordosis of the neck ('straight neck') is seen, although the significance of this finding has been disputed.[3]

Treatment is analgesia, neck support and early mobilization. Initially NSAIDs, narcotics, trigger point injections or cervical epidural steroid injec-tion may all be required. Support of the neck should be with a soft collar or, in severe cases associated with subluxation, a brace. Physiotherapy, with heat treatment and stretching exercises, should be used as soon as the acute damage to muscle and ligaments has settled, after 2–4 weeks. In over 33% of cases, however, symptoms may persist beyond 2 years, particularly in the elderly, or when associated with disc damage. The persistence of symptoms at 8–12 months is of poor prognostic significance.

### Myofascial pain

Myofascial pain is covered in depth in Chapter 6, but in the neck may be part of a general or localized process. Posteriorly pain arises most commonly (from cephalad to caudad) from multifidus, splenius, levator scapulae, trapezius, infraspinatus, and anteriorly from sternocleidomastoid, posterior digastric and the medial pterygoid. Pain can be localized within the neck or referred to the head.

### Cervical dystonia (torticollis)

Cervical dystonia or spasmodic torticollis is a condition characterized by an intermittent abnormal posturing of the head due to painful involuntary contraction of the neck muscles. It may rarely be secondary to cerebral injury, neurodegenerative diseases such as Wilson's disease, or trauma. Onset is most common in middle-aged adults. Rotation of the head commonly occurs due to contraction of sternocleidomastoid, trapezius or splenius, but lateral flexion and extension may also occur.[4] The muscle posture relaxes during sleep. Tremor is also common, in 70% of one series. The disease remits and recurs. Eventually contractures develop, and there is risk of a secondary radiculopathy or myelopathy.

Treatment with anticholinergics reduces muscle tone, and surgery can be used to release contractures. However specific treatment with botulinus toxin (which prevents acetylcholine release and so causes temporary muscle weakness) has been shown to cause a marked improvement in 76% of patients in one study.[5] The effects lasted on average 9 weeks, but have been successfully repeated many times.[6]

### Referred pain

Pain can be referred to the neck from almost any of the structures in the upper body, in particular from the heart, temporomandibular joints and teeth, or due to malignancy. Differential diagnosis must be made on clinical grounds, with referral to the appropriate specialist. However, proven referred pain may still present difficult management problems and result in re-referral to the pain specialist.

## Summary

Neck pain often arises from structural components or nerves within the neck, and is very common, in part due to the unique relationship between structure and function. Degenerative conditions and trauma are the most frequent causes. Treatment is aimed at symptom relief and improvement of functional ability, with NSAIDs and physiotherapy being mainstays of management, although patient participation in any treatment programme may be important.[7] Many conditions have a remitting and relapsing course, and may present intermittently to a pain clinic over many years. Here in particular the preservation of function to as near a normal level as possible is vital.

## Pain-relieving injection therapies for neck pain

Like other pain-relieving techniques in the lumbar spine, pain-relieving injections in the neck are best viewed as a prelude to restoration of function of the spine using physiotherapy techniques rather than a means of permanent relief of symptoms.

### Cervical epidural

Cervical epidural may be of use in many forms of neck pain, and also possibly with cervical root pain.[8] While the procedure has not been subjected to randomized clinical trials it is commonly performed in pain clinics.

Cervical epidural can be done at any level of the cervical spine. The procedure should be done under image intensification in view of potential spinal cord injury. The best X-ray images can be obtained in the mid cervical levels as the shoulders make imaging of the lower cervical vertebrae difficult. Both anteroposterior and lateral views are needed. The patient can be placed prone with pillows under the chest so that the cervical spine is flexed. A Tuohy needle (18 G) or spinal needle (22 G) can be used with loss of resistance to air or saline. The loss of resistance will not be as marked as in the lumbar spine. Contrast medium will demonstrate the cervical epidural space and is unmistakable (Figure 9.3). There must be no aspiration of fluid

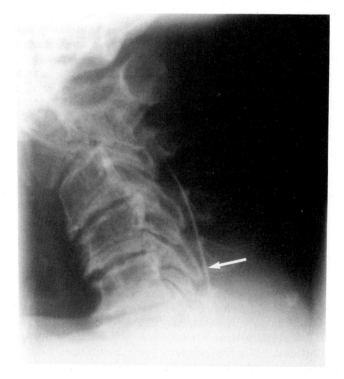

**Figure 9.3** Cervical epidural. X-ray of lateral view of cervical spine. The line of contrast outlines the epidural space (arrow). The needle is inferior to the X-ray and not seen in this view.

through the needle. A solution of local anaesthetic (bupivacaine 0.25% 3 ml) and steroid (methylprednisolone 40 mg in 1 ml or triamcinolone 40 mg in 1 ml) can then be injected. A patent intravenous line and adequate monitoring and resuscitation facilities must be available. Sedation is generally not required as the procedure is only minimally stimulating. Intrathecal injection is a remote possibility and careful technique and the use of imaging and contrast should make this avoidable. The use of modest doses of local anaesthetic is also advised.

### Radiofrequency cervical posterior primary ramus rhizolysis

This procedure is useful for the treatment of whiplash injury where facet joint injury is thought to be a mechanism of persistent neck pain. It may also have a role to play in treatment of chronic neck pain of degenerate or inflammatory origin. Randomized clinical trials of the technique are underway but had not been published at the time of going to press.

The procedure is generally done in the mid cervical levels. C2 is best avoided as rhizotomy of this nerve can result in denervation of the greater occipital nerve. C3–C5 are most commonly done, although other levels can also be lesioned. The patient is positioned supine. A line is marked on the skin along the posterior border of sternomastoid. Using an image intensifier oblique view (45°) the C3 level is readily identified as the first vertebra with an intervertebral foramen. A radiofrequency needle (22 G, 5 cm, 4 mm active tip) is advanced from the posterior border of sternomastoid to contact the transverse process of C3. It is then advanced, maintaining contact with bone, to a position posterior and lateral to the intervertebral foramen on the oblique view. Care must be taken not to place the needle too close to the anterior nerve root. Placement can be verified by stimulation using sensory stimulation (100 Hz, threshold up to 0.5 V); this should produce sensations only in the posterior neck, and not in the arm. Following correct placement a small amount of local anaesthetic should precede the radiofrequency lesion. Radiofrequency partial rhizotomy of the posterior nerve roots can be achieved by heating the electrode to 75°C for 90 s.[9] This procedure may be unpleasant for the patient and may require sedation, but sedation will need to be reversed for the stimulation. Possible side-effects include partial effects on the anterior nerve root which may manifest as temporary and usually incomplete sensory and even motor deficit in the arm. This will usually settle spontaneously but is best avoided by careful technique.

### Selective radiofrequency lesion of the dorsal root ganglion

This technique may have a place in the treatment of cervical nerve root pain. It should only be considered after a thorough diagnostic work-up which should include CT and MRI to exclude an underlying cause. Diagnostic nerve blocks of the relevant nerve roots should be carried out in advance to determine which nerve root is involved.

The patient is placed supine and the intervertebral foramina of the cervical spine imaged by image intensifier using an oblique view (45°). A radiofrequency needle (22 G, 5 cm, 4 mm active tip) is advanced under X-ray vision to be placed in the posterior and caudal corner of the intervertebral foramen. An anteroposterior X-ray view is obtained. The tip of the needle should be in the middle of the projection of the facetal column. Sensory stimulation (100 Hz, threshold less than 0.5 V) should produce sensations in the territory of the nerve in the shoulder or arm. Motor stimulation (2 Hz, thresholds two to three times greater than sensory) should also be tested and will demonstrate twitching in muscle groups supplied by the relevant nerve. Once a satisfactory position has been obtained and a small amount of local anaesthetic has been injected, a modest lesion 67–70°C for 60 s will produce a partial lesion of the dorsal root ganglion. This should result in diminution of pain without producing sensory deficit.[10]

### Cervical epidural catheter

Indwelling cervical epidural catheter with infusions of bupivacaine alone (0.125% 1–4 ml per hour) or bupivacaine (0.125%) plus morphine (0.05 mg per ml, 1–4 ml per hour) can provide analgesia for neck and arm pain. It is feasible to leave the catheters in place for several days up to one week. This will allow physiotherapy to occur under pain free conditions and may allow rapid rehabilitation of neck or arm pain. Although this technique is in use in a number of pain clinics, no outcome data has been published to date, but the technique may offer unique opportunities and is certainly free of possible side effects of alternative neurolytic techniques. Titration of the rate should allow analgesia without sensory or motor deficits and appears to be free of respiratory depression, although careful and frequent monitoring of vital signs is essential to the success of this technique.

## References

1. Wilson PR. Chronic neck pain and cervicogenic headache. *Clin J Pain* 7: 5–11, 1991
2. Robinson DD, Cassar-Pullicina VN. Acute neck sprain after road traffic accident: a long-term clinical and radiological view. *Injury* 24: 79–82, 1993
3. Helliwell PS, Evans PF, Wright V. The straight cervical spine: does it indicate muscle spasm? *J Bone Joint Surg Br* 76: 103–106, 1994
4. Jankovic J, Leder S, Warner D, Schwartz K. Cervical dystonia: clinical findings and associated movement disorders. *Neurology* 41: 1088–1091, 1991
5. Anderson TJ, Rivest J, Stell R *et al*. Botulinum toxin treatment of spasmodic torticollis. *J R Soc Med* 85: 524–529, 1992
6. Poewe W, Schelosky L, Kleedorfer B, Heinen F, Wagner M, Deuschl G. Treatment of spasmodic torticollis with local injections of botulinum toxin. One year follow-up in 37 patients. *J Neurol* 239: 21–25, 1992
7. Sweeney T. Neck school: cervicothoracic stabilisation training. *Occup Med* 7: 43–45, 1992
8. Castagnera L, Maurette P, Pointillart V, Vital JM, Erny P, Senegas J. Long-term results of cervical epidural steroid injection with and without morphine in chronic cervical radicular pain. *Pain* 58: 239–243, 1994
9. Sluitjer ME, Koesteld-Baart CC. Interruption of pain pathways in the treatment of the cervical syndrome. *Anaesthesia* 35: 302–307, 1980
10. Vervest ACM, Stolker RJ. The treatment of the cervical pain syndromes with radio-frequency procedures. *Pain Clin* 4: 103–112, 1991

# Further reading

Bonica JJ. *The Management of Pain*. Philadelphia: Lea & Febiger, 1990

Maddison PJ, Isenbeig DA, Woo P, Glass DN (eds) *Oxford Textbook of Rheumatology*. Oxford: Oxford University Press, 1993

Weatherall DJ, Ledingham JGG, Warrell DA. *Oxford Textbook of Medicine*. Oxford: Oxford University Press, 1984

# 10

# Thoracic pain

**J. Kent**

A wide variety of disorders may present with pain in the thoracic region. Most of these disorders, however, rarely present to a pain clinic. Clinical entities affecting intrathoracic organs, such as angina, myocardial infarction, aortic dissection, pneumothorax and pulmonary embolus, or thoracic manifestations of systemic disease are seldom treated by pain specialists. Nevertheless, all clinicians should be familiar with the presenting signs and symptoms of such disorders and be aware of their incidence in the community (including in pain patients) so that appropriate investigations are ordered, treatments initiated, and referrals made when they are suspected. It should also be remembered that some syndromes, especially cardiac and cancer pain, may be uppermost in the patient's mind.

The following is a review of thoracic pain syndromes likely to present to pain specialists for management. They include pain of musculoskeletal origin, cancer pain and pain of neuropathic origin.

## Musculoskeletal pain

### Costochondritis

Costochondritis presents as pain in the anterior chest, usually involving multiple chondral levels, with the second to fifth being most commonly affected.[1] This syndrome usually occurs in patients over 40 years of age, with females significantly outnumbering males (3 : 1).[2] On examination, involved sites are tender to palpation but not swollen. The pain in this condition is often confused with cardiac pain and the diagnosis of costochondritis is usually made following negative cardiac evaluation. It is a benign self-limiting disorder that usually responds to non-steroidal anti-inflammatory drugs (NSAIDs), mild analgesics, local heat and reassurance.

### Tietze's syndrome

Tietze's syndrome is a rarer condition which should be contrasted with costochondritis. It presents as pain and swelling at a single chondral level. The second or third costal cartilages are most commonly affected.[3] Tietze's

syndrome is usually seen in young teenagers and adults and is evenly distributed between the sexes. Often a recent history of respiratory straining or
manual labour can be elicited as a precipitating factor, and there are associated respiratory symptoms. Treatment is similar to that of costochondritis
– NSAIDs, local heat and reassurance – and resolution does occur, although
sometimes it takes several months.

### Xiphodynia

Xiphodynia is another rare cause of anterior chest pain.[4] Patients present
with low substernal or epigastric pain, but wide radiations are possible.
The pain is often quite severe and is aggravated by bending and large
meals. It may mimic pain of cardiac or gastrointestinal origin, and can be
associated with these conditions. Xiphodynia is self-limiting over a period
of months, and treatment is mainly conservative. Injection of local anaesthetic plus steroid into the xiphisternal joint will benefit some patients
with persistent pain. Surgical resection of the xiphoid is reserved for
severe cases.

### Sternal arthritis

Sternal arthritis may involve either the sternoclavicular or the manubriosternal joints. It usually develops in association with signs of systemic
rheumatological disease (rheumatoid arthritis, psoriatic arthritis, ankylosing
spondylitis, etc.). Patients present with joint pain, tenderness and sometimes overt inflammation. Sternoclavicular disease is suggested when pain
is increased in response to shrugging of the shoulders. Manubriosternal
pain is aggravated by deep breathing and coughing. These conditions are
usually managed conservatively and local joint injection is appropriate for
severe localized cases.

### Slipped rib syndrome

Slipped rib syndrome is a painful disorder of the lower anterior costal
margin. In this condition the costal cartilage of the eighth, ninth or 10th
rib does not articulate with the cartilage above it. The pain is often sharp,
associated with postural changes, and can be reproduced by manipulation
of the involved rib,[5] or by lifting the arms above the head. Treatment
includes NSAIDs and injection of local anaesthetic with steroid. In recalci-
trant cases surgical resection of the distal rib may rarely be required.

### Myofascial pain syndrome

Myofascial pain is a commonly treated disorder in pain clinics. Any muscle
of the chest may develop trigger points and their existence should be
pursued during physical examination. The locations of common trigger
points and their associated pain referral patterns are described in detail in
Travell and Rinzler's text[6] regarding myofascial pain. Treatment of myofascial pain syndrome includes heat, spray and stretch, and trigger point

injections.[6] Please refer to Chapter 6 for more details regarding myofascial pain.

### Other painful disorders of the thoracic skeleton

Many other primary disorders of the thoracic skeleton can result in chest pain (e.g. vertebral deformities, dislocations, fractures, arthritis). An individual discussion of each of these is beyond the scope of this text. However, most of these disorders respond to conservative interventions such as NSAIDs, mild analgesics and physiotherapy. Rib fracture pain is well-managed with either epidural or intercostal nerve blocks. Epidural blockade can also be used as an adjunct to conservative therapy in patients with acute vertebral fractures.

Pain from intervertebral discs or apophyseal facet disease may develop in the thorax, but is more common in the cervical and lumbar regions. Presentation of facet joint disease is typically a history of aching pain which is worse on hyperextension, with loss of mobility and reduction in thoracic curvature due to associated muscle spasm. The level of vertebral involvement is irrelevant to the management of these disorders. Please refer to Chapter 13 for specific management options.

## Cancer pain

Cancer is a common cause of severe thoracic pain (Figure 10.1). The most common primary thoracic tumours include lung and breast cancer. Lung cancer is more common in males, but the gender difference has narrowed in recent years secondary to the increased prevalence of cigarette smoking among females. Breast cancer is predominantly a disease of females and will currently affect 1 in 10 females during the course of their lives. In addition to these primary thoracic tumours, the chest is also frequently involved by metastatic disease from extrathoracic lesions. Common sites of metastatic involvement include the lungs, ribs and vertebral column.

The management of thoracic cancer pain, like cancer pain at any other anatomical site, begins with the maximization of anticancer therapies (e.g. surgical resection, radiation treatment, chemotherapy). Pharmacological management of pain includes the initial use of NSAIDs and weak opiates with addition of more potent opiates with disease progression, according to the World Health Organization analgesic ladder. Tricyclic antidepressants and anticonvulsants are indicated in the treatment of deafferentation pain. Additional management strategies may be required in the treatment of specific cancer pain syndromes, as described below.

### Costopleural syndrome

Costopleural syndrome is the most common cancer-related thoracic pain syndrome, usually secondary to lung cancer. Pain results from direct tumour invasion of the parietal pleura, ribs or other thoracic cage structures.[7] This process usually results in sharp, well-localized pain.

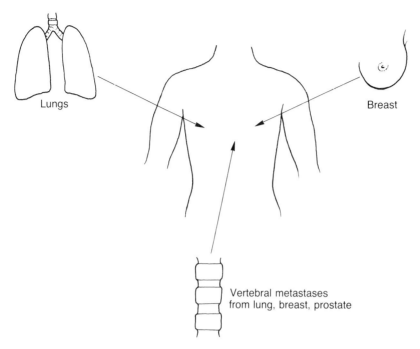

**Figure 10.1** Common cancers giving rise to thoracic pain.

If tumour growth causes invasion or compression of intercostal nerves, symptoms of neuropathic pain may develop (e.g. burning pain, bouts of lancinating pain, allodynia). With advancing disease, progressive neural injury results in sensory loss distal to the lesion, and there may be a reduction in neuropathic pain when the nerve is completely destroyed. Diaphragm involvement may also occur, often with referred aching pain to the ipsilateral shoulder, or the back.

Continuous epidural infusions can offer superior analgesia to this patient population.[8] Local anaesthetics, opiates, and $\alpha_2$-agonists can be used in combination and in relatively low doses in order to optimize analgesia and minimize undesired side-effects. Subcutaneous tunnelling of the catheter allows for several weeks of safe drug delivery provided it is monitored closely for evidence of infection. Permanent implantable infusion pumps (usually connected to intrathecal catheters) have been found to be efficacious and cost-effective in cancer patients with life expectancies of greater than 3 months.[9,10]

Patients with severe pain responsive to a diagnostic local anaesthetic blockade can also be considered for neurolytic procedures. Subarachnoid neurolysis is an effective, easily administered and low-cost procedure. Alcohol is preferred by most practitioners, but phenol can also be used. Patients commonly require a brief series of two or three injections before effective analgesia is obtained. Epidural neurolysis using phenol has also been described.

Several other nerve blocks may be effective in selected patients. Intercostal blocks can be useful with unilateral chest pain as commonly seen in the costopleural syndrome. Stellate ganglion block should be considered in patients experiencing burning pain or allodynia in the upper chest and arm. Recent research suggests that interpleural local anaesthetics are safe and effective in terminally ill patients.[11]

### Pain associated with apical chest tumours (Pancoast's tumour)

Apical chest tumours often invade the inferior aspect of the brachial plexus, resulting in the development of neuropathic pain in the medial hand and forearm (C8–T1 distribution).[12] Shoulder and arm pain are often the first presenting complaints, with weakness, atrophy and sensory changes occurring with disease progression. The triad of apical chest tumour, shoulder/ arm pain and Horner's syndrome is commonly known as Pancoast's tumour. Involvement of the superior plexus is less common but can occur (sometimes seen with metastatic breast cancer). Then involvement of C5–6 will result in shoulder pain radiating to the lateral forearm and thumb.

Early recognition of this syndrome and referral for radiation, surgery and chemotherapy are essential in limiting the development of permanent neurological sequelae. The pain associated with this process is in part due to extensive inflammation surrounding areas of tumour invasion. This explains why many patients experience significant reductions in pain following brachial plexus block with local anaesthetic plus steroid.

Subarachnoid neurolysis has been described in the management of continuing severe pain in patients with apical chest tumours.[13,14] Careful consideration, however, should be given to the risks versus benefits of this procedure when performed in the upper thorax as upper-extremity weakness, and are common sequelae. Given this, upper thoracic neurolysis is usually reserved for patients with such severe pain that potential paralysis would be preferable to persistent pain.

### Radiation plexopathy

The findings in this syndrome should be contrasted with those of apical chest tumours. Radiation-induced injury tends to predominate in the upper plexus (C5–6); the lower plexus tends to be shielded from damage by the clavicle.[15,16] Numbness and paraesthesiae are often present in the thumb and first finger and weakness may be identified in the deltoid and biceps. These symptoms usually develop soon (i.e. within 1 year) after high-dose (> 6000 rad) radiation therapy. Pain is less prominent than that associated with tumour invasion, and Horner's syndrome is rarely seen with radiation plexopathy. Careful clinical and radiological evaluation, possibly including computed tomography and magnetic resonance imaging scan, may be necessary to differentiate these two entities.

### Pain associated with vertebral column involvement

The vertebral column is the most common site of bone metastasis secondary to the unique anatomy of the vertebral venous (Batson's) plexus

(Figure 10.2).[17,18] Batson's plexus is a valveless, low-pressure system that allows free flow of venous blood in both cranial and caudal directions. Acts of coughing, lifting and straining force cancer cells out of structures in the thoracoabdominal cavity and into Batson's plexus. The most common tumours to metastasize to the vertebral column are lung, breast and prostate.[19]

Pain of vertebral origin is often localized and associated with tenderness upon palpation. Compression of the spinal cord or nerve roots may occur as disease progresses, and will result in neuropathic pain and neurological dysfunction. This syndrome represents an oncological emergency which is acutely treated with parenteral steroids and bedrest.[20] Additional treatment options, including radiotherapy, are determined following consultation with the involved specialists.

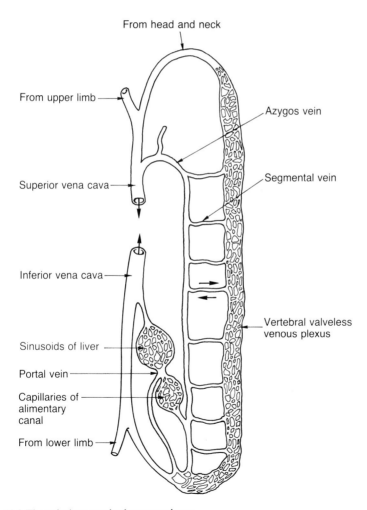

**Figure 10.2** The valveless vertebral venous plexus

## Other thoracic pain syndromes

### Postmastectomy syndrome

This neuropathic pain syndrome occurs in 4–6% of mastectomy patients.[21] The intercostobrachial nerve (the lateral cutaneous branch of the second intercostal nerve supplying the arm) and the lateral cutaneous branches of intercostal nerves T3–5 are the most commonly affected (Figure 10.3). Nerve damage may be secondary to surgical trauma or postsurgical fibrosis. Complaints of unilateral chest tightness or constriction are common in addition to other neuropathic symptoms. Conservative therapy includes physiotherapy, analgesics and tricyclic antidepressants. Limb disabilities, such as frozen shoulders and reflex sympathetic dystrophy, can result following mastectomy. Given this, neural blockade with local anaesthetics (epidural, paravertebral, intercostal) is indicated to facilitate physiotherapy in severe cases.

### Postthoracotomy pain

This condition is very similar to postmastectomy syndrome except that the injury (secondary to surgical trauma or fibrosis) involves the main trunk of the intercostal nerve. It is one of the operations most likely to result in

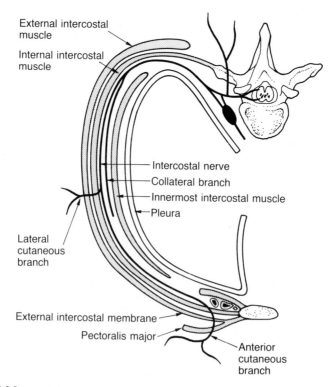

**Figure 10.3** Intercostal nerve.

chronic postoperative pain (along with nephrectomy and inguinal herniorrhaphy). Pain is of neuropathic quality and follows a dermatomal distribution. Management is similar to that of postmastectomy syndrome. Antidepressants and anticonvulsants are more useful than conventional analgesics. Diagnostic local anaesthetic block may be followed with cryotherapy to the affected nerves, giving prolonged analgesia. In both of these syndromes it is important to consider recurrent carcinoma in the differential diagnosis of patients followed oncological surgery.[22] Careful physical examination and radiological evaluation are often indicated to determine the precise aetiology of the patient's pain complaints.

### Chronic mastalgia

In this condition patients complain of chronic diffuse breast pain in the absence of any identifiable pathological process. The majority of patients experience discomfort preceding menses (cyclic pain).[23,24] These patients often respond favourably to treatment with oral contraceptive agents or the onset of menopause. Patients with non-cyclical mastalgia are less likely to respond to hormonal manipulation.

### Adiposa dolorosa (Dercum's disease)

In this rare syndrome patients complain of well-localized pain in subcutaneous adipose tissue or in discrete lipomas.[25,26] This condition is predominantly seen in females (30 : 1) and is associated with obesity and emotional instability. No specific treatment has produced consistently satisfactory results in these patients.

### Herpes zoster

The majority of cases of acute herpes zoster occur in the thoracic region. Aggressive management including antiviral drugs and regional anaesthetic blockade is indicated in elderly and immunocompromised patients, who are at the greatest risk for developing postherpetic neuralgia. (Please see Chapter 17 for more details regarding this disorder.)

## References

1. Calabro JJ, Jeghen H, Miller KA *et al.* Classification of anterior chest wall syndromes. *JAMA* **243:** 1420, 1980
2. Bonica J. Chest pain caused by other disorders. In: (Bonica JJ, ed.) *The Management of Pain.* vol II. Malvern, PA: Lea & Febiger, 1990, p. 1114
3. Motulsky A, Rohn FJ. Tietze's syndrome: cause of chest pain and chest wall swelling. *JAMA* **152:** 504, 1953
4. Lipkin M, Fulton LR, Wolfson EA. Xiphoidalgia syndrome. *N Engl J Med* **253:** 609, 1955
5. Heins GJ, Zavala DC. Slipping rib syndrome. Diagnosis using the 'hooking maneuver'. *JAMA* **237:** 794, 1977
6. Travell JG, Rinzler SH. Pain syndromes of the chest muscles: resemblance of effort angina and myocardial infarction and relief by local block. *Can Med Assoc J* **59:** 333, 1948

7. Bonica J. Chest pain related to cancer. In: (Bonica JJ, ed.) *The Management of Pain*. vol II. Malvern, PA: Lea & Febiger, 1990, p. 1083

8. Raj PP. Local anesthetic blockade. In: (Patt RB, ed.) *Cancer Pain*. Philadelphia: JB Lippincott, 1993, p. 329

9. Bedder MD, Burchiel K, Larson A. Cost analysis of two implantable narcotic delivery systems. *J Pain Symptom Management* **6:** 368, 1991

10. Lanning RM, Hrushesky WJ. Cost comparison of wearable and implantable drug delivery systems. Presented at American Society of Clinical Oncology, 1990

11. Myers DP, Lema MJ, de Leon-Casasola OA, Bacon DR. Interpleural analgesia for the treatment of severe cancer pain in terminally ill patients. *J Pain Symptom Management* **8:** 505, 1993

12. Pancoast HK. Superior pulmonary sulcus tumor. *JAMA* **99:** 1391, 1932

13. Ventafridda V, Martino G. Clinical evaluation of subarachnoid neurolytic blocks in intractable cancer pain. In: (Bonica J, Albe-Fessard D, eds) *Advances in Pain Research and Therapy*. vol 1. New York: Raven Press, 1976, p. 699

14. Swerdlow M. Spinal and peripheral neurolysis for managing Pancoast's syndrome. In: (Bonica J, Ventafridda V, Pagni CA, eds) *Advances in Pain Research and Therapy*. vol 4. New York: Raven Press, 1982, p. 135

15. Berger PS. Neurological complications of radiotherapy. In: (Silberstein A, ed.) *Neurological Complications of Therapy: Selected Topics*. Mount Kisco, NY: Futura, 1982, p. 137.

16. Kori SH *et al*. Brachial plexus lesions in patients with cancer: 100 cases. *Neurology* **31:** 45, 1981

17. Galasko CS. The anatomy and pathways of skeletal metastases. In: (Weiss L, Gilbert HA, eds.) *Bone Metastasis*. Boston, MA: GK Hall, 1981, p. 49

18. Posner JB. Back pain and epidural spinal cord compression. *Med Clin North Am* **71:** 185, 1987

19. Gilbert RW, Kim JB, Posner JB. Epidural spinal cord compression from metastatic tumor: diagnosis and treatment. *Ann Neurol* **3:** 183, 1978

20. Ladd-Smith J. Oncologic emergencies. In: (Patt RB, ed.) *Cancer Pain*. Philadelphia, PA: JB Lippincott, 1993, p. 527

21. Granek I, Ashikari R, Foley KM. Postmastectomy pain syndrome: clinical and anatomic correlates. *Proc Am Soc Clin Oncol* **3:** 122, 1983

22. Kanner R, Martini N, Foley KM. Nature and incidence of postthoracotomy pain. *Proc Am Soc Clin Oncol* **1:** 152, 1982

23. Mansel RE, Preece PE, Hughes LE. A double-blind trial of the prolactin inhibitor bromocriptine in painful nodular benign breast disease. *Br J Surg* **65:** 724, 1978

24. Mansel RE, Wisbey JR, Hughes LE. Controlled trial of the antigonadotropin danasol in painful nodular benign breast disease. *Lancet* **2:** 928, 1982

25. Dercum FX. Three cases of a hitherto unclassified infection resembling in its grosser aspects obesity, but associated with special nervous symptoms: adiposis dolorosa. *Am J Med Sci* **104:** 521, 1982

26. Foster DW. Lipodystrophies and other rare disorders of adipose tissue. In: (Braunwald E *et al.*, eds) *Harrison's Principles of Internal Medicine*, 11th edn. New York: McGraw-Hill, 1987, p. 1680

# 11

# Abdominal pain

**N. L. Padfield**

Abdominal pain may be acute or chronic and classified as nociceptive (somatic or visceral), neuropathic or psychogenic. Since patients will often be referred after extensive investigation not only must the pain clinician be aware of medical and surgical causes of disease but also understand the pathophysiology of the production of abdominal pain. Thus a knowledge of the relevant anatomy and the neurophysiology of nociception in this part of the body is essential.

## Anatomy

### Innervation of abdominal viscera

The abdominal viscera receive their innervation from the sympathetic nervous system via the coeliac plexus. This is the largest of the sympathetic plexi. It consists of a variable number of ganglia (usually 1–5), each of which is between 0.5 and 4.5 cm in diameter. There is an extensive network of interconnecting nerve fibres. It receives its primary innervation from the greater, lesser and least splanchnic nerves which arise from the fifth to 12th thoracic sympathetic ganglia. These preganglionic fibres synapse in the ganglia of the coeliac plexus and their postganglionic fibres are distributed to the abdominal viscera. Each thoracic sympathetic ganglion is connected to the corresponding spinal nerve by preganglionic (white) and postganglionic (grey) rami communicantes.

In addition to carrying afferent sympathetic fibres to the coeliac plexus, the splanchnic nerves also carry efferent fibres which pass via the grey rami communicantes from the sympathetic ganglia to the corresponding somatic nerves.

The coeliac plexus also has parasympathetic fibres, predominantly from the left vagus nerve, which pass through the plexus *en route* to supplying the abdominal viscera down to the splenic flexure.

### Relations of the coeliac plexus

The coeliac plexus lies on the anterior surface of the aorta, superolateral to the origin of the coeliac artery at the level of the body of the 12th thoracic or first lumbar vertebral body. The pancreas lies anteriorly, the kidneys lie laterally and the inferior vena cava lies anterolaterally to the right.

### Principal organs and their segmental innervation

- Pancreas            T5–11
- Stomach             T6–9
- Duodenum            T6–8
- Jejunum             T9–11
- Gallbladder         T6–9 mostly (some from T10 to T12)
- Liver               T6–11
- Kidney and ureter   T10–12 and L1–2

## Pathophysiology

The first distinction that must be made is whether the pain complained of is visceral or somatic.

- Visceral pain arises from organs with a sympathetic innervation. The pain is poorly localized and often described as deep, dragging or squeezing. It may be paroxysmal and colicky, especially when acute.
- Somatic pain arises from activation of peripheral nociceptors. It is well-localized and usually constant. Aching, throbbing and gnawing are terms often used to describe the pain which is opioid-responsive and can be relieved by proximal neural blockade.

Pain referred to the abdomen arises from sources within and outside the abdominal cavity. The commonest causes are listed in Table 11.1.

**Table 11.1** Causes of abdominal pain

EXTRA-ABDOMINAL
Angina/myocardial infarction
Vertebral column disease
Fractured ribs
Spinal tumours
Pleuritic pain
Haemolytic crisis
Acute porphyria
Lead poisoning

INTRA-ABDOMINAL
*Hollow organ dysfunction*
Oesophageal disease
Gastric ulceration/cancer
Biliary disease
Bowel obstruction
Diverticular disease
Renal pelvic or ureteric calculus or blood
Irritable bowel
  Toxins/pharmacological
  Environmental
  Pharmacological

**Table 11.1** (*cont.*)

*Solid organ dysfunction*
Hepatic tumour, inflammation, distension
Pancreatic (acute or chronic)
Pancreatic tumour
Renal tumour or inflammation

*Abdominal wall*
Scar pain/nerve entrapment
Postherpetic neuralgia
Hernias
Myofascial syndrome
Rib tip syndrome

*Vascular*
Occlusion
  Superior mesenteric artery syndrome
  Sick-cell anaemia
  Splenic infarct

*Miscellaneous*
Diabetic autonomic neuropathy
Tabes dorsalis
Vitamin deficiencies
Porphyria

## History and examination

In order to build a picture of the pain it is worth starting with Ryle's 10 questions (Table 11.2).

Following this, any history of previous and current illnesses must be elicited. Family history and social history, including alcohol intake, may also indicate non-organic causes. Previous psychiatric treatment should also be elicited. Current medication and any history of allergy may indicate a reversible iatrogenic cause.

**Table 11.2** Ryle's 10 questions

Site
Radiation
Character
Severity
Duration
Frequency
Description
Precipitating factors
Relieving factors
Associated problems

Inspection of the abdomen will reveal any previous surgical scars, cachexia, visible peristalsis, distension, vascular abnormalities. Gentle palpation may cause reproduction of the pain in instances of nerve entrapment or elicit tenderness or guarding if there is underlying visceral disease. Organ enlargement or masses may also be discovered. Carnett's test is useful in differentiating pain of abdominal wall origin from intra-abdominal causes. The point of maximum tenderness is elicited with the patient lying supine; the patient then folds the arms across the chest and tenses the abdominal wall muscles by raising the head. If palpation of the tender spot then produces increased pain, the test is positive and the pain deemed to originate from the abdominal wall. Conversely, if the pain is diminished then the test is negative, the implication being that the abdominal viscera are protected from the palpating hand by the tensed abdominal muscles.

A useful algorithm has been developed to facilitate the diagnosis in abdominal wall pain[1] (Figure 11.1), although it must be appreciated that false-positive results can occur.

## Investigations

The patient should have some routine baseline screening tests performed, if only to exclude serious systemic disease. These would include:

- full blood count
- erythrocyte sedimentation rate
- urea and electrolytes
- blood glucose
- liver function tests
- serum calcium
- serum amylase
- urine analysis

Further investigation then depends on the findings of such tests and may indicate further investigation with referral to another specialist, though it is usual for these to have already been performed prior to referral to the pain clinic. They are summarized in Table 11.3.

**Table 11.3** Further investigations in undiagnosed abdominal pain

| Suspected origin of pain | Investigation |
| --- | --- |
| Upper gastrointestinal tract | Oesophagoduodenoscopy<br>Barium swallow/meal/follow-through |
| Renal tract | Plain abdominal X-ray, intravenous urography<br>Cystoscopy/ureteroscopy |
| Liver and bilary tree | Ultrasound<br>Cholangiography/cholecystogram<br>Endoscopic retrograde choledochopancreatogram (ERCP) |
| Pancreas | Computed tomography<br>ERCP |
| Abdominal vasculature | Angiography |

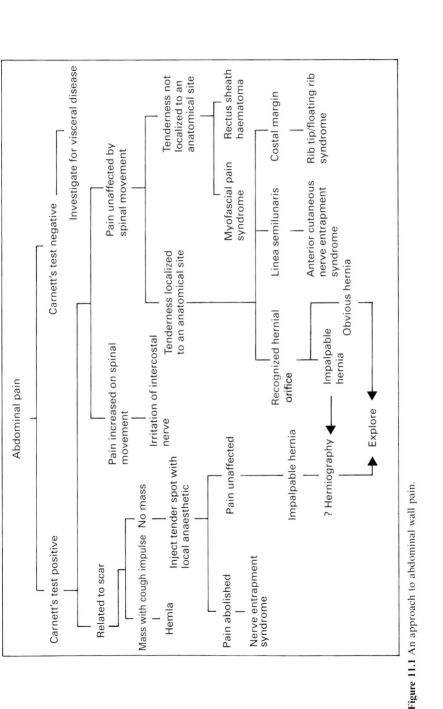

**Figure 11.1** An approach to abdominal wall pain.

## Pancreas

### Clinical features

- Pain associated with either pancreatitis or pancreatic carcinoma is usually described as sharp, boring, often knife-like, excruciating epigastric pain which radiates to the upper quadrants of the abdomen and laterally to the left back. However, it may also present as diffuse hypogastric pain or radiate into the flank, anterior or lower abdomen.

### Pathophysiology

- Pain as a result of pancreatic pathology has been little investigated. However, a positive correlation between the pressure in the pancreatic duct and the presence of pain has been demonstrated,[2] and there is the suggestion that, as a result of the destruction of an intact perineural barrier, peripheral nerve endings are exposed to inflammatory mediators and pancreatic enzymes, including lysolecithin, which is known to break down cell membranes. This is supported by the findings of raised levels of substance P and calcitonin gene-related peptide (CGRP) in sensory nerves of patients with chronic pancreatitis.[3]
- Pain associated with pancreatic carcinoma is even less well-understood, although one might postulate that the above processes are occurring distal to the obstructing tumour mass. One group has demonstrated perineural infiltration of the pancreatic nerve plexus as a postmortem finding in patients with carcinoma of the pancreas.[4] The relationship between local spread and the severity of the pain is unclear. Pressure on the coeliac plexus from the tumour will produce excruciating pain. This pressure is relieved on standing and bending forwards and explains why the supine position often intensifies the pain in patients with pancreatic carcinoma.

### Acute pancreatitis

The presentation of acute pancreatitis can vary from severe upper abdominal pain with little systemic upset to a life-threatening condition with circulatory collapse, respiratory, renal and haemostatic failure. Treatment is aimed at analgesia, reduction/suppression of pancreatic secretion and tissue damage limitation by selective inhibition of inflammatory mediators.

- Analgesia is best managed by pethidine, because of its lack of effect on the sphincter of Oddi, given by a patient-controlled analgesia system at a dose of 10–20 mg per bolus with a lock-out of 5 min. Norpethidine toxicity can occur and close observation of the patient is required to detect this complication.[5] This can be supplemented with regional anaesthesia techniques like epidural anaesthesia[6] and interpleural anaesthesia.[7] It is important to exclude any coagulopathy first.
- Reduction of secretions by octreotide may have a role, but this has yet to be established.[8]

### Chronic pancreatitis

Once this has become chronic it is important to exclude surgically correctable structural abnormalities by appropriate investigations.

- Dietary advice should be given to reduce the size and increase the frequency of meals where carbohydrate content is increased and fat and protein content decreased.
- A reduction in the acid load presented to the duodenum by proton pump inhibitors like omeprazole or $H_2$ antagonists like ranitidine is also recommended.
- Oral pancreatic enzyme preparations to reduce endogenous pancreatic secretion have not been successful as a measure to reduce pain.[9-12] An explanation for this has been demonstrated in animal studies, but not confirmed in humans, and involves a trypsin-sensitive cholecystokinin-releasing peptide. In the resting state there is insufficient pancreatic release of trypsin to inactivate the enzyme. In chronic pancreatitis, however, there is insufficient trypsin released by the pancreas, with a resultant increase in cholecystokinin and hence an increase in pancreatic secretion.[13-15]
- Oral anticholinergic agents have been suggested to block the neurally mediated release of pancreatic secretions, but the side-effects usually preclude success.[16]
- Somatostatin and octreotide have yet to be shown to be of significant benefit.
- Pharmacological treatment with non-narcotic analgesics and tricyclic antidepressants, whilst useful, may not be sufficient to control the pain. Strong narcotic analgesics are best prescribed by one clinician alone to minimize the risk of abuse.
- Acupuncture, transcutaneous electrical nerve stimulation (TENS) and hypnosis all have their advocates, but generally have limited success.
- Coeliac plexus block with local anaesthetic and depo-steroid preparations, which can be performed repeatedly, can bring relief to patients with chronic pancreatitis and pancreatic cancers. This latter group may benefit from having this block performed with neurolytic solutions. Splanchnic nerve blocks are now replacing coeliac plexus blocks as they are associated with far fewer serious side-effects. Both techniques will be detailed further on in this chapter.
- A number of surgical approaches have been advocated. In the presence of a dilated main pancreatic duct, lateral pancreaticojejunostomy has been associated with significant pain relief. Unfortunately, pain recurs in a high percentage of patients, usually relating to a continuous disease process in the head of the pancreas. For these patients and those with disease confined to the head of the pancreas without duct dilation, a number of procedures are available which are successful in relieving pain. These include a Whipple's operation, or more recently described, resecting the head of the pancreas without resecting the duodenum.[17,18] If disease activity is confined to the tail of the pancreas, a limited resection of the tail of the pancreas provides good pain relief. In the presence of diffuse pancreatic disease without duct dilation, surgical

procedures directed at the pancreas have been abandoned because they are largely unsuccessful in providing pain relief and are associated with severe metabolic and nutritional consequences. However, two surgical approaches to denervate the pancreas have been described.[19,20]

### Carcinoma of the pancreas

Carcinoma of the pancreas carries a very poor prognosis with a 2% 5-year survival. Clinical deterioration is often accompanied by poorly controlled pain and therefore effective analgesia is a priority and progression up the analgesic ladder should be expedited with a minimum of delay. In addition, significant benefit may be gained by using alternative routes of administration, such as continuous subcutaneous or intravenous infusions or the use of the epidural route.

- Neurolytic coeliac plexus block is commonly described as the most effective form of palliative therapy for the pain of carcinoma of the pancreas and recent evidence seems to support this claim.[21] It may not be successful in eliminating all pain, but is usually associated with a reduction in opioid intake. This may be the cause for a reduction in nausea and vomiting and improvement in food intake and bowel motility. If there is an unacceptable rise in opioid intake it may be appropriate to repeat the block.
- Comparative studies of the complication rates of the two common approaches (antero- and retrocrural) to the coeliac plexus are not available. Both appear to achieve a satisfactory result, but the potential for causing paraplegia has driven some clinicians away from the antero-crural approach. Details of the complication of neurolytic retrocrural approach (splanchnic nerve block) are awaited.[22]
- Surgery may well have been performed. Early reports of peroperative coeliac plexus block have been disappointing. This may be due to an inadequate volume of neurolytic solution or disruption, at dissection, of the restraining layer of peritoneum, resulting in loss of neurolytic solution. A more recent study indicates that a successful block can be achieved.[23]

### Pancreas divisum

A proportion of patients complaining of upper abdominal pain will be found to have this variant. The relationship of this anatomical variant to pancreatic pain is uncertain and opinions vary as to whether it can be the cause of pancreatitis.

- Management should begin by endoscopic stenting of the minor dorsal papilla. This has the added advantage of being a diagnostic test, in addition to being therapeutic.[4,24,25] It may then progress to endoscopic sphincteroplasty, open drainage of the caudal segment or resection of the minor duct.

# Stomach

## Clinical features

Pain from erosions, gastritis or peptic ulceration is referred to the epigastrium and is described as persistent oppressive pain that can radiate to either the left or right quadrant. The intensity changes with food. In cases of gastric carcinoma, as the tumour spreads and invades surrounding structures, the pain becomes constant and is described as boring, dull and aching, radiating to the upper quadrants and to the interscapular region. When the coeliac plexus itself is invaded the pain becomes excruciating and unrelenting.

## Management

This starts with analgesics, antacids and tricyclic antidepressants. As the pain progresses, other forms of non-invasive therapies may be tried, such as acupuncture, TENS and biofeedback. But if these measures fail to control the pain then opiate analgesics and splanchnic nerve blocks may be useful. If nausea and vomiting are a particular feature of the patients' pain then intrathecal opiates may be indicated. This is dealt with elsewhere in this book (see Chapters 23, 24 and Appendix).

# Small intestine

## Clinical features

Intestinal pain varies from colicky, crampy pain to dull, continuous and severe. Pain is referred to different parts of the abdomen and can cause diagnostic confusion. Ileitis can be referred to the epigastric, periumbilical and/or right lower quadrant regions and thus can be confused with acute appendicitis. When the caecum and colon are involved the pain tends to be suprapubic or pelvic. Two conditions in particular are referred to the pain clinic: Crohn's disease and irritable bowel syndrome. Crohn's disease is characterized by discontinuity of lesions, which 'skip' from one part of the bowel to another. Thus symptoms will vary depending on which part of the bowel is affected. Most frequently there is a history of right upper quadrant pain, weight loss, loss of appetite and psychological stress. If the ileum is involved then the symptoms can mimic acute appendicitis and there may be a palpable mass in the right lower quadrant.

## Management

- Pharmacological therapy includes non-opioid and opioid analgesics, antispasmodics and antidepressants.
- Non-pharmacological treatment includes biofeedback, TENS and acupuncture.
- Strong psychological support and support from family and friends help these sufferers enormously.

## Irritable bowel syndrome

### Clinical features

This condition affects 8–17% of the population. It is characterized by diffuse aching and cramping pain of the lower quadrants mostly but can occur over the epigastrium. Stools may be looser and more frequent with the onset of the pain and defaecation often leaves a feeling of incomplete evacuation, though constipation and abdominal distension can also occur.

### Management

- Antispasmodics
- Tricyclic antidepressants
- Biofeedback

## Gallbladder

### Clinical features

- Biliary colic is characterized by sudden severe epigastric or right upper quadrant pain which radiates to the interscapular region, the right scapula or shoulder. It causes nausea and vomiting and is often unresponsive to strong narcotic analgesics.
- Postcholecystectomy pain, however, will be the pain most likely to be referred to the clinic. Up to 40% of patients continue to have symptoms or develop recurrent symptoms. Whilst it is important to exclude other pathology in the tract, the possibility of further biliary or pancreatic pathology demands exclusion. A strategy for investigating these cases has been developed and is shown in Figure 11.2.

### Causes of postcholecystectomy pain

- common bile duct (CBD) calculi
- biliary stricture
- pancreatitis
- ampullary stenosis
- carcinoma – ampullary
            – pancreatic
            – cholangio

### Management

- pharmacological treatment with analgesics and antispasmodics
- epidural or paravertebral sympathetic blockade
- biofeedback, TENS and acupuncture may also have a role in relieving the suffering

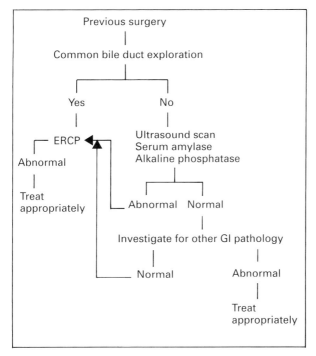

**Figure 11.2** Algorithm for postcholecystectomy pain. ERCP = Endoscopic retrograde choledochopancreatogram GI = gastrointestinal.

## Liver

### Clinical features

Pain due to hepatitis, abscess or carcinoma is usually described as a discomfort in the right upper quadrant which radiates to the back. It is rarely excruciating and often only requires mild analgesics.

### Management

Pharmacological and non-pharmacological treatments are similar to those for other upper abdominal organ pain.

## Kidney and ureters

### Clinical features

- Renal colic is excruciating flank pain that radiates into the groin, genitalia and thigh on the affected side. It gradually builds up in intensity and then wears off, leaving the sufferer with an immense sense of relief.

## Management

- Antispasmodics have been used but more success has been claimed with sublingual nifedipine 20 mg.
- Anti-inflammatory drugs and prostaglandin synthesis inhibitors can help.
- Opioid analgesics, whilst useful, are often insufficient to control the pain during severe attacks.
- Paravertebral or epidural blocks may be required.

## Abdominal wall pain (Figure 11.1)

### Clinical features

Carnett's test is useful in confirming that the origin of the pain lies in the abdominal wall. The point of maximum tenderness is located with the patient living supine. The arms are then folded across the chest and the head raised to tense the abdominal musculature. The test is positive if this manoeuvre amplifies the pain and negative if it diminishes it; the implication is that the abdominal viscera are protected from the palpating hand by the tensed abdominal muscles. In the rectus abdominis syndrome the pain starts from a localized point, then spreads to become a diffuse pain involving the whole quadrant.

### Management

- Injection into the point of maximum tenderness with local anaesthetic and a steroid suspension (e.g. 0.5% bupivacaine + triamcinolone 20 mg/ml) will in most cases relieve if not abolish the pain. This may need to be repeated.
- Occasionally, if such injections have been helpful, neurolytic agents such as 50% alcohol or 5% aqueous phenol may be employed. The attendant risk of development of neuropathic pain after the use of neurolytics can be lessened by instilling a little bupivacaine and depo-steroid mixture after each injection of the neurolytic agent.
- The use of cold spray and stretch procedures has also been shown to be beneficial (see Chapter 6).

## Superior mesenteric artery syndrome

### Clinical features

This condition presents as recurrent acute attacks of diffuse colicky abdominal pain. The abdomen may be tense and distended and the development of symptoms follows meals minutes to hours later. If the condition does not require surgery or balloon angioplasty, which it usually does, it may progress into an abdominal causalgia syndrome with ischaemic neuritis to the nerves supplying the abdominal viscera.

**Management**

- Calcium channel blockers are initially helpful.
- Antidepressants are used when calcium channel blockers are no longer beneficial because ischaemic neuritis has developed.
- Psychotrophic agents like fluphenazine in small doses can complement antidepressant therapy.
- Repeated splanchnic nerve blockade may also provide some temporary relief.

## Pain following intra-abdominal surgery

### Clinical features

The presence of intra-abdominal adhesions may give rise to chronic post-operative pain. Conventional treatment with spasmolytics (e.g. Buscopan) is often unsuccessful. Diagnostic laparoscopy may have a role to play as treatment is often unsatisfactory.[26]

### Management

- Splanchnic nerve block affords relief occasionally.
- Biofeedback, TENS and acupuncture may be more effective.

## Technical details

### Coeliac plexus block (Figure 11.3)

This is sometimes referred to as the anterocrural approach to the coeliac plexus. Numerous techniques have been described, including the posterior, the transaortic, and the anterior approach with ultrasonic and computed tomographic guidance (Figure 11.4).

The posterior approach is most commonly used and will be described here. The patient may be prone, lateral or sitting for this procedure.

The surface markings are similar to those used for a splanchnic nerve block (retrocrural coeliac plexus block). The differences are that the apex of the triangle, point A, lies between the spinous processes of T12 and L1. The point of needle insertion lies along the line of BC, which is as previously described, but only 5–8 cm from the midline. The needles are inserted at an angle of 45° to hit the vertebral body of L1 (Figure 11.3). The needle is then withdrawn to the subcutaneous tissue and redirected at a more acute angle to glance just past the vertebral body.

On the left side, the tip of the needle should lie approximately 1.5–2 cm in front of the anterior margin of the body of L1 (on the lateral X-ray). If this needle is advanced gently, the aortic pulsation can be felt being transmitted through the needle before the aorta is entered. Once this pulsation can be felt, the needle is withdrawn a couple of millimetres and the needle aspirated in four quadrants (to exclude intravascular or intrathecal placement of the needle) before the injection of contrast medium. Having determined the

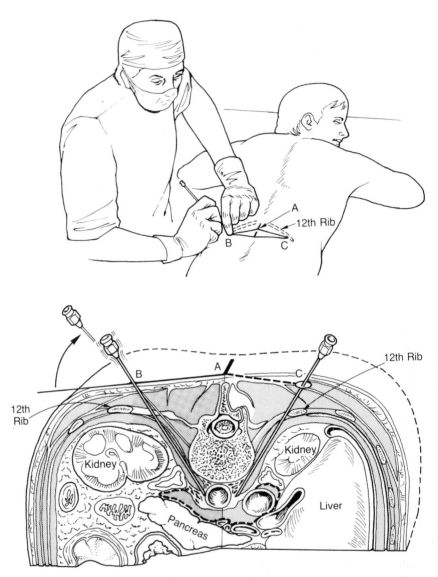

**Figure 11.3** Coeliac plexus block. Top: skin markings, position of patient and initial insertion of needle. Note: Triangle formed by skin marks on lower border of 12th ribs (B and C) in line with inferior border of L1 spinous process and joined to inferior border of T12 (A). Bottom: needle insertion and deep anatomy. Skin markings and triangle (A, B, C) are still shown. Needle initially directed in the plane of the line BA or CA, and at 45° to the horizontal axis of the body, to contact the lateral aspect of the L1 vertebral body. It passes inferior to the 12th rib and medial to the kidney. The angle of insertion of the horizontal axis of the body is then increased until the needle slips past the lateral aspect of the vertebral body, still in the line BA or CA to reach to the anterolateral aspect. On the left side the aortic pulsations will be detected at the needle hub before puncturing the artery.

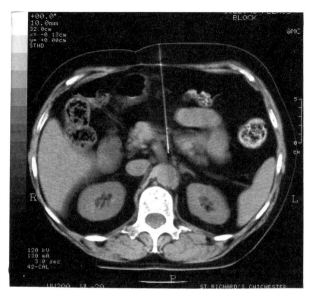

**Figure 11.4** Anterior approach to the coeliac plexus under computed tomographic guidance. The needle tip lies next to the coeliac axis and anterior to the aorta. The components of the coeliac plexus can be clearly seen.

depth on the left, the approach on the right is made in the same way, but the needle is inserted an additional 0.5–1 cm. When viewed on an antero-posterior X-ray, the needles should overlie the body of the vertebra by 0.5–1 cm.

If either needle moves with respiration, it has passed through the kidney and it should be withdrawn and a new approach made. This is likely to occur if the original point of insertion through the skin is made more than 8 cm from the midline.

There should be minimal resistance to injection, although it is possible to achieve a bilateral spread of solution from a unilateral injection.[27] Radiographic confirmation of the needle tip and spread of contrast medium are used to improve the accuracy of the injection. Once the needles are in a satisfactory position 20 ml of 0.5% bupivacaine is injected each side. The addition of steroid is of debatable value.

A neurolytic solution can be used and there is debate, but no clinical trials, as to what volume of which neurolytic agent should be used. Most published studies of coeliac plexus block in pancreatic cancer use a volume of 20–50 ml of 50–75% alcohol, although some have used as little as 16 ml of absolute alcohol and others have used 6% aqueous phenol.[28] It would seem that 25 ml of 50% alcohol injected bilaterally provides a satisfactory response.

In the event of an unsatisfactory result, it is worth repeating the block with 75% alcohol.

Complications of the procedure include postural hypotension,[29] intra-vascular injection and aortic pseudoaneurysm formation. In addition, if a neurolytic solution is used, persistent diarrhoea, posterior spread of the neurolytic solution to cause neuropathic pain in the region of the lower rib cage and upper thigh,[30,31] paraplegia[32,33] and retroperitoneal fibrosis[34] may occur.

The use of sedation is at the preference of the clinician, but a low-dose propofol infusion provides very satisfactory conditions for performing the block.

## Splanchnic nerve block

This can be by either the interpleural approach or the retrocrural approach.

### Interpleural approach

For a left-sided block the patient is placed in the right lateral position and prepared in an aseptic manner.

The intrapleural space is identified 8–10 cm from the posterior midline at the level of the seventh and eighth ribs using a passive loss of resistance technique with an epidural needle connected to a loss of resistance syringe. Once the space is identified and epidural catheter is inserted 5–6 cm and secured in place. 30 ml of 0.25% or 0.5% bupivacaine with 1:200 000 adrenaline is injected every 8–12 h. There are as yet no studies comparing strengths of solution or dosage intervals.

The technique has the advantage over other forms of neural blockade in that it is safe with a low complication rate and is easy to perform without the need for image intensification.[35,36]

### Transcutaineous approach

This is sometimes described as the retrocrural approach to the coeliac plexus The technique blocks the splanchnic nerves above the diaphragm before they reach the coeliac plexus. It has replaced coeliac plexus block in some centres because it is perceived to have a lower incidence of complications, although comparative data are not available. In addition, the effectiveness and duration of analgesia have yet to be fully established.

The patient is placed prone on a radiolucent table, intravenous access is secured and 1 litre of compound sodium lactate solution infused. Standard monitoring of non-invasive blood pressure, electrocardiography and pulse oximetry are employed.

Three points are made on the patient's back. Point A lies over the superior aspect of the spinous process of T12. Points B and C lie on the inferior margin of the 12th ribs on a line running through the inferior margin of the spinous process of L1 (Figure 11.5).

A 15-cm 20-gauge needle is then inserted along lines BA and CA to lie on the anterolateral border of the body of T12. Placement of the needle at the level of T11 may give better spread of solution over all three splanchnic nerves. Contrast medium is then injected to confirm that there is no movement of dye on respiration (indicating that the needle tip lies within the crus of the diaphragm).

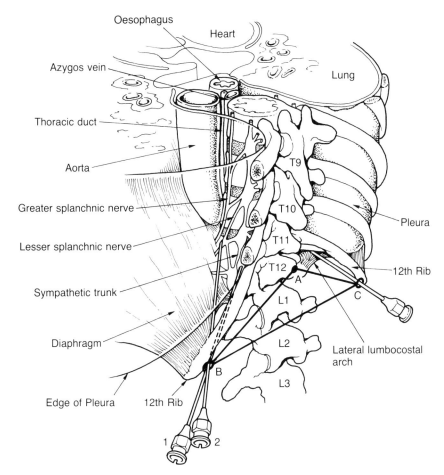

**Figure 11.5** Splanchnic nerve block, posterolateral view. Skin markings B and C are described. A is marked at the superior aspect of T12 spinous process.

Studies comparing the volume of local anaesthetic and the benefits conferred by the addition of steroid are not available. However, a volume of 10–20 ml of 0.25% bupivacaine solution is appropriate, to which Depo-Medrone (methylprednisolone acetate) 40 mg can be added.

Hypotension and pneumothorax are potential complications of this technique. Hypotension can be minimized by volume preloading but vasopressors may be required. Pneumothorax is even less common, but should it occur, formal drainage is rarely required. Overnight observation in hospital would, however, be prudent.

A neurolytic block can be performed using as little as 3–4 ml of 50% alcohol injected on each side.

# References

1. Gallegos NC, Hobsley M. Abdominal wall pain: an alternative diagnosis. *Br J Surg* **10:** 1167–1169, 1990
2. Beger HG, Bulcher M, Bittner R. The duodenum preserving resection of the head of the pancreas in patients with chronic pancreatitis and an inflammatory mass in the head – an alternative surgical technique to the Whipple operation. *Acta Chir Scand* **156:** 309–315, 1990
3. Nagakawa T, Mori K, Nakano T *et al.* Perineural invasion of carcinoma of the pancreas and biliary tract. *Br J Surg* **80:** 619–621, 1993
4. Lans JI, Geenen JE, Johanson JF, Hogan WJ. Endoscopic therapy in patients with pancreas divisum and acute pancreatitis: a prospective, randomized, controlled clinical trial. *Gastrointest Endosc* **38:** 430–434, 1992
5. Stone PA, Macintyre PE, Jarvis DA. Norpethidine toxicity and patient controlled analgesia. *Br J Anaesth* **71:** 738–740, 1993
6. Browne RA, Ashworth EJ. The use of epidural block in acute pancreatitis: a report of eight cases. *Can Anaesth Soc J* **16:** 416–424, 1969
7. Murphy D. Interpleural analgesia. *Br J Anaesth* **71:** 426–434, 1993
8. Ladas SD, Raptis SA. Conservative treatment of acute pancreatitis: the use of somatostatin. *Hepato-Gastroenterology* **39:** 466–469, 1992
9. Saksson G, Ihse I. Pain reduction by oral pancreatic preparation in chronic pancreatitis. *Dig Dis Sci* **28:** 97–102, 1983
10. Slaff J, Jacobsen D, Tillman CR *et al.* Protease-specific suppression of pancreatic exocrine secretion. *Gastroenterology* **87:** 44–52, 1984
11. Halgreen H, Pederson NT, Worning H. Symptomatic effect of pancreatic enzyme therapy in patients with chronic pancreatitis. *Scand J Gastroenterol* **21:** 104–108, 1986
12. Ramo OJ, Puolakkainen PA, Seppala K *et al.* Self-administration of enzyme substitution in the treatment of exocrine pancreatic insufficiency. *Scand J Gastroenterol* **24:** 688–692, 1989
13. Lu I, Louie D, Owyang C. A cholecystokinin releasing peptide mediates feedback regulation of pancreatic secretion. *Am J Physiol* **256:** G430–G435, 1989
14. Myasaka K, Guan D, Liddle RA *et al.* Feedback regulation by trypsin: evidence for CCK-releasing peptide. *Am J Physiol* **256:** G175–G181, 1989
15. Cantor P, Petronijevic L, Worning H. Plasma cholecystokinin concentrations in patients with advanced chronic pancreatitis. *Pancreas* **1:** 488–493, 1986
16. Adler G, Reinshagen M, Koop I *et al.* Differential effects of atropine and a cholecystokinin receptor antagonist on pancreatic secretion. *Gastroenterology* **96:** 1158–1164, 1989
17. Beger HG, Bulcher M, Bittner RR. Duodenum-preserving resection of the head of the pancreas in severe chronic pancreatitis. *Ann Surg* **209:** 273–278, 1989
18. Frey CF, Smith GJ. Description and rationale of a new operation for chronic pancreatitis. *Pancreas* **2:** 701–707, 1987
19. Stibe HH, Chauvin EJ. Pancreatic denervation for pain relief in chronic alcohol associated pancreatitis. *Br J Surg* **77:** 303–305, 1990
20. Hiroka T, Watanabe E, Katoh T *et al.* A new surgical approach for control of pain in chronic pancreatitis: complete denervation of the pancreas. *Am J Surg* **152:** 549–551, 1986
21. Mercadante S. Coeliac plexus block versus analgesics in pancreatic cancer pain. *Pain* **52:** 187–192, 1993
22. Ischia S, Ischia A, Polati E, Finco G. Three posterior percutaneous coeliac plexus block techniques. A prospective, randomized study in 61 patients with pancreatic cancer pain. *Anaesthesiology* **76:** 534–540, 1992
23. Sharp KW, Stevens EJ. Improving palliation in pancreatic cancer: intraoperative coeliac plexus block for pain relief. *South Med J* **84:** 469–471, 1991
24. Cooperman AM, Seigel J, Hammerman H. Pancreas divisum – advocates and agnostics. *J Clin Gastroenterol* **11:** 489–491, 1989

25. Kalkay MN, Derman A. Pancreatitis of pancreas divisum. *N Jersey Med* **86**: 281–285, 1989
26. Easter DW, Cuschieri A, Nathanson LK, Lavelle-Jones M. The utility of diagnostic laparoscopy for abdominal disorders. *Arch Surg* **127**: 379–383, 1992
27. Hankemeier V. Neurolytic coeliac plexus block for cancer-related upper abdominal pain using the unilateral puncture technique and lateral position. *Pain* **4** (suppl): S135
28. Lebovits AH, Lefkowitz M. Pain management for pancreatic carcinoma: a review. *Pain* **36**: 1–11, 1989
29. Black A, Dwyer B. Coeliac plexus block. *Anaesth Intensive Care* **1**: 315, 1973
30. Gorbitz C, Leavens ME. Alcohol block for the control of upper abdominal pain caused by cancer and pancreatitis. *J Neurosurg* **34**: 575, 1971
31. Cherry DA, Lamberty J. Paraplegia following coeliac plexus block. *Anaesth Intensive Care* **1**: 59–61, 1984
32. Galizia EJ, Lahiri SK. Paraplegia following coeliac plexus block with alcohol. *Br J Anaesth* **46**: 539–540, 1987
33. Pateman J, Williams MP, Filshie J. Retroperitoneal fibrosis after multiple coeliac plexus blocks. *Anaesthesia* **45**: 309–310, 1990
34. Ebbehoj N, Borly L, Bulow J *et al*. Pancreatic tissue fluid pressure in chronic pancreatitis. Relation to pain, morphology, and function. *Scand J Gastroenterol* **25**: 1046–1051, 1990
35. Reiestad F, McIlvanine WB, Kvalheim L *et al*. Successful treatment of chronic pancreatitis pain with interpleural analgesia. *Can J Anaesth* **36**: 713–716, 1989
36. Ahlburg P, Noreng M, Mølgaard J, Egebo K. Treatment of pancreatic pain with inter-pleural bupivacaine: an open trial. *Acta Anaesthesiol Scand* **34**: 156–157, 1990

# 12

# Pelvic pain

**J. P. O'Dwyer**

Chronic pelvic pain (CPP) has been defined as non-cyclical abdominal and pelvic pain of at least 6 months' duration. Many authors discuss CPP with reference to pain affecting females, but there are other causes of pelvic pain which are not gender-specific, arising from bowel, the urinary tract and the musculoskeletal system. Some of these will also be discussed briefly.

## Incidence and aetiology

Chronic pelvic pain has a prevalence of about 12% in the USA, with a lifetime incidence of 33%.[1] It accounts for 10% of gynaecological consultations, and up to 33% of laparoscopies,[2] while in the UK it accounts for up to 40–52% of laparoscopies.[3] It also accounts for 12–16% of hysterectomies, with questionable efficacy since it is reported that 25% of CPP referrals have had hysterectomies previously for CPP.[4] CPP has been attributed to a variety of conditions, including pelvic congestion, uterine retroversion, uterine prolapse or broad ligament defects, but laparoscopy has led to the more frequent diagnosis of endometriosis and pelvic adhesions. However, controlled trials have shown that the prevalence of these conditions is similar for CPP patients and painfree controls (e.g. women undergoing laparoscopy for tubal ligation).[5] Thus these too may be incidental findings in some cases.

The following should be borne in mind when dealing with chronic pelvic pain:

- Often no cause is found.
- Where a 'cause' is found it may be an incidental finding.
- Where a 'cause' is treated there may be no improvement.
- Many cases are inextricably tied to psychosexual problems.

## Causes of chronic pelvic pain (Table 12.1)

### Psychological factors

Following appropriate surgical and medical investigation, many patients with CPP may continue to search for an organic cause in the face of negative

**Table 12.1** Causes of chronic pelvic pain

| Gynaecological | Urological | Gastrointestinal | Musculoskeletal |
| --- | --- | --- | --- |
| Endometriosis | Chronic urinary | Irritable bowel | Low back pain |
| Pelvic inflammatory | tract infection | Crohn's disease | Scar pain |
| disease | Urethral syndrome | Ulcerative colitis | Myofascial pain |
| Adhesions | Prostadynia | Diverticulitis | Tumour |
| Pelvic congestion | Cystitis | Hernia | |
| Retroverted uterus | Calculi | Tumour | *Psychological* |
| Prolapsed uterus | Testicular pain | Constipation | Somatization |
| Broad ligament | Tumour | Malabsorption | Depression |
| defect | | Abdominal angina | Anxiety |
| Dysmenorrhoea | | | Eating disorders |
| Dyspareunia | | | Posttraumatic |
| Mid-cycle pain | | | |
| Fibroids | | | |
| Malignancy | | | |
| Intrauterine device | | | |

investigations, often resulting in further unnecessary investigation and surgery. While it is important to exclude organic causes, an integrated approach looking for the influence of both physical and psychological factors may be more satisfactory in managing the problem. Many studies have shown that patients with CPP are psychologically distressed, though not necessarily differing in this respect from other chronic pain patients. The expression of pain is also influenced by social and cultural factors.

The following psychological factors may be relevant.

- Depression: Often pain and depression coexist, and patients with CPP have a significantly greater prevalence of lifetime major depression and of current major depression than controls. In one study of CPP patients with depression, the depression predated the pain in 75% of cases.[6]
- Physical and sexual abuse: Many patients with CPP are from disturbed backgrounds, which they may perpetuate into adulthood by choosing partners who abuse them physically, sexually or emotionally.[7] Previous sexual abuse appears to be a significant factor for somatisation and for CPP without identifiable organic cause.[8] It also increases the risk of life-time psychiatric illness, especially mood and anxiety disorders. Although sexual abuse is not specific to CPP, it may be associated with CPP to a greater degree than other abuse syndromes.[9] It is important to look for other forms of abuse as well, since at least one study has shown significantly greater incidence of childhood physical abuse in CPP compared to other chronic pain or controls.[10]
- Somatisation disorders: CPP patients have an increased incidence of abdominal pain outside the pelvis, diarrhoea, constipation, low back pain, dyspareunia, dysmenorrhoea, nausea, bloating, shortness of breath, dizziness, weakness and menstrual irregularity.[1,6] Nevertheless, most CPP patients, while showing some features of somatisation, do not fulfil the criteria for such a diagnosis.[7] The few who do are dramatic, and require ongoing psychiatric therapy.

## Pathology

Various pain models have been described to explain the generation and perception of pain. These include the Cartesian model, the gate theory and the biopsychosocial model of pain. This last suggests that the occurrence and maintenance of adverse clinical and social outcomes are the result of the complex interaction between chronic nociceptive stimuli and social and psychological determinants.[11] All chronic pain has a psychosocial dimension, but it is particularly important to emphasize psychosocial factors in the genesis of CPP.

The elucidation of CPP may be helped by an understanding of the innervation of the pelvic organs, which is complex, and briefly outlined here:

- The descending ureter is progressively innervated by sympathetic fibres via the renal, aortic, and the superior and inferior hypogastric plexuses.
- The bladder receives sympathetic motor fibres for bladder relaxation and sensory fibres for light touch, pain and temperature via the superior and inferior hypogastric ganglia from T11 to L2. It also receives parasympathetic motor fibres for contraction, and sensory fibres for stretch sensation via inferior hypogastric plexus from S2 to S4.
- The uterus, ovarian tubes and ovaries receive sympathetic sensory innervation via Frankenhauser's plexus from the sympathetic chain at T11–L1, passing through superior, middle and inferior hypogastric plexuses *en route*. The parasympathetic motor supply is via nervi erigentes from S2 to S4.
- The vagina, vulva, distal urethra and perineum are supplied by the pudendal nerve (S2–4). Small areas of vulva and perineum also receive sensory supply from the ilioinguinal, iliohypogastric and genitofemoral nerves.
- In the male the testes receive sympathetic innervation via the renal plexus, and the epididymis via the hypogastric plexus. The scrotum is innervated by the pudendal nerve, and also ilioinguinal and hypogastric nerves, while the penis receives autonomic supply from S2 to S4 via the hypogastric plexus, and sensory supply from the pudendal nerve.

## Clinical features

### History

A good history is essential, and should include a chronological account of the referrals, investigations and treatments, with outcomes thereof. It should include a detailed description of the pain and its impact on the patient, and a psychological assessment, which if possible should be done by a psychologist experienced in the area of sexual function.[12] The assessment should include self-report questionnaires, such as the Beck depression inventory, and a detailed interview, during which issues such as sexuality, past and current sexual abuse, any history of genital injuries, etc., should be explored, in addition to a general psychosocial assessment. This calls for great skill and patience, and relies upon gaining the patient's trust.

It can be difficult to decide whether pain is gynaecological in origin, but the following may be useful (adapted from Renaer[13]):

- Site – Pain arising from gynaecological causes is usually experienced in a ventral area not higher than the anterior superior iliac spine, and a dorsal area located over the upper half of the sacrum extending laterally over the gluteal zones. The pain may be in both zones or a part of them, more commonly in the lower abdominal zone. Rarely it is felt deep in the pelvis. Lumbar, lumbosacral and low lumbar pain are usually orthopaedic and iliac fossa pain extending higher is usually musculoskeletal or gastrointestinal in origin.
- Radiation – Pain radiating higher in the abdomen is not usually gynaecological though it may coexist with a gastrointestinal condition. Uterine pain may radiate to the thigh anteriorly, less commonly medially or laterally, but not posteriorly. Sciatic pain is not usually associated with pelvic disorders.
- Relationship to menstrual cycle – chronic painful gynaecological conditions usually show fluctuations of pain intensity during the cycle; mid-cycle pain is classic of this. Endometriosis is associated with pain worsening towards the end of menstruation. Orthopaedic pain can also show menstrual fluctuation.
- Hyperalgesia – the presence of trigger points in the abdominal wall or more commonly the back makes it likely that the pain has a parietal source. Also, pain that increases or remains constant during voluntary tightening of the abdominal wall is usually parietal.

### Examination

Examination is focused on the area of pain and detailed with regard to motor and sensory systems. Most patients will already have had a full gynaecological (or urological, depending on symptoms) investigation, including laparoscopy, by the time they reach the pain clinic, and repeat pelvic examination is unlikely to be helpful, especially if the pain specialist is unaccustomed to performing them regularly. A rectal examination should be performed in males.

### Investigations

Investigations which should have been completed prior to pain clinic referral include full blood count, urine and electrolytes, urine for microscopy and culture, cervical smear for culture and cytology, plain abdominal film, ultrasound, and possibly magnetic resonance imaging or computed tomographic scan of the pelvis and lumbosacral spine.

## Management

As with other chronic pains, the aim of treatment is to maximise function and improve the quality of life. The choice of treatment strategy will depend on the likely cause of the pain, the influence of psychological factors and the investigations and treatments already undertaken.

Therapy should be aimed at a multidisciplinary approach from the outset. It is important to establish a rapport with the patient who may feel that no one believes in the pain, in the face of negative investigation. There is a need to treat the physical and emotional aspects, and reassure the patient of the lack of a sinister cause, or of the pain indicating progressive disease. In common with other chronic pain sufferers, the patient should be discouraged from taking medication which proves ineffective.

- Antidepressants may be particularly useful when there is a pattern of poor sleep, or when the patient is clinically depressed, despite a lack of objective evidence that they are effective in CPP. In clinically depressed patients with CPP, psychiatric referral has been recommended, while acknowledging that patients will often be ambivalent to this.[14] It also appears that antidepressants may be less effective in patients who have a history of prior sexual victimisation.
- If other medications have not been tried, then a stepwise approach, from paracetamol to NSAIDs (which are particularly effective with dysmenorrhoea) to tricyclics and anticonvulsants can be made.
- A transcutaneous electrical nerve stimulation (TENS) machine may be effective and is worth a trial, as is acupuncture.
- Where the pain is in the distribution of a peripheral nerve, a local anaesthetic block may be employed, and if effective, repeated blocks or cryotherapy may be used. Where there are abdominal trigger points, an alternative is to infuse local anaesthetic continuously following placement of an abdominal catheter. It is also possible to do serial blocks of the nerves supplying the perineum to see which may be involved; however, this requires a thorough knowledge of the anatomy, and the availability of sufficient time for the series of blocks.
- Surgical exploration of an abdominal scar may reveal a trapped nerve or a neuroma. The results from this are often disappointing, however, even where a lesion has been found.
- If it seems that the pain is sympathetically mediated or there is little response to the above, blockade of the sympathetic ganglia can be attempted. This is achieved by the lumbar approach, but may need to be bilateral.
- Sympathectomy may also be achieved by a lumbar epidural block using a low concentration of local anaesthetic without steroid. It is possible to do repeated epidural blocks, or to place a catheter and infuse opiate into the epidural space.
- Neurosurgical procedures such as spinothalamic cordotomy and dorsal root entry zone lesions have been described in the management of particularly difficult cases, but have no proven benefit with possible morbidity. Cordotomy is only 80% successful in the best hands, and carries a significant risk for anaesthesia dolorosa, so should be avoided where possible in the therapy of benign pain.[15] Presacral neurectomy has been used for endometriosis, dyspareunia and dysmenorrhoea, but long-term results are poor, and it is not often performed.
- Ovarian cycle suppressants may be useful for a functional cycle pain.

- In cases where there is a positive culture demonstrating infection, antibiotic treatments may help the pain. However, empirical treatment in the absence of proof of infection is not indicated.

The importance of involvement of the psychologist has already been referred to. The basic strategy of psychotherapy is to develop a therapeutic alliance with patients:

- Take them seriously.
- Assess their quality of life.
- Lay out the expectations for therapy and enlist their help.
- Emphasize that the aim of treatment is not cure, but to maximize function and improve quality of life.

These patients are often resistant to psychotherapy and any suggestion that the pain is not organic. It is often necessary to spend much time listening to the history of pain and investigation before they will agree to talk about any other problems. Once they talk about these problems, they may sense a benefit to airing their problems and it becomes easier for them to make the link between their pain and the stresses in their life. When they accept that one influences the other, behavioural changes can be suggested. This may include setting limits on demands from others, setting realistic and attainable goals, and developing appropriate assertiveness.[7]

Patients with deeply buried painful memories of sexual abuse will need skilled psychotherapy to help them to alter their defence mechanisms built against such memories. The painful memories may return as nightmares, flashbacks or as an exaggerated reaction to stimuli, such as surgery. Two therapeutic approaches may be used. Hypnosis seeks to bring these feelings to the surface and confront them. This approach has been somewhat discredited of late, with claims that patients may 'recall' events that never happened. The other approach seeks to engender confidence and coping skills and discourage dissociative experiences by allowing the patient to choose the speed and intensity for dealing with the painful repressed memories.

There may also be benefit to be gained from seeking marital and/or sex therapy in some cases.

## Prognosis

- Reduced distress and increased life satisfaction are more realistic and likely outcomes than total pain relief. Most patients with CPP will still have some pain at 5 years.
- Non-surgical therapy is likely to be more beneficial than hysterectomy (orchidectomy), etc.[16]
- The success rates for most therapies fall with time.
- There is a significant reduction in utilization of hospital services over 1–2 years following a pain management programme, in patients with chronic pain. It is not clear whether this applies to patients with CPP.

## Specific conditions

### Endometriosis

#### Aetiology

Endometriosis has been estimated to be present in 4–65% of women with CPP in various studies.[17] Looking only at pain of greater than 6 months' duration, it seems that endometriosis is found about twice as commonly at laparoscopy in CPP patients compared to controls, with rates varying from 15 to 32%.[18,19] The implanted endometrial tissue causes local peritoneal inflammation and infiltrative tissue damage, both of which lead to the release of chemical mediators of pain.

#### Clinical features

There is a poor correlation between clinical symptoms and the laparoscopic demonstration of endometriosis. Endometriosis is said to be three times as likely if a woman has two of the following three: dyspareunia, dysmenorrhoea and pelvic pain, though some people with endometriosis are free of these symptoms.[20] However, an unpublished study by Overton found no difference in premenstrual tension, dyspareunia and pelvic pain between 49 patients with and 51 patients without endometriosis, in a group of 100 patients undergoing laparoscopy for either infertility or pelvic pain.[15]

#### Management

Medical therapy can be undertaken with medroxyprogesterone, danazol (a synthetic steroid derivative of ethisterone) or nafarelin (a potent agonistic analogue of gonadotrophin-releasing hormone). In a controlled trial danazol and nafarelin have been shown to be 80% effective in reducing disease as judged by second-look laparoscopy, with a reduction in severe pain from 40 to 5–10%.[21] In all gonadotrophin-releasing hormone therapy, symptoms of oestrogen deficiency are prominent and therapy should be supervised by someone experienced in these matters. It is also worth remembering that other studies have shown disappointing levels of pain relief in CPP following therapy for endometriosis. The 5-year recurrence of pain following conservative medical and surgical treatment is quoted as 50%.[22]

Surgical therapy revolves around laparoscopic laser ablation and excision of affected tissue, with some studies suggesting that complete excision of affected tissue may be needed. Randomized controlled trials of efficacy are not available.[23] Where fertility is not an issue, and the pain is the dominant problem, laparotomy ± oophorectomy has been advocated, but needs careful consideration and counselling. There is up to 10% recurrence of pain if ovaries are preserved.[15]

Patients with endometriosis are usually referred to the pain clinic because of failure of the above therapies. This may have been failure to respond to therapy, or it may indicate the pain has a different cause. Usually such patients will have been fully investigated, however, and further investigations should only be undertaken if specifically indicated. The choice of therapy is as set out in the general section of the chapter. It is worth empha-sizing that if hormonal therapy has not been tried, then this should be tried first, and if a nerve block is indicated then the choice should be an epidural block. If epidural local anaesthetic is of no benefit, then it is possible to try epidural opiates and/or clonidine.[15] Presacral neurectomy has been shown to be ineffective in the long-term treatment of endometriosis pain.

## Pelvic inflammatory disease (PID)

### Aetiology

The incidence of CPP following PID is estimated at up to 23%.[24] Contro-versy exists as to whether the CPP results from the formation of adhesions following peritoneal inflammation, since adhesions are noted as commonly at laparoscopy in patients without CPP[4] (one study[19] did find an increased incidence of adhesions in CPP) and prior PID does not lead to an increased incidence of adhesions in patients with CPP.[25] Evidence of benefit from division of adhesions is inconclusive. Therefore in any patient with previous PID it is important to look for other causes of CPP rather than assume it is due to adhesions.

### Clinical features

There may be a past history of PID or surgical procedures. There may be adnexal tenderness on internal examination. Such patients will present to the pain clinic already having seen and investigated by the gynaecologist. It is probable that they will also have had laparoscopy, and may well have undergone surgery for division of adhesions.

No specific therapy is indicated, in the absence of evidence of ongoing inflammation, and treatment is for CPP as set out above.

## Urethral syndrome

This usually presents in postmenopausal women with symptoms of a urinary tract infection, but with a sterile culture. Various proposed causes include chronic low-grade infection with periurethral inflammation, urethral spasm, hypo-oestrogenism and trauma from intercourse, causing bacteria to be massaged into the periurethral glands.[26] Dyspareunia is frequently present, but dysmenorrhoea is uncommon. In one group of 8 women, 7 had post-coital voiding dysfunction.[27] On examination there may be tenderness over urethral and bladder base. It is occasionally helped by prolonged treatment with nitrofurantoin and/or oestrogen cream. Also, urinary analgesics such as Pyridium may help.[28]

## Chronic prostatitis

This is commonest in the third and fourth decades, and associated with a nervous personality and a history of urethritis.[28] The symptoms include painful micturition, frequency and nocturia, and pain on ejaculation. The pain is referred to many sites, including testes, groin, and low back.

Alcohol, spicy foods and irregular sexual activity may exacerbate the symptoms and hot baths may provide some relief. The prostate is tender, and prostatic secretions copious on massage. Culture is usually sterile but occasionally yields *Chlamydia* or *Mycoplasma*, in which case antibiotic therapy is appropriate.

It is reassuring for patients to know that there is no serious underlying disease, although they may have recurring symptoms.

## Irritable bowel syndrome

### Aetiology

Irritable bowel syndrome (IBS) is defined as symptoms of abdominal pain and disturbance of bowel function lasting more than 3 months without organic cause. It is more common in women, with a peak incidence in the third decade.

### Pathology

There is no demonstrable physical abnormality in these cases. The gut has its own neuroplexus and there are many gut hormones which exert effects locally that may be independent of central control. It may be that IBS sufferers have an altered pain threshold for otherwise normal sensations since studies of balloon distension of the sigmoid colon in IBS and controls led to pain in 55% of IBS and 6% of controls.[29] Also the controls experienced pain in the nerve distribution of the distended colon, while the IBS patients experienced pain anywhere in the abdomen, and even the back or thighs.[30] There is a higher incidence of negative life events and psychopathology in IBS patients.[31]

### Clinical

Pain occurs most commonly in the left iliac fossa in adults (periumbilical in children), and varies from dull ache to excruciating in intensity, lasting from minutes to several hours.[32] It rarely disturbs sleep at night. Most sufferers complain of constipation and/or diarrhoea, usually worse in the morning. Where diarrhoea predominates, there may be several watery stools in the morning followed by normal motions later in the day. Defecation relieves the pain in 50% of cases; eating aggravates pain, as does stress, but weight loss is unusual.

Associated features include nausea without vomiting, dyspepsia, bloating, tenesmus, urinary symptoms, gynaecological symptoms and headache. Dyspareunia can occur, but usually indicates a gynaecological cause. Many of these patients have features of anxiety and/or depression.

On examination there is little to find, apart from localized abdominal tenderness over an area of colon which is also palpable. The presence of perineal fistula or abscess indicates an inflammatory bowel disorder.

### Management

Medical treatment alone is unlikely to be as effective as a multidisciplinary approach, and few drugs have been shown to be better than placebo. Of these, the best are bulk-forming agents. Therapy should consist of re-assurance, education about the disorder, stress reduction, bulk-forming agents and low-dose tricyclic antidepressants.[31]

## References

1. Walker EA, Katon WJ, Jemelka R *et al.* The prevalence of chronic pain and irritable bowel syndrome in two university clinics. *J Psychosom Obstet Gynaecol* **12** (suppl): 65, 1991
2. Reiter RC, Gambone JC. Demographic and historical variables in women with idiopathic chronic pelvic pain. *Obstet Gynecol* **75**: 428, 1990
3. Campbell F, Collett B. Chronic pelvic pain. *Nr J Anaesth* **73**: 574–578, 1994
4. Slocumb JC. Operative management of chronic abdominal pelvic pain. *Clin Obstet Gynecol* **33**: 196, 1990
5. Rapkin AJ. Adhesions and pelvic pain: a retrospective study. *Obstet Gynecol* **68**: 13, 1986
6. Walker EA, Katon WJ, Harrop-Griffiths J *et al.* Relationship of chronic pelvic pain to psychiatric diagnoses and childhood sexual abuse. *Am J Psychiatry* **145**: 75–80, 1988
7. Rosenthal RH. Psychology of chronic pelvic pain. *Obstet Gynecol Clin North Am* **20**: 627–642, 1993
8. Reiter RC, Shakerin LR, Gambone JC *et al.* Correlation between sexual abuse and soma-tisation in women with somatic and nonsomatic chronic pelvic pain. *Am J Obstet Gynecol* **165**: 104–109, 1991
9. Walker EA, Stenchever MA. Sexual victimisation and chronic pelvic abuse in women with chronic pelvic pain. *Obstet Gynecol Clin North Am* **20**: 795–807, 1993
10. Rapkin AJ, Kames LK, Darke LL *et al.* History of physical and sexual abuse in women with chronic pelvic pain. *Obstet Gynecol* **79**: 92–96, 1990
11. Milburn A, Reiter RC, Rhomberg AT. Multidisciplinary approach to chronic pelvic pain. *Obstet Gynecol Clin North A,* **20**: 643–662, 1993
12. McDonald JS. Management of chronic pelvic pain. *Obstet Gynecol Clin North Am* **20**: 817–838, 1993
13. Renaer M. Gynaecological pain. In: (Wall PD, Melzack R, eds.) *Textbook of Pain*, 1st edn. London: Churchill Livingstone, 1984, pp. 359–376
14. Walker EA, Sullivan MD, Stenchever MA. Use of antidepressants in the management of women with chronic pelvic pain. *Obstet Gynecol Clin North Am* **20**: 743–751, 1993
15. Barlow DH, Glynn CJ. Endometriosis and chronic pain. *Clin Obstet Gynecol* **7**: 775–789, 1993
16. Peters AAW, van Dorst E. A randomised clinical trial to compare two different approaches in women with chronic pelvic pain. *Obstet Gynecol* **77**: 740, 1991
17. Mahmood TA, Templeton AA. Prevalence and genesis of endometriosis. *Hum Reprod* **6**: 544–549, 1991
18. Mahmood TA, Templeton AA *et al.* Menstrual symptoms in women with endometriosis. *Br J Obstet Gynaecol* **98**: 558–563, 1991
19. Kresch AJ, Seifer DB *et al.* Laparoscopy in 100 women with chronic pelvic pain. *Obstet Gynecol* **64**: 672–674, 1972
20. Fedele L, Stefano B *et al.* Pain symptoms associated with endometriosis. *Obstet Gynecol* **79**: 767–769, 1992
21. Henzel MR, Corson SL *et al.* Administration of nasal nafarelin as compared with oral danazol for endometriosis. *N Engl J Med* **318**: 485–489, 1990
22. Evers JL, Dunselman GA *et al.* Is there a solution for recurrent endometriosis? *Br J Clin Pract* **72** (suppl): 45–50

23. Ripps BA, Martin DC. Endometriosis and chronic pelvic pain. *Obstet Gynecol Clin North Am* **20:** 709–717, 1993
24. Lipscomb GH, Ling FW. Relationship of pelvic infection and chronic pelvic pain. *Obstet Gynecol Clin North Am* **20:** 699–708, 1993
25. Stovall T, Elder R, Ling F. Predictors of pelvic adhesions. *J Reprod Med* **34:** 345–348, 1989
26. Summitt RL. Urogynecologic causes of chronic pelvic pain. *Obstet Gynecol Clin North Am* **20:** 685–698, 1993
27. Summitt RL, Ling FW. Urethral syndrome presenting as chronic pelvic pain. *J Psychosom Obstet Gynaecol* **12** (suppl): 77, 1991
28. Elhilali MM, Winfield HN. Genitourinary pain. In: (Wall PD, Melzak R, eds) *Textbook of Pain*. London: Churchill Livingstone, 1989, pp. 500–508
29. Ritchie J. Pain in IBS. *Pract Gastroenterol* **3:** 16, 1979
30. Dawson AM. Origin of pain in irritable bowel syndrome. In: (Read NW, ed.) *Irritable Bowel Syndrome*. Philadelphia: Grune & Stratton, 1985, p. 155
31. Rapkin AJ, Mayer EA. Gastroenterologic causes of chronic pelvic pain. *Obstet Gynecol Clin North Am* **20:** 663–683, 1993
32. Blendis LM. Abdominal pain. In: (Wall PD, Melzak R, eds) *Textbook of Pain*. London: Churchill Livingstone, 1989, pp. 455–465

# 13

# Back pain: the medical viewpoint

**M. G. Ridley**

Low back pain (LBP) remains an increasing source of disability and loss of time from work and the commonest musculoskeletal reason for consulting doctors. In the UK in 1993 there were almost 120 million lost days from work through back pain. The vast majority of these will be associated with acute or subacute LBP which resolves over 1–2 months without sequelae. However, the burden of chronic LBP within this number has also dramatically increased and it is the assessment and management of this problem that have to be addressed in the pain clinic and which concern the rest of this chapter.

## Aetiology

In the context of the pain clinic the aetiology of chronic LBP is rather different from the full spectrum of diseases (Table 13.1) that need to be considered when seeing a patient with new back pain. Most patients will fall into one of two categories: non-specific mechanical LBP or postdisc surgery LBP. Both of these groups will have varying degrees of associated leg pain. Many patients with so-called mechanical back pain will have little or any radiologically demonstrable pathology. Such X-ray changes as exist will consist of combinations of varying degrees of lumbar disc degeneration and/or facet joint arthritis. As will probably be only too apparent, the aetiology of chronic LBP remains as much a question of pain as of the back. Thus it includes those factors which are so important in all chronic pain: psychological distress, the destructive combination of fear and avoidance of provocative activity, coping difficulties, depression and the development of the sick role. Whatever can be achieved in purely nociceptive terms with specific treatment will only be successful in the longer term if it is combined with a thorough assessment of these other factors. With this in mind it is important to remember, whatever the possible aetiology in anatomical terms, that what the patient believes to be the aetiology of his or her pain is even more important. It is unfortunately all too easy for a patient to have acquired numerous conflicting explanations for the physical basis of the problem from the various practitioners they

**Table 13.1** Causes of low back pain

Non-specific mechanical back pain
Facet joint syndrome ± facet joint arthritis
Lumbar disc degeneration (lumbar spondylosis)
Lumbar disc prolapse
Spondylolisthesis
Spinal stenosis

Osteoporosis
Seronegative spondarthritis (including ankylosing spondylitis)
Vertebral infection
Disc space infection
Malignancy
  Secondary
  Myeloma
  Primary
Paget's disease
Referred – visceral, pancreatic/pelvic, etc.

will have seen, both orthodox and heterodox. Once the patient reaches the pain clinic, it is important that any future explanations given are consistent, simple and in language readily understood. They should emphasize function rather than anatomy so that they can be rationally incorporated into a positive approach towards a rehabilitation programme.

## Clinical assessment

At the initial consultation in the pain clinic of a patient with chronic LBP it is important that a realistic allocation of time is given to this assessment since patients often have long multifaceted histories. Furthermore the consultation is an important first step in the reassurance and re-education that are such an important part of patient management. It cannot be emphasized too strongly that this is an important part of the treatment of this condition – this principle is common to most chronic diseases. The consequent development of a rapport between doctor and patient may go a long way to open up the path to a better understanding. Time spent at this point will be saved many times over later on.

The history should establish:

- characteristics of pain, including using pain diagram[1] and McGill pain questionnaire[2]
- patients' beliefs about their LBP
- previous treatment in chronological order
- functional impact of condition on daily life
- functional impact of condition at work (sadly, most will not be at work)
- whether litigation is involved

## Examination

This should include assessment of:

- pain behaviour
- lumbar spinal movement/muscle tone/tenderness
- neurology, including nerve root tension or dural tensions signs

### Pain behaviour

The assessment of this begins as the patient enters the consultation room but specifically includes noting the presence or absence of signs that indicate emotional distress and illness behaviour. Waddell in particular has drawn attention to these signs and a useful assessment can now be made to gauge them more objectively[3] (Table 13.2).

### Spinal signs

Assessment should begin with inspection, looking specifically for deformity and scoliosis, both structural and due to muscle spasm, and pelvic tilt. With the patient standing, movements of the lumbar spine can be assessed making allowance for age. Lumbar spinal flexion can be measured by the modified Schöber test. Palpation for muscle spasm, tenderness and trigger points can also be performed but can be usefully reassessed with the patient on the couch.

**Table 13.2** Comparison of symptoms and signs of physical disease and illness behaviour in chronic low back pain sciatica

| Symptoms/signs | Normal illness behaviour | Abnormal illness behaviour |
|---|---|---|
| Pain drawing | Localized neuroanatomical proportionate | Non-anatomical regional magnified |
| Pain adjectives | Sensory | Affective emotional |
| *Symptoms* | | |
| Pain | Localized | Whole leg pain |
| | | Tail bone pain |
| Numbness | Dermatomal | Whole leg |
| Weakness | Myotomal | Whole leg gives away |
| Time pattern | Varies | Never free of pain |
| Response to treatment | Variable benefit | Intolerance of treatment |
| | | Emergency admission for back pain |
| *Signs* | | |
| Tenderness | Localized | Superficial, widespread, non-anatomical |
| Axial loading | No lumbar pain | Lumbar pain |
| Simulated rotation | No lumbar pain | Lumbar pain |
| Straight leg raising | Limited on distraction | Improves with distraction |
| Sensory | Dermatomal | Regional |
| Motor | Myotomal | Regional/Jerky/Giving way |
| General response | Appropriate | Overt pain behaviour |

Modified from Waddell.[3]

**Neurology**

Assessment of power must include assessment while the patient is standing as minor S1 weakness in particular can otherwise be missed. Standing and walking on tiptoe tests the S1 root, walking on heels the L5 root. On the couch quadriceps strength tests L4. Nerve root tension signs should now be addressed. Straight leg raising (SLR) assesses dural tension in the lower lumbar nerve roots L5 and S1. It requires muscle relaxation and involves passive elevation of the leg by the examiner. It is often helpful as a preliminary to gain the patient's cooperation and good muscle relaxation, to flex the hip and knee passively first before then elevating the straightened leg. The test is positive if it produces buttock or leg pain, but not just back pain or mild tightness behind the knee due to shortening of the hamstrings. Elicitation of leg pain/buttock pain on the symptomatic side when performing SLR on the contralateral leg (crossed positive sciatic nerve stretch) is powerful evidence of dural tension and frequently indicates an often large lumbar disc prolapse. With the patient prone, high lumbar nerve root tension can be assessed using the femoral nerve stretch test. This tests dural tension in association with L3/4 and sometimes L5 roots. Thus it is less frequently positive since most lumbar nerve entrapment syndromes affect L5 or S1 but particularly it should be borne in mind in patients with atypical leg pain, possibly indicating a high lumbar disc lesion. The patient lies prone and the symptomatic leg is passively flexed at the knee. A positive test produces anterior thigh pain. Again reproduction of back pain alone is not indicative of dural tension. Finally elicitation of deep tendon reflexes and sensory examination complete the neurological assessment. The ankle reflex is usually subserved by S1 but can include L5. The knee reflex is subserved by L3 or L4 but occasionally includes elements of L5. In the sensory examination it is important to ascertain whether there is true dermatomal loss, including the saddle area. Whole-leg anaesthesia tells the doctor more about the patient's illness behaviour than his or her neuropathology.

**Differential diagnosis**

At the initial assessment, the referring diagnosis should be reconsidered and positively confirmed if appropriate. Conditions that can lead to confusion with chronic LBP even at this stage include:

• Seronegative spondarthritis (typified by ankylosing spondylitis; AS). Typically, patients with AS should have experienced their first symptoms before the age of 40. They will usually have suffered continuous symptoms for several months at a time; early morning and post-immobility stiffness should be prominent features with relative relief by exercise. They may experience marked night pain. There is usually a good response to anti-inflammatory drugs, but sometimes side-effects or concern about using the drugs in the right way will have precluded an adequate trial of therapy. The presence of human leukocyte antigen (HLA)-B27 supports but is not absolute confirmation of the diagnosis. Similarly, the absence of B27 does not totally exclude the diagnosis. HLA-B27 is carried by 98% of patients with classical AS but between only 60 and 80% of patients with other sero-negative spondarthritides, and by 8–10% of the healthy Caucasian population.

- Metabolic bone disease: sometimes osteoporotic vertebral collapse will have occurred without typical acute pain and limitation and can enter the differential diagnosis of chronic LBP. Osteomalacia causes spinal and more generalized musculoskeletal pain and needs to be considered in the relevant at-risk population, especially females originating from the Indian subcontinent. Serum alkaline phosphatase should be elevated.
- Infections: tuberculosis and brucellosis are the two chronic indolent infections that can elude diagnosis for some months and hence find their way to the pain clinic. Both are likely to be associated with systemic symptoms, including weight loss. They need particularly to be considered in the relevant at-risk populations – those working with animals for brucellosis and the immunosuppressed, alcoholics or immi-grants for tuberculosis.
- Tumours: these are unlikely to remain undiagnosed prior to referral to a pain clinic. Unremitting localized pain should arouse suspicion. Myeloma in particular can have an indolent course and cause diag-nostic problems, especially in those patients lacking a serum protein band and only excreting light chains in the urine. Bone scanning will frequently be negative since myeloma deposits do not excite an osteo-blastic reaction around them, hence appearing as cool spots or normal tracer intensity rather than the hot spots so typical of metastatic bony secondaries from carcinomas.

Clearly associated leg pain widens the differential diagnosis which will then include potentially surgically correctable lumbar nerve root entrap-ment syndromes. These require careful clinical assessment combined with review of the relevant computed tomographic or magnetic resonance imaging scans (and occasionally still radiculograms) and consideration for reinvestigation if the clinical evidence of nerve root entrapment is strong. This reassessment can usefully be undertaken in a combined clinic with the relevant orthopaedic and rheumatological colleagues.

## Management

We need to consider:

- physical treatment
- injection treatment
- drug treatment
- transcutaneous electrical nerve stimulation (TENS)
- psychosocial management
- patient education

## Physical treatment

The basic principle that mobilization and strengthening exercises are helpful has been supported by studies.[4,5] The relevance of any logical theoretical basis for specific exercises however is lacking. The self-help aspect of rebuilding patients' confidence in their physical abilities and the realization that exercise can be done without producing more acute pain are probably all part of the reason for the success of exercise. There is evidence to suggest[6] that chiropractic manipulation is superior to a conventional physiotherapy approach, including Maitlands mobilizations and Cyriax manipulative techniques. Although the results of this large study have been much discussed, perhaps the important principle to remember is that manipulation does help chronic as well as acute LBP.

## Injection treatment

The evidence for long-term benefit of injection therapy alone is limited. However, this should not and does not nullify its value as an adjunct to treatment.

- Epidural local anaesthetic injections with or without corticosteroids do have useful short- and medium-term benefits in the relief of sciatica and some patients with LBP.[7] These procedures buy useful time, sometimes simply to allow the natural history of the problem to be followed more comfortably – as when they are used in acute or recurrent sciatica related to lumbar nerve root entrapment. Sometimes they allow mobilization of a patient in an intractable cycle of pain, immobility and depression, when the use of an indwelling epidural catheter infusing low-dose local anaesthetic can be highly effective. Patients' concerns regarding epidural steroid injections have recently been inappropriately fuelled by further speculation about the possible role of Depo-Medrone (methylprednisolone) in causing arachnoiditis. As has been pointed out by the British Society for Rheumatology (BSR) clinical affairs committee, these allegations followed the use of intrathecal steroids to treat myelogram contrast reactions and in multiple sclerosis.[8] It is thought that the polyethylene glycol used as a dispersant in the Depo-Medrone may be responsible for the intrathecal reaction. The large body of evidence regarding epidural steroid injections confirms their general safety.[9,10] The BSR has recommended to its members that individual informed consent is required if Depo-Medrone is used epidurally. Triamcinolone and the other non depot steroid preparations do not contain polyethylene glycol.
- Facet joint injections with local anaesthetic and steroid are applied on the principle that the facet joint is richly innervated, in contrast to the intervertebral disc itself, and hence a likely source of back pain. Facet joint pain is clinically said to be characterized by pain in the low back which is often lateralized and associated with pseudoradicular radiation to the leg, mostly the thigh. Pain is often worse on spinal extension with rotation. Most studies have shown benefit for several months only and, like epidurals, they cannot be used as treatment in isolation (Figure 13.1).

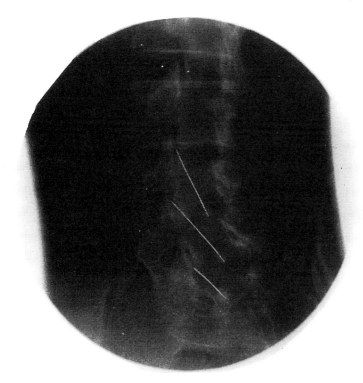

**Figure 13.1** Lumbar facet joint injection (25° rotation).

- Facet joint rhizolysis (Figures 13.2 and 13.3): Lumbar facet denervation using a radiofrequency induced nerve lesions can provide long-
  lasting relief of back pain once a diagnosis of facet syndrome has been
  made. Facet pain is often unilateral in the younger age group following
  injury and may warrant a unilateral procedure. In the older age group,
  symptoms are more likely to be due to degenerative change and may be
  bilateral. Insulated radiofrequency needles (22 G 100 mm with 5 mm
  active tip) are placed at the junction of the transverse process and
  articular facet of the lowest three lumbar vertebrae. At the S1 level
  the needle is placed at the superior edge of the sacrum at the point
  where it joins the superior articular process of S1. The aim is to place
  the active tip of the needle against the articular branch of the posterior
  primary ramus. Needle placement can be confirmed by stimulation at
  100 Hz with thresholds up to approximately 0.5 V, but is not always
  used. A radiofrequency probe with a thermistor in the tip can be
  placed down the needle and a current generated by a radiofrequency
  lesion generator (Radionics, Rocket). A radiofrequency lesion at 75°C
  for 90 s is then made and the electrode removed. As long as the
  needle tip remains in contact with the transverse process, the anterior
  nerve root itself will be shield from the effects of the radiofrequency
  lesion. There may be some soft-tissue pain and local muscle tenderness for up to 1 week afterwards. Follow-up activating physiotherapy

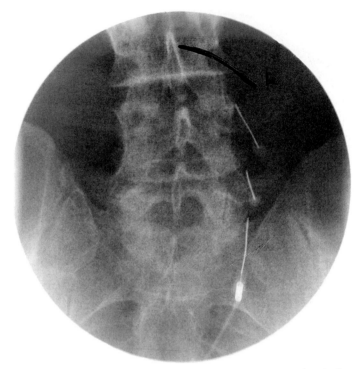

**Figure 13.2** Lumbar radiofrequency facet joint rhizolysis (anteroposterior view).

programmes are an essential sequel to this procedure to maintain best results in the long term.

- Sclerosants applied to the ligaments in the lumbar spine and pelvis have enthusiastic support. However, there are few controlled studies of their benefit[12] and the duration of benefit is uncertain.

### Drug treatment

- Non-steroidal anti-inflammatory drugs (NSAIDs) are likely to have been used extensively before the patient comes to the pain clinic. However their full potential should be explored before they are abandoned as unhelpful in an individual case. They are often helpful for night pain and morning stiffness and a slow-release preparation is often the most logical form of treatment. Pharmacological gastroprotection should be considered in patients over the age of 60, especially those who would tolerate the effects of a gastrointestinal bleed poorly. Whether misoprostol or $H_2$ antagonists are most appropriate remains an open question.
- Tricyclic antidepressants in low to medium dosage have a definite effect in chronic pain which is independent of their antidepressant action.[13] Patients should be reassured about their lack of addictive potential and the specific reason for their prescription.

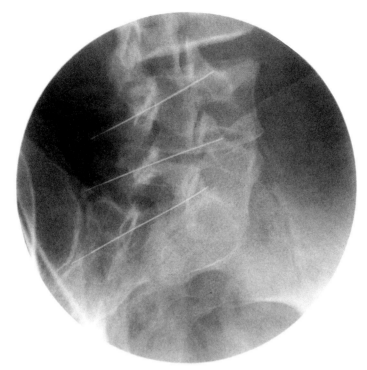

**Figure 13.3** Lumbar radiofrequency facet joint rhizolysis (45° rotation).

## Transcutaneous nerve stimulation

Some physiotherapists maintain that responsiveness or otherwise to inter-ferential therapy on a short-term basis predicts the responsiveness of the patient's back pain to TENS. Nevertheless, whatever this relationship, TENS is valuable and, apart from the expense of the individual machine to the patient, an acceptable and safe form of treatment. It can often reduce a patient's dependence on oral analgesia, which is a worthwhile end in itself. In patients with LBP its use can be limited by difficulty with electrode placement unless the patient has a partner or carer to help.

## Psychosocial management

The background stresses and strains which aggravate and potentiate the patient's distress in LBP may be difficult to clarify and it may take some time before the pain team is able to explore this aspect. Once the patient's confidence has been gained and the purely physical aspects of management have begun to be addressed, then the patient is better able to accept the involvement of the psychologist. The importance of addressing pain in all its aspects should be emphasized. Reassurance regarding the acceptance of the reality of the patient's pain is often repeatedly necessary. Behavioural methods of treatment are useful in those with marked illness behaviour and the psychologist can help by guiding other therapists as well as the patient in applying these. To be successful, all these treatments need to be applied as part of a team approach, often most usefully to patients in groups where patients gain insight and confidence by shared experiences. Whether this is equally successful when done on an outpatient or inpatient basis probably relates more to the local logistics of organization but studies have shown a greater benefit for inpatient-based rehabilitation regimes.[14]

### Patient education

The most important aspect of this is consistency – consistency of the information provided to patients by all therapists in the team. Patients must learn to understand the basic dos and don'ts of back pain and in particular lifting technique. It is important to educate doctors in primary care also to be able to pass on the same sort of information to patients presenting with acute LBP in order to increase the general body of knowledge amongst the public regarding how to use their backs, and thus to try and minimize the risks of recurrent problems. Putting the patient in control again of his or her own body and the illness is the key to successful management of chronic LBP.

## References

1. Ransford AO, Cairns D, Mooney V. The pain drawing as an aid in the psychological evaluation of patients with low back pain. *Spine* **1:** 127–134, 1976
2. Melzack R. The McGill pain questionnaire: major properties and scoring methods. *Pain* **1:** 277–299, 1975
3. Waddell G. A new clinical model for the treatment of low back pain. *Spine* **12:** 632–644, 1987
4. Manniche C, Bentazen L, Hesselsoe G, Christiensen I, Lundberg E. Clinical trial of intensive muscle training for chronic low back pain. *Lancet* **ii:** 1473–1476, 1988
5. Deyo RA, Walsh NE, Martin DC, Schoenfeld LS, Ramamurthy S. A controlled trial of TENS and exercise for chronic low back pain. *N Engl J Med* **322:** 1627–1634, 1990
6. Meade TW, Dyer S, Browne W, Townsend J, Frank AO. Low back pain of mechanical origin: randomised comparison of chiropractic and hospital outpatient treatment. *Br Med J* **300:** 1431–1437, 1990
7. Ridley MG, Kingsley GH, Gibson T, Grahame R. Outpatient lumbar epidural corticosteroid injection in the management of sciatica. *Br J Rheumatol* **27:** 295–299, 1988
8. Nelson DA. Intraspinal therapy using methyl prednisolone acetate. *Spine* **18:** 278–286, 1993
9. Corrigon AB, Carr G, Tulwell S. Intraspinal corticosteroid injections. *Med J Aust* 224–225, 1982
10. Benzon HT. Epidural injections for low back pain and H.R. lumbo sacral radiculopathy. *Pain* **24:** 277–295, 1986
11. Bogduk N, Long DM. Percutaneous lumbar medial branch neurotomy: a modification of facet denervation. *Spine* **5:** 193–200, 1980
12. Mathews JA, Miles SB, Jenkins VM *et al.* Back pain and sciatica: controlled trials of manipulation, traction, sclerosant and epidural injection. *Br J Rheumatol* **26:** 416–423, 1987
13. Ward NG. Tricyclic anti-depressants for chronic low back pain: mechanisms of action and predictors of responses. *Spine* **11:** 661–665, 1986
14. Harkapaa, Mellin G, Jarvikoski A *et al.* A controlled study on the outcome of inpatient and outpatient treatment of low back pain, disability and compliance. *Scand J Rehab Med* **22:** 181–188, 1990

# 14

# Back and leg pain: the surgical perspective

**L. J. Taylor and J. Bell**

## Glossary of terms

- Low back pain: This is pain occurring between the ribcage and gluteal folds, it may be associated with radiation to the posterior thigh and greater trochanter but it is unusual distal to the knee. The referred pain is poorly localized and varies from an acute pain to a deep ache in character.
- Sciatica is a sharp pain, often described as electric shock-like in nature, radiating down the leg into the dermatome of the affected nerve root. It is well-localized and in the majority of cases radiates below the knee. It may be associated with dermatomal reduction in sensation, paraesthesia or hyperaesthesia.
- Spinal claudication is a deep, poorly localized pain in the legs. It is exacerbated by walking, and may be associated with increasing weakness. Sensory features are rare. The symptoms are often relieved by spinal flexion.
- Nerve root claudication: This is a well-defined pain in the leg (occasionally bilateral) usually without sensory or motor deficit. It is often exacerbated by walking and relieved by rest and spinal flexion.
- Lateral recess stenosis is a degenerative disorder leading to a reduction in the dimensions of the anterolateral limit of the spinal canal (lateral recess) in which the nerve root lies. It may also be congenital in origin.
- Spinal stenosis: This is a narrowing of the spinal canal, lateral recess and/or nerve root canal which is due to developmental, degenerative or deforming disorders of the spinal column.
- Spondylolysis is a defect in one or both pars interarticulares and may be the precursor of spondylolisthesis. In its own right it is a significant cause of back pain.
- Spondylolisthesis is sagittal translation of one vertebral body on another. The more rostral slips anteriorly with respect to the next one in line (in retrolisthesis, the opposite applies). The most commonly affected levels are at L5/S1 (congenital) and L4/L5 (degenerative).
- Spondylosis is the commonest cause of low back pain. It describes a degenerative arthritic process that may affect any of the joints in the spinal column, but predominantly the facet joints. It may be associated with degenerative disc disease.

- Spinal instability (an ill-understood concept): This is loss of the ability of the spine under normal physiological conditions to maintain the relationship between the vertebrae, such that there is neither damage to the spinal cord or nerve roots, nor is there development of incapacitating deformity or severe pain.

## Introduction

The surgical treatment of low back pain and sciatica was originated by Mixter and Barr in 1934.[1] Since then disc surgery has become commonplace, with excellent results in some patients and equally disappointing failures in others. Improvements in imaging, patient selection and a better understanding of the pathology have helped improve the results of surgery. Psychological profiles may help in the assessment of back pain but a clear history root pain supported by physical signs and radiographic imaging[2] is all that is required for the treatment of sciatica.

Surgical back pain/leg pain can be described as follows:

- nerve root pain due to disc protrusion or stenosis  ⎫  Root pain
- back pain alone                                      ⎬  almost always radiates below
- back pain and root pain                              ⎭  the knee

It is useful to think in this way as patients with root pain have a more predictable response to surgery.

### Lumbar spine pain

Pain originating in the disc is felt in the lumbar region.

Pain from facet joints/ligaments/dura is felt in the lumbar region. It may also be referred to the sacroiliac joint, buttock, posterior thigh and around the greater trochanter. Pain is rarely felt beyond the upper calf.

Referred pain is perceived as being a deep, diffuse ache and poorly localized (cf. root pain).

Paravertebral muscle spasm is caused by a sensorimotor reflex.

### Root pain

Spinal nerve roots are more sensitive to mechanical deformation than peripheral nerves.

Nerve root compression or traction *per se* does not cause pain. A nerve already compromised by either ischaemia or mechanical/chemical irritation will give rise to characteristic root pain if then squeezed or pulled.

## Anatomy

The vertebrae articulate at the intervertebral disc and the paired facets joints. The lumbar nerve roots exit the spinal canal via the intervertebral foramen (IVF). The IVF is enclosed by the facet joints, pars interarticularis, pedicles, disc and part of the vertebral bodies (Figures 14.1 and 14.2).

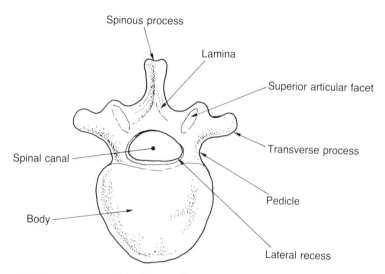

**Figure 14.1** Transverse view of lumbar vertebrae.

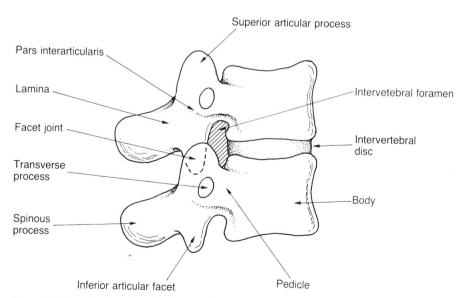

**Figure 14.2** Lateral view of two lumbar vertebrae.

- Nerve roots pass beneath the pedicle of the vertebra, from which its name is derived (Figure 14.3).
- Nerve root canal: this is a tubular canal arising at the lateral aspect of the dural sac. It forms a sleeve around the spinal nerve as it passes obliquely downwards and laterally towards the IVF. The upper lumbar nerve roots are at almost a right angle to the dural sac, passing almost immediately from the dural sac into the IVF. The nerve root canals in the lower lumbar spine are more oblique and the nerve roots have a longer intraspinal course.
- Disc: The intervertebral disc consists of a nucleus pulposus contained by the concentric lamellae of the annulus fibrosus and with the cartilage end-plates of the vertebra above and below. The disc is avascular with pain fibres in the outer annulus.

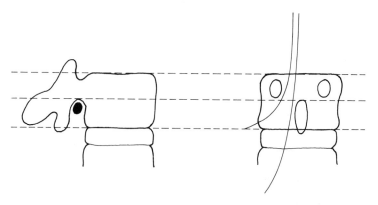

**Figure 14.3** Two nerve roots and their relationship to the lumbar vertebra. The nerve root with the same number as the vertebra emerges laterally through the intervertebral foramen. The next lower nerve root passes through the spinal canal to the next lowest level.

## Investigation of surgical back pain

Imaging is not a substitute for poor clinical technique. It should be used to differentiate the underlying pathology. As a rule special investigations are not performed unless surgery is indicated on clinical grounds.

### Plain X-ray

This is of limited use in the diagnosis of low back pain.

Between 20 and 50 years, plain X-rays are unlikely to discover pathology not already clinically suspected. Plain films will confirm spondylosis, spondylolysis or spondylolisthesis.

More sinister pathology is likely to be discovered outside this age group, for example, Paget's disease or malignant deposits.

No quantitative information regarding the space available for the neural elements can be obtained.

Oblique views are of value in excluding spondylolysis, but are not performed routinely.

## Myelography

Myelography has been largely superseded by computed tomography (CT) and magnetic resonance imaging (MRI), but it still has a role in the diagnosis of tumours, intradural lesions, multiple sclerosis and occasionally, when combined with CT, in the previously operated back.

## CT

CT was a major advance, enabling cross-sectional imaging. Disc prolapse cannot be reliably diagnosed on plain CT. It is of particular value for the diagnosis of spinal stenosis, lateral nerve root entrapment and the far-out disc prolapse. For resolution of disc and soft tissues, MRI is superior. Absolute measurements of the cross-sectional area of the canal are not as useful as the overall impression of space available for the neural elements (Figure 14.4). The interpretation of CT in spondylolisthesis requires experience and observation of the scout film is essential before interpreting any cuts.

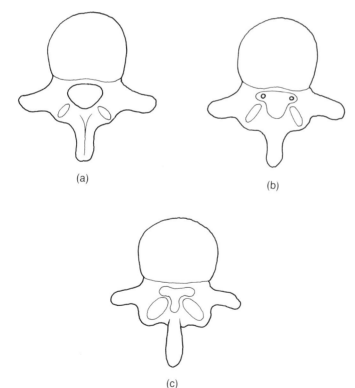

(a)

(b)

(c)

**Figure 14.4** Transverse section through (a) a normal lumbar vertebra; (b) lateral recess stenosis and (c) severe spinal stenosis of degenerate origin.

## MRI

MRI is rapidly establishing itself as the modality of choice when imaging the spine, but the authors still prefer CT where bone overgrowth is suspected.

### Advantages of MRI

- lack of ionizing radiation
- superior soft-tissue resolution and tissue characterization
- gadolinium (diethylebetriaminepentaacetic acid; DTPA) helps differentiation of scar tissue from disc prolapse; this is useful in the previously operated spine.

Manipulation of the field and data can alter the appearance of specific tissues on a hard copy of the image. Therefore images with different tissue characteristics can be obtained. As scanners become more sophisticated the specificity of tissue characterization is improved. T1 and T2 images are most commonly used.

### Disadvantages of MRI

Some patients find lying in the tunnel claustrophobic. Counselling is advisable.

### Tissue characteristics with MRI

- Vertebral body: T1/T2 a low signal, apart from high signal from the marrow fat on T1.
- Normal disc: A high signal on T2 due to water content of the nucleus pulposus. Desiccation, as seen in degeneration, shows clearly on the T2 image.
- Nerve root: T1 a high signal from the epidural fat outlines the root. If epidural fat is obliterated, cerebrospinal fluid in root sleeves contrasts with the root.
- Bone: Cortical bone or sclerotic osteophytes give no signal, which is relevant in bony entrapment.

**Table 14.1** Information obtainable from magnetic resonance imaging

|    | High signal | Intermediate signal | Low signal |
|----|-------------|---------------------|------------|
| T1 | Epidural and marrow fat | Ligamentum flavum<br>Normal disc | Water/CSF annulus/ALL/ PLL/compact bone/theca |
| T2 | Normal pulposus Fat/water/CSF |  | ALL/PLL |

CSF = Cerebrospinal fluid; ALL/PLL = anterior/posterior longitudinal ligament.

Any implant, especially metallic, can be a contraindication to MRI. Patients who have had surgery for a cerebral aneurysm should not have an MRI scan.

### Electromyography

Electromyography can provide useful information concerning root dysfunction in the previously operated back, but an experienced clinical neurophysiologist is required for interpretation.

### Facet joint injection

The use of provocation tests or, more accurately, provocation/relief tests can be used to identify the source of pain. The clinician attempts to reproduce the patient's symptoms by direct stimulation of selected areas followed by attempting to abolish the pain by subsequent introduction of local anaesthetic.

Selective facet joint injection under local anaesthetic can help localize the site of pain and identify capsular tears.

### Selective nerve root sleeve injection

This is a technically demanding procedure. Abolition of leg pain following infiltration of local anaesthetic around a nerve root sleeve is good evidence of it begin a source of pain. It can be useful when, despite investigation, the level (or levels) of pathology cannot be convincingly demonstrated; it is also useful in the previously operated back.

### Discography

Discography can be used in isolation or in combination with CT. Opinion is divided on its value but it can be used to identify levels for fusion. Discitis is a recognized complication.

## Root pain

### Aetiology

The commonest causes of root pain are:

- disc prolapse
- bony entrapment
  - central spinal stenosis
  - lateral recess stenosis

Although there are similarities in the presentation, they can usually be distinguished clinically.

Spondylolisthesis is a well-recognized cause of low back and, less commonly, root pain.

In the child or adolescent primary tumour must be considered (especially if night pain is present); in the elderly, metastatic deposits must be excluded. Many unrelated conditions may mimic sciatica.[3]

### Disc prolapse

Disc prolapse is a degenerative process. For a disc prolapse to occur there must be a fissure in the annulus fibrosus and a fragment of nucleus pulposus to herniate into the defect. The different stages of prolapse (Figure 14.5) can sometimes be identified on imaging and at operation.[5] Usually it is the nerve root passing to the level below that is affected but a sequestrated disc prolapse may migrate. The prolapse may be 'far out', when the nerve root at the same level is affected (Figure 14.6). Rarely a cauda equina syndrome may result.

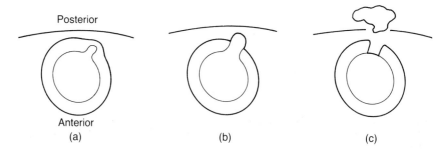

**Figure 14.5** Transverse section through a lumbar intervertebral disc showing different types of disc prolapse. (a) Annular tear; (b) protrusion: critically weakened annulus; (c) sequestration.

### Bone entrapment

Root entrapment can occur in:

- central spinal canal
- lateral recess
- root canal
- any combination

Degenerative spondylosis is the commonest cause.[7]

In degenerative central spinal stenosis there is hypertrophy of the facet joints and ligamentum flavum. Degenerative changes in the disc result in loss of height or prolapse. Degenerative spondylolisthesis may produce spinal stenosis, although many levels may be affected, L4/5 is the most frequent site.

In lateral recess stenosis the main pathology is in the facet joint and often a solitary root is involved with loss of disc height – a secondary factor.

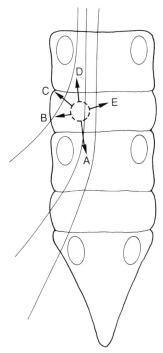

**Figure 14.6** Possible routes of migration for prolapsed intervertebral discs. Disc herniations may migrate (A) to pedicle of segment below; (B) far out; (C) foraminal; (D) to the pedicle of the same level; (E) midline.

## Clinical assessment of patients with disc prolapse (Figure 14.7)

### History

Most patients are 20–50 years old. Often there is a history of a minor twisting or lifting injury. The severity of low back pain is variable; it may predate the onset of sciatica by a few days. Sciatica is exacerbated by forward flexion of the lumbar spine, coughing or sneezing. Duration and severity of the pain are important, as are previous episodes. The proportion of the total pain that is due to sciatica must be clearly established, as sciatica responds to surgery, back pain is less predictable. Previous treatment should be noted, particularly surgery.

### Examination

There is often paravertebral muscle spasm, a scoliosis and loss of lardosis. Forwards flexion is grossly restricted by pain. Lateral flexion away from the scoliosis is painful. Extension is usually comparatively painfree.

Root tension signs indicate irritability of the nerve root. They may be used to monitor a patient's response to conservative treatment.

- Straight leg raise: Raise the affected leg off the couch with the knee extended until the patient indicates the onset of the sciatic pain. Record the elevation in degrees. Pain felt in the low back does not

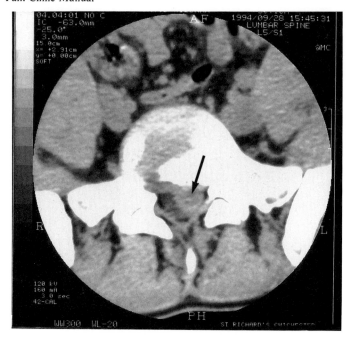

**Figure 14.7** Computed tomographic scan showing prolapsed intervertebral disc (arrow).

confer a positive result. Raising the unaffected leg may cause sciatica to be felt in the symptomatic leg – cross-over sign – which is highly suggestive of disc prolapse.

- Sciatic stretch test: Elevate leg until sciatica is just brought on; dorsiflex the foot. If positive, the pain is exacerbated. It should then be relieved by flexing the knee.
- Femoral stretch test: Patient lies prone, the leg is extended at the hip with the knee at 90°. Reproducing the patient's anterior thigh pain indicates an L3/4 disc prolapse.

The presence of a sensorimotor deficit is useful confirmation of root compression and helps to identify the affected nerve root. Neurological signs are indicative of significant root compression but may not be always present (Table 14.2).

**Table 14.2** Neurological signs

|  | L4 | L5 | S1 |
|---|---|---|---|
| Muscle wasting | Quadriceps | Extensor digitorum brevis | Calf, buttocks |
| Reduced power | Quadriceps | Extensor hallucis longus | Plantar flexors |
| Reflex | Decreased knee jerk | Jerks intact | Decreased ankle jerk |
| Sensation (Figure 14.8) | Anteromedial skin | Lateral calf, dorsum of foot, great toe | Lateral border of foot and midline of calf |

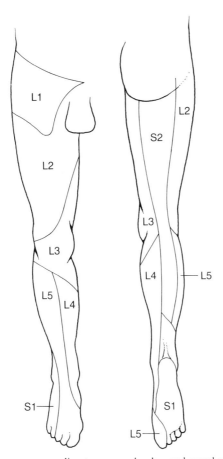

**Figure 14.8** Dermatomes corresponding to sensory lumbar and sacral nerves.

*Cauda equina syndrome must be excluded, therefore an assessment of sphincter function and perineal sensation is mandatory.*

## Assessment for surgery of disc prolapse

The history and clinical examination will be all that is needed to make the diagnosis in most cases and investigations should be used to confirm the clinical suspicion, not as a basis for treatment. The results of surgery for sciatica are more predictable than for back pain.

### Psychosocial problems/litigation

Psychosocial problems or pending litigation do not exclude a patient from having a genuine indication for surgical intervention but can make assessment of these patients extremely difficult. Psychological assessment is of particular value in surgery for back pain. Waddell *et al.*[10] defined a series of non-organic signs in patients with low back pain.

- superficial or non-anatomical tenderness
- simulation tests causing low back pain
  - axial loading of the skull
  - rotation of the shoulders/pelvis as one unit
- inappropriate straight leg raise
- regional weakness and/or sensory deficit
- overreaction

Three or more of these features are highly significant.[10]

## Treatment of disc prolapse

### Natural history

Patients with sciatica have a good prognosis; 90% recover within 6 weeks. Spontaneous resolution becomes less likely with increasing age. Fewer than 10% of patients with sciatica come to surgery. Five per cent of patients have significant neurological deficit. Delay in treatment does not affect the outcome unless there is significant neurological deficit. Acute cauda equina syndrome is rare but an emergency.

In many instances, especially in patients over 35 years, in addition to disc protrusion there may be associated lateral recess stenosis.

### Conservative treatment

- Bedrest – 1–2 weeks' strict bedrest (i.e. up to toilet only) should be tried initially. Bedrest may be intolerable and often indicates a sequestrated disc prolapse.
- Analgesics in severe cases have little benefit.
- Muscle relaxants may reduce associated muscle spasm.
- Epidural corticosteroids (lumbar or caudal) can have a dramatic effect on sciatica but not all reports agree on their efficacy. Their use may shorten the clinical course.[9] However, they can make the result of an MRI scan impossible to interpret.
- Indwelling epidural catheter may provide good analgesia for up to 1 week, if needed, while surgical assessment is made.

### Indications for surgical treatment of sciatica (Figure 14.9)

- Failed conservative treatment – ideally followed for 6 weeks. This is the commonest indication for surgery. Prolonged pressure may cause an extraneural fibrosis.
- Progressive or persistent neurological deficit – if there is no improvement in straight leg raise or motor/sensory deficit.[8] Recurrent sciatica is less likely to respond to conservative treatment.
- Cauda equina syndrome – this is rare but represents a surgical emergency.

A patient may choose to live with the symptoms.

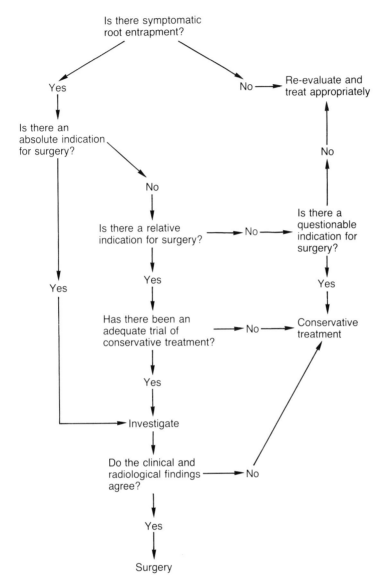

**Figure 14.9** Algorithm for management of root pain.

## Surgery for disc prolapse

Formal laminectomy to gain access to the disc has been largely replaced by less destructive procedures. Currently the standard technique is a limited fenestration and discectomy. The success rate of discectomy should be 85–90% and it should only rarely be combined with fusion.

### Fenestration and discectomy/microdiscectomy

This technique uses a small incision and may be aided by an operating microscope or magnifying loops and a headlight.

*Advantages*

- high-power magnification and improved illumination
- less dissection, therefore less scar tissue
- lower postoperative morbidity
- earlier mobilization and discharge

*Disadvantages*

- limited access and field of view; pathology may be missed
- more likely to have wrong level
- higher incidence of recurrence
- even a small amount of bleeding may obscure the view
- higher incidence of contamination and postoperative infection/discitis

Many of the advantages of microdiscectomy can be obtained by using better lighting (e.g. head-light/operating loupes), and minimal dissection/removal of bone.

### Percutaneous discectomy

This is only appropriate for a non-sequestrated disc prolapse. The technique does achieve good results in a highly selected group of patients.

### Chemonucleolysis

This involves instillation of chymopapain to digest and hence shrink the disc.

*Advantages*

- percutaneous, performed under local or neuroleptic anaesthesia
- can be performed as a day case

*Disadvantages*

- patient selection more difficult
- not suitable for many patients, contraindicated in sequestration
- high incidence of complications
- may give rise to markedly increased back pain for a number of months before recovery
- hypersensitivity or anaphylaxis unacceptably high risk
- intrathecal introduction of chymopapain is hazardous, resulting in sub-arachnoid haemorrhage, transverse myelitis or cauda equina syndrome
- discitis occurs in approximately 2%

- the reported success rate is approximately 75%
- the effect is not limited to the nucleus and does affect the annulus with significant disc space narrowing

## Complications of surgery for prolapsed disc

Some 5–15% of patients require reoperation following discectomy. Poor patient selection remains the commonest cause for failure and look-and-see surgery should be obsolete.

In addition to the usual complications of major surgery, anaesthesia and recumbency, those specific to the procedure include the following.

### Technical problems

Poor access may be due to inexperience, poor surgical technique, obesity or the increasing desire for minimally invasive procedures. Bad lighting can be largely overcome by the use of head-lamp or operating microscope.

Bleeding can quickly obscure the operating field; meticulous attention to the coagulation of small epidural veins is essential; this is especially true when using the operating microscope.

### Surgical error

- wrong levels – accurate identification by X-ray if there is any doubt. It is important to have the scan available in theatre and for the surgeon to interpret it him- or herself
- migration of sequestrated prolapse
- associated bone entrapment
- far-out prolapse
- neurological damage and cerebrospinal fluid leakage are rare in primary surgery
- vascular injury is rare but can be fatal

### Extradural haematoma (very rare and should be a diagnosis of exclusion)

This may cause cauda equina syndrome and requires emergency re-exploration.

### Recurrent symptoms

Clearly there are a group of patients who have a recurrent disc prolapse at the same level (1–2%). The risk of this diminishes after the first year following discectomy.

A small number sustain a second disc prolapse at a new level and should be treated on the merits of the new symptoms.

A particularly difficult group of patients to deal with are those whose initial result is satisfying but have recurrent symptoms due to scarring around the nerve root. Repeat surgery in these patients is disappointing.

### Discitis

This may follow surgery or any instrumentation of the disc. There is a sudden increase in back pain a few days following the procedure. It quickly becomes non-mechanical in nature, being unrelenting and particularly bad at night. The patient has a pyrexia, raised erythrocyte sedimentation rate (ESR) and white blood cell count (WBC).

If a limited discectomy has been performed, then a plain X-ray may show dramatic disc space narrowing. A labelled WBC scan may be helpful as it quickly becomes positive. MRI is also sensitive in the diagnosis of discitis. Exploration is only indicated for those who fail to respond to antibiotics and prolonged conservative treatment (1 year plus) or develop an abscess or neurological signs. Anterior disc clearance and fusion should be performed. Treated discitis usually progresses to spontaneous fusion. Today, where prophylactic antibiotics may have been used, the presentation is often less acute.

## Bony entrapment (Figure 4.10)

Nerve root entrapment due to spondylosis is the primary cause of root entrapment in patients over 50 years.

Spinal stenosis may be congenital but is most frequently degenerative. Its onset is often preceded by a long history of low back pain. Stenosis is less frequently seen in degenerative spondylolisthesis (L4/5), and rarely in scoliosis, after spinal fusion and in Paget's disease.

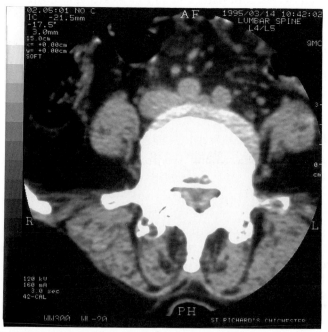

**Figure 14.10** Computed tomographic scan showing spinal stenosis.

## Central spinal stenosis

Central spinal stenosis[13] is suggested by a history of neurogenic claudication.

Pain is often felt in both legs and described as a dull ache or heavy feeling, affecting the whole leg. It is frequently brought on by walking. Flexing the spine increases the volume of the spinal canal so that stooping or sitting down relieves pain; standing is usually not enough, as when standing the spine remains extended. The patient may stoop when walking or standing. The flexed position of the spine when going uphill is preferred, in contrast to a patient with ischaemic claudication where leg pain would be exacerbated. Similarly, riding a bicycle can be done with ease.

Subjective sensory changes may be seen but dermatomal changes are rare. Motor weakness is also uncommon. Sensorimotor signs may be induced by exercise.

Sphincter disturbance is very rare, but must always be considered.

## Lateral recess stenosis

Patients with lateral recess stenosis[13] may present at a younger age than those with central spinal stenosis. Sensory symptoms are more common. Root irritation, and claudication are less frequent.

The pain tends to be unremitting and worse at night.

Similar to central spinal stenosis, clinical signs are often unremarkable; there may be no root tension signs and neurology is often normal. When there is abnormal neurology, it tends to be confined to a single nerve root, unlike multiple root pathology in central spinal stenosis.

## Differential diagnosis of bony entrapment

The diagnoses most easily confused are disc prolapse and vascular disease (Table 14.3).

**Table 14.3** Comparison of disc prolapse with bone entrapment

|  | Prolapsed intervertebral disc | Bone entrapment |
|---|---|---|
| Age | <40 years | >40 years |
| Duration of low back pain | Short or absent | Long |
| Pain | Increases with cough | Neurogenic claudication |
| Straight leg raise | Decreased | Unrestricted |
| Reflexes | Often reduced | Often normal |
| Power | Often reduced | Usually normal |
| Sensory deficit | Common | Unusual |
| Number of roots involved | 1–2 | 1–2 (if unilateral) |
| Spinal movement | Restricted | Good |

### Clinical features favouring peripheral vascular disease

- patient over 60
- slow onset of leg pain, rapid relief with rest
- smoking or evidence of atherosclerosis
- cramping dull ache in calf/buttock
- induced by exercise/cycling
- normal neurology

### Treatment of bony entrapment

#### Natural history

The prevalence of spinal stenosis is unknown. It is probably more common than was previously thought. Less is known about the natural history of untreated spinal stenosis than for prolapsed intervertebral disc.

Once the syndrome of neurogenic claudication is well-established, the symptoms rarely improve with conservative treatment.[14] Although symptoms tend not to resolve, they also rarely deteriorate quickly. Patients with lateral recess stenosis may improve over a 2-year period without surgery.

#### Conservative management of spinal stenosis

The symptoms of spinal stenosis are often not severe enough to justify surgical treatment. A trial of conservative treatment is justified but of limited value.

- Bedrest is of no benefit.
- Epidural corticosteroids – Response to epidurals is unpredictable but can occasionally be dramatic.
- Physiotherapy – Heat, ultrasound and gentle isometric exercises to strengthen paraspinal and abdominal musculature are of limited benefit in the majority of patients.
- Non-steroidal anti-inflammatory drugs – These may be helpful, though there is a high incidence of side-effects in the elderly.
- Calcitonin can reduce the vascularity of bone. In cases of Paget's disease of the vertebral column associated with spinal stenosis, there may be a dramatic reduction in symptoms. There may be some benefit in patients with lateral recess stenosis.[15]

#### Indications for surgical treatment of spinal stenosis

The decision to operate is a clinical one. Special investigations help to localize the site of pathology and its severity.

The decision on which levels to operate is based on a consideration of the radiographic imaging and clinical examination. Careful patient selection is mandatory.

- failed conservative treatment – root pain or neurogenic claudication that has failed to respond to conservative measures and is interfering with daily activities
- significant or progressive neurological abnormality
- cauda equina syndrome (very rare)

### Laminectomy

Between one and three levels are usually decompressed in central spinal stenosis; in lateral recess stenosis frequently only a single-level procedure is all that is necessary. The commonest levels decompressed are the L4/5 and L5/S1.

In the past extensive laminectomies were combined with fusion – a procedure which today is rarely indicated.

More recently, with a better understanding of the pathoanatomy, surgery is confined to the motion segment (i.e. the facet joint/disc), thus preserving as much of the lamina and facet as possible.

This involves undercutting the facet joint to remove as much of the hypertrophied joint as it necessary to decompress the root as it passes down the root canal. Anterior vertebral body osteophytes, degenerate ligamentum flavum and, if required, removal of disc material may be necessary.

## Complications of surgery for bony entrapment

### Technique

The surgeon runs a thin line between performing an inadequate decompression and destabilizing the spine. If the spine is rendered unstable it should be fused over the unstable levels. This should wherever possible be recognized at the original procedure; failure to do so will leave the patient in a great deal of pain.

An inadequate decompression may lead to a poor early result or recurrence of symptoms.

### Persistent back pain

Patients must be warned preoperatively that surgery may not help – and may even aggravate – their back pain.

This may be due to facet joint arthrosis, segmental instability, infection, malignancy or symptomatic spondylosis at another level. Also other unrelated pathology may have been overlooked or found to have been contributing to the patient's back pain. In patients with degenerative spondylolisthesis and a significant element of low back pain a combined decompression and fusion may be carried out successfully.

### Persistent or recurrent root pain

In patients with no relief of symptoms at all, reconsider whether the original diagnosis was correct.

In the presence of a more pronounced neurological deficit the nerve root may have been damaged. If there has been no change then possibly the wrong level or an inadequate number of levels were decompressed. If a new deficit appears then consider a haematoma, missed fragment or instability.

Some patients deteriorate after an initial improvement; the reason is rarely obvious and can be difficult to elucidate.

## Surgical treatment of back pain without root pain

Back pain may be the presenting feature of a variety of conditions including malignancy, infection, genitourinary or aortoiliac disease.

A full blood count, ESR and plain X-ray will exclude most cases of more sinister spinal pathology.

Plain films often reveal findings that are as common in asymptomatic individuals.

The vast majority of patients with low back pain alone should be treated conservatively.[2]

### Spondylolysis and spondylolisthesis

The classification of spondylolysis and spondylolisthesis is well-documented.[16]

#### Isthmic spondylolisthesis

- commonest cause of spondylolisthesis below the age of 50
- an acquired defect in the pars interarticularis, a spondylolysis (Figure 14.11)
- genetic predisposition: seen in active young athletes, especially gymnasts and bowlers

#### Degenerative spondylolisthesis

- commonest
- usually L4/5
- pars intact, listhesis due to degenerative changes in facet joint and disc
- rarely greater than 30% slip

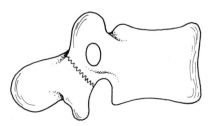

**Figure 14.11** Lateral view of lumbar vertebra showing fracture through the pars interarticularis, known as spondylolysis.

- reduction in space for thecal sac and roots may contribute to development of central spinal stenosis or lateral recess stenosis
- not always symptomatic

## Malignancy

Malignancy should always be considered as a cause for back pain in a patient over the age of 50. Secondary deposits are the commonest; primary tumours of the spine are rare. Primary tumours should be considered in children, especially if night pain is present.

Secondary malignant deposits often arise in the vertebral bodies and the pedicles. Destructive lesions may thus lead to instability. Expanding lesions may cause neurological embarrassment. The presence of symptomatic instability or neurological compromise will require surgical stabilization, often over many levels, with internal fixation and decompression. Unfortunately, the resolution of neurological change is frequently unpredictable.

## Infection

Primary infection is most likely to be tuberculosis. Despite improved chemotherapy, decompression of the spinal cord or stabilization of the spine is still occasionally necessary. The posterior elements are often spared in tuberculosis and thus surgery is usually anterior.

Secondary infection is most commonly discitis following instrumentation of the disc. These patients usually spontaneously fuse the affected segment and thus rarely require surgical intervention.

## Postsurgical back pain

This may follow failed fusion or iatrogenic instability. Rarely, a discectomy may lead to instability if performed in the presence of a degenerate spondylolisthesis.

## Isolated disc resorption (L4/5–L5/S1)

This is a specific form of degenerative change in the intervertebral disc. It is rarely a cause of root pain. It is characterized by marked narrowing of a disc space. Radiographically there may be gas in the disc.

Isolated disc resorption can remain asymptomatic but may give rise to a syndrome of bilateral buttock pain and thigh pains. The pain may be quite severe and may be accompanied by sciatica.

Spinal fusion may be indicated with or without decompression.

## Spinal instability

Spinal instability can be defined as a state where, under physiological conditions, the normal structures conferring stability fail. This loss of stiffness allows abnormal movements and abnormal range of movement to occur.

There is no universally agreed classification of spinal instability.

### Chronic segmental spinal instability

The diagnosis of segmental spinal instability remains a difficult problem and is largely based on experience rather than a reproducible test or investigation.

The symptoms and signs remain controversial. The diagnosis is suggested by a history of recurrent episodes of low back pain, often following minor lifting or twisting injuries. The pain may be aggravated by standing and often relieved by lying down or walking. The pain is made worse by changing position. Sometimes the patient describes a locking of the back. There is often a great deal of paravertebral spasm and tenderness. There will be an absence of nerve root tension signs. A high proportion of these patients exhibit non-organic features.

Investigation of these patients is again controversial, there being no recognized test of instability. Many of the tests are interventional or painful.

## Surgery for stabilization of the spine

Approaches to the lumbar spine may be posterior, which is the least traumatic, anterior, which is more complicated, combined which is very extensive surgery.

The advantage of instrumentation of the spine is that it confers immediate rigidity to the spine. This is obviously a benefit where the spine is grossly unstable, as in trauma. Postoperative morbidity and the numbers developing a pseudoarthrosis of the spinal fusion may be reduced. Implants may be applied to the anterior or posterior aspect of the spine. They consist of malleable wires, screws through the facets, rods, rigid loops, or plates in combination with spinal screw or pedicle screw fixation to the vertebra. Internal fixation increases the complication rate particularly with infection, neurological injury and implant failure.

Methods of fusion are largely dictated by the pathology being treated. However, complication of certain techniques and surgical preference are also important.

## Back pain service

It is now appreciated that the treatment of back pain warrants a multidisciplinary approach. Particularly important is the prevention and early detection of back problems at the place of work. Aggressive rehabilitation through 'back schools' and early consultation with the 'pain team' is necessary to avoid the slide into a chronic pain syndrome. The orthopaedic surgeon plays a small but valuable part in this service.

## References

1. Mixter WJ, Barr JS. Rupture of the intervertebral disc with involvement of the spinal canal. *N Engl J Med* **211:** 210–215, 1934
2. Frymoyer JW. Medical progress: back pain and sciatica. *N Engl J Med* **318:** 291–300, 1988

3. McCulloch JA. Modern lumbar disc surgery. *Curr Orthop* **6:** 13, 1992

4. Porter RW, Hibbert C, Wicks M. The spinal canal in symptomatic lumbar disc lesions. *J Bone Joint Surg* **60B:** 485–487, 1978

5. Spengler DM. Lumbar discectomy. Results with limited disc excision and selective foraminotomy. *Spine* **7:** 604–607, 1982

6. Arnoldi CC, Brodsky AE, Cauchoix J *et al*. Lumbar spinal stenosis and nerve root entrapment syndromes: definition and classification. *Clin Orthop Res* **115:** 4–5, 1976

7. Edgar MA. The pathogenesis of low back and leg pain. In: (Nixon JE, ed.) *Spinal Stenosis* Chapter 3, pp. 36–54

8. Weber H. Lumbar disc herniation: a controlled prospective study with 10 years of observation. *Spine* **8:** 131–140, 1983

9. White AH, Derby R, Wynne G. Epidural injections for the diagnosis and treatment of low back pain. *Spine* **5:** 78–86, 1980

10. Waddell G, McCulloch JA, Kummel E, Venner RM. Non-organic physical signs in low back pain. *Spine* **5:** 117–125, 1980

11. Williams RW. Microlumbar discectomy. A 12 year statistical review. *Spine* **11:** 851–852, 1986

12. Nixon JE. Clinical diagnosis (of spinal stenosis). In: (Nixon JE, ed.) *Spinal Stenosis* Chapter 5, pp. 61–81

13. Getty CJM, Johnson JR, Kirwan E, Sullivan MF. Partial undercutting facetectomy for bony entrapment of the lumbar nerve root. *J Bone Joint Surg* **63b:** 330–335, 1981

14. Wiltse LL, Kirkaldy-Willis WH, McIvor GWD. The treatment of spinal stenosis. *Clin Orthop Rel Res* **115:** 83–90, 1976

15. Porter R, Hibbert C. Calcitonin treatment for neurogenic claudication. *Spine* **8:** 585–592, 1983

16. Wiltse LL, Newman PH, Macnab I. Classification of spondylolisis and spondylolisthesis. *Clin Orthop Rel Res* **117:** 23–29, 1976

# Coccydynia

**J. E. Williams**

Coccydynia or coccygodynia are names used to describe pain in the region of the coccyx.[1] These terms refer to symptoms rather than pathological diagnoses. A painful coccyx can be the result of many different underlying disease processes, but in many cases no organic cause is found. Patients normally have considerable pain when sitting or lying in the supine position. Usually the pain will gradually subside within a few months but in a minority of patients the condition becomes intractable. Coccydynia usually responds to conservative measures but occasionally when this is ineffective it may be necessary to consider more aggressive approaches such as chemical neurolysis or surgery.

## Aetiology

### Acute coccydynia

This occurs more commonly in women than in men. Sprained coccygeal ligaments, fractures and dislocations commonly occur as a result of falls exposing the coccyx to direct trauma. Childbirth may result in such damage, and is a common cause of acute coccydynia.

### Chronic coccydynia

Pain that has persisted for some time may be related to osteoarthritis of the sacrococcygeal joint, or be due to repetitive microtrauma.

### Neoplastic disease

Pain may arise from direct metastatic involvement or external compression or oedema.

### Referred pain

Pain may be referred from spinal cord disease (lumbar disc), anorectal disease (abscesses, fistulae), pelvic inflammatory disease or, rarely, osteomyelitis.

### Idiopathic coccydynia

In up to 50% of patients no specific cause is found despite extensive investigation. In such cases the pain has been attributed to a variety of conditions, including spasm of the muscles of the pelvic floor and functional neurosis.

## Clinical features

Patients complain of deep aching or throbbing pains with episodic stabbing in the vicinity of the lower end of the sacrum and coccyx and also of pain radiating to the buttocks and posterior aspect of the thigh. There is often a history of pain on sitting, and patients may have made arrangements to allow them to stand whilst at work or at home.

Physical examination by external palpation or per rectum will reveal an exquisitely tender coccyx. Occasionally coccygeal deformity may be felt. Muscular spasm of all pelvic floor muscles is common.

## Management

### Investigations

A full history and examination are necessary to exclude any of the underlying causes of the pain mentioned above. X-rays may be necessary to detect abnormalities such as fractures and dislocations, though often X-rays are completely normal.[2] Magnetic resonance imaging or computed tomography may also be useful in excluding disc disease.

### Treatment

Conservative measures should be commenced prior to more invasive treatment.

- Heat pads and warm baths may be useful in relaxing the pelvic musculature. Rubber cushions or doughnuts may be useful in redistributing weight away from the painful area.
- Mild analgesics, non-steroidal anti-inflammatory drugs and muscle relaxants may be required.
- Percutaneous and per rectum local anaesthetic and steroid injections into the sacrococcygeal joint have been used with some success,[3] or caudal epidural local anaesthetic and steroid injections.
- Neurolytic injections using phenol and ammonium chloride are directed towards the lower sacral and coccygeal nerves.[4]
- Coccygectomy. This should only be considered for persistent and intractable pain when all conservative measures have failed and when it is considered that the pain is confined to the coccyx. Success rates of 50–70% in patients with traumatic or idiopathic coccydynia have been reported.[5] (Though Bailey and Love[6] warn that 'excision of the

coccyx does not usually relieve the symptoms completely, if at all, and the patient should be warned of this before going ahead with surgery.')
- Psychological approaches may be beneficial in helping patients deal with their pain.

## References

1. Simpson JY. On coccydynia and the diseases and deformities of the coccyx. *Med Times Gazette* **40:** 1–7, 1859
2. Postacchini F, Massobrio M. Idiopathic coccygodynia. *J Bone Joint Surg* **65:** 1116–1124, 1983
3. Kersey PJ. Non-operative management of coccygodynia. *Lancet* **1:** 318, 1980
4. Wright BD. Treatment of intractable coccygodynia by transacral ammonium chloride injection. *Anesth Analg* **50:** 519–525, 1971
5. Eng JB, Rymaszewski L, Jepson K. Coccygectomy. *J R Coll Surg Edin* **33:** 202–203, 1988
6. Bailey and Love. Fractures and dislocations. Pelvis and lower limb. In: *Short Practice of Surgery*. Chapman and Hall, London, 1992

16

# Postspinal surgery pain

**C. J. Fairley**

There are many long-term follow-up studies after spinal surgery which variably estimate success rates at between 19 and 90% with an average of 30–40%, although criteria for success are broad.[1] Therefore many patients continue to be disabled by back pain following lumbar spine surgery. Such patients form the majority of admissions to chronic pain treatment programmes.[2] Since the failed back surgery syndrome (FBSS) is, in part, an iatrogenic complaint and the original operation cannot be undone, prevention must assume priority. The patient with established FBSS, however, often presents a complex diagnostic and therapeutic problem. The syndrome impinges on the patient's entire life; self-esteem is often low, owing to unemployment and breakdown of relationships and many fail to return to their previous activities, including employment, following surgery. In addition, management of physical symptomatology is often complicated by learned chronic pain behaviour and by the possibility of secondary financial gain through litigation.

Many authorities agree that spinal surgery has been previously over-prescribed.[3,4] It is to be hoped that increased appreciation of the problem with stricter application of operative criteria will reduce the future occurrence of FBSS.

## Aetiology

### Surgical procedures

The most commonly performed spinal operations aim either to stabilize the spinal column or to relieve pressure on the contents of the spinal canal:

- Spinal fusion is undertaken for degenerative disc disease or spondylolisthesis. Success depends on the creation and maintenance of a structural and functional fusion with resulting spinal stability.
- Lumbar decompression: Successful relief of pressure on neural components depends on accurate diagnosis and appropriate treatment of the cause.

## Causes of failure

- Inappropriate patient selection: Many patients with FBSS have undergone surgery with dubious operative criteria. In the presence of major psychiatric or psychosocial abnormalities, this may be a major cause of the maintenance of pain.
- Inappropriate or inadequate surgery: Incomplete removal of a prolapsed disc may result in persistence of symptoms. Surgery may have been performed at the wrong level or on the wrong side, or one level treated in the presence of multilevel pathology.
- Missed diagnosis: The most common example is lumbar spinal stenosis which is frequently missed in patients with nerve root symptoms operated on for coincidental disc pathology and is the primary cause of FBSS in 57% of patients.[5]
- Iatrogenic complications may follow any spinal surgery and include nerve injuries,[6] epidural fibrosis, retained foreign body and adhesive arachnoiditis.[7]
- Coincidental pathology: Disorders unrelated to the original surgery, such as a spinal tumour or intra-abdominal or pelvic pathology, may cause back pain.
- Non-organic causes: Many patients have no physical abnormalities to explain their complaint.

## Organic causes

These can be grouped into:

- those in which nerve root compression, irritation or damage predominate, causing neurological deficits in the lower limbs
- those in which back pain is the main complaint, suggesting musculoskeletal disease without neural involvement

The two may coexist, however, and operations originally to alleviate leg pain, i.e. for nerve root symptoms, may lead to disorders causing back pain and vice versa. In addition, back pain frequently radiates to the lower limbs.

Organic causes commonly, but not exclusively, associated with the FBSS include:

- Lateral spinal stenosis: The advent of computed tomographic (CT) scanning may decrease the likelihood of this frequently missed diagnosis. Bone encroachment on the spinal canal results in compression and ischaemia of spinal nerve roots, causing dysfunction. Pain may be unilateral or bilateral. It is experienced in the legs, thighs, buttocks and low back and is heavy and cramping in quality. Forward flexion of the spine relieves pain unless the stenosis is severe, when it may be continuous. Because symptoms may increase with exercise, and are often similar to those associated with peripheral vascular disease, the latter must be excluded by demonstration of peripheral pulses and by lower-limb arteriography if doubt remains. Central spinal stenosis may result from bone overgrowth following spinal fusion.

- Lumbosacral adhesive arachnoiditis: This condition is estimated to account for between 6 and 16% of all cases of FBSS.[5] It usually occurs secondary to physical injury. Contrast media, particularly those which are oil-based, and surgery for prolapsed intervertebral disc and laminectomy account for the majority of cases.[8] Damage to the pia mater of the cauda equina results in the formation of fibrinous bands which constrict the surrounding neural tissues. Symptoms may vary markedly between patients and may include pain in the back, the legs or both, anaesthesia or hypoaesthesia in the affected distribution with reduced muscle power and hyporeflexia, paraspinal muscle atrophy, contracture or spasm and sphincter dysfunction. The pain is typically burning, tingling or gripping in nature, and is usually unrelieved by posture or rest. Its severe and unrelenting nature causes severe psychological complications in most patients. As there is no proven cure for adhesive arachnoiditis, treatment centres on alleviation of symptoms, psychological support and on rehabilitation.[9]
- Epidural fibrosis: Postoperative fibrosis and scarring result in neural entrapment causing neuropathic symptoms. It frequently accompanies arachnoiditis.[10]
- Facet joint disruption: Disruption of the disc space, particularly after discectomy or spinal fusion, may result in misalignment of the facet joints. Stress on the joints results in synovial changes with capsular thickening. Pain is felt in the back and radiates to the buttocks. Morning stiffness is common. The pain is exacerbated by extension and rotation and relieved by flexion and can often be reproduced accurately by palpation over the affected joints. Straight leg raising is normal.
- Paraspinal muscle atrophy: This is an important and often overlooked cause of FBSS. Lesions of the dorsal rami during surgery may result in denervation atrophy of the corresponding paraspinal muscles, particularly the extensors, leading to loss of functional support of the spine.[11] Over time, secondary arthritic changes occur in stressed joints leading to further pain and loss of function. Generalized muscle disuse can cause atrophy of back muscles at unoperated levels. Symptoms of muscle fatigue and backache are precipitated by exercise and stationary activities in which spinal muscular support is needed.

## Assessment

The initial assessment aims to eliminate a surgically remediable cause of pain, to ascertain the presence or absence of an organic lesion, and to gauge the contribution of compounding factors which may potentially hinder rehabilitation, including drug dependence, and psychological disorders, particularly anxiety, depression and maladaptive personality. Previous medical records, including details of preoperative symptoms, diagnostic investigations and surgical treatment may indicate the need for further investigations, and provide an indication of the contribution of organic pathology to the original complaint.

### History

The diagnosis may be suggested by the patient's description of the pain. The history should include an assessment of psychological status, the impingement of the pain on the patient's lifestyle, and drug usage.

### Examination

This includes full neurological examination of the lower limbs and an assessment of the degree of spinal mobility and functional impairment. The absence of objective findings and inappropriate reactions or signs during examination may suggest a functional component.[12]

### Diagnostic investigations

These may be indicated if the history and examination suggest a specific diagnosis.

- Magnetic resonance imaging (MRI) scanning allows images to be made in both the sagittal and coronal planes and is therefore of benefit in multiple-level investigations. An additional advantage is the absence of ionizing radiation. It is useful in the detection of fibrosis, arachnoiditis,[13] disc herniation,[14,15] stenoses of the canal and foramina and the functional integrity of spinal fusions.[16]
- CT scanning allows accurate measurement of the dimensions of the canal and visualization of the site and scale of the encroachment of the bony canal and nerve root foramina on neural tissue. It is useful in differentiating the causes of lumbar spinal canal stenosis and in determining the causes of failure of spinal fusion.[17] Disc protrusion, scar tissue and nerve root displacement following lumbar disc surgery[18] and paraspinal muscle atrophy can be detected.
- X-rays: Anteroposterior and lateral films can demonstrate degenerative disease, facet joint abnormalities, loss of disc space, spondylolisthesis, fractures, infection and tumour. Flexion/extension X-rays may be of value in demonstrating the functional and structural integrity of spinal fusions. The place of X-rays in establishing an accurate diagnosis, however, is of limited value.
- Myelography: This technique has been largely superseded by the non-invasive techniques of CT and MRI scanning.
- Electromyography: When combined with selective nerve root blocks this may be of value in determining the level or number of involved roots.
- Bone scanning: This may be indicated if tumour, fracture or infection is suspected.

### Diagnostic local blockade

Facet joint injections with local anaesthetic agents under X-ray guidance may be used as a diagnostic or therapeutic procedure. Permanent facet joint denervation procedures may be considered if temporary blockade relieves the pain.

Paravertebral blocks may elucidate the contribution of single or multiple nerve roots.

## Conservative management

In the absence of a surgically correctable lesion, management centres on:

- symptomatic relief
- prevention of further damage
- restoration of function
- eliminating dependence on anxiolytic and analgesic medication
- assisting the patient in coping with and minimizing the disability and disruption to activities of daily living
- reduction of depression, anxiety and insomnia

FBSS patients may share many common disabilities, irrespective of the diagnosis or lack of one. The long-term physical, psychological and social problems are often best managed in a multidisciplinary setting. Patients should be made aware from the outset that a programme is not intended to cure their pain, but to reduce its impact on their life through improvement of physical and psychological function.

Rehabilitation programmes for the patient with FBSS may be conducted on an inpatient or outpatient basis.[19]

- Inpatient programmes allow rapid assessment and intensive treatment under continuous supervision. They allow the use of invasive analgesic techniques while rehabilitation takes place, and may remove the patient temporarily from a destructive domestic environment. They obviate the need for continuous trips to and from outpatient departments. Drug detoxification may be more easily achieved as an inpatient. Few centres, however, run such programmes owing to the prohibitive cost of several weeks of inpatient care.
- Outpatient programmes are widely used in most hospitals. They are cheaper to run and have the potential advantage of allowing the patient to remain in a normal social environment.

## The rehabilitation team

This usually comprises a physician with overall responsibility for assessing the patient and coordinating a management plan working in conjunction with other professional input. This includes:

- Occupational therapist: The occupational therapist assists the patient in coping with the activities of daily living, including domestic organization, hobbies and relaxation, and transport. Attention is paid to developing coping strategies and setting and achieving goals.
- Physiotherapist: Patients usually have poor general fitness with weak muscles, particularly those of the lower back and abdomen, and stiff

joints through chronic underuse. Pain, and the belief that movement of the painful back will result in further damage, perpetuates the vicious cycle. Intensive and sustained back training can result in dramatic improvement in pain.[20] After an assessment of power and tone, posture and range of movement and ability to walk, sit and stand, an individually tailored exercise plan is formulated. A graded exercise programme under supervision improves well-being and demonstrates to the patient that such exercise is not harmful. Pain-related behaviour, work capacity and self-rated disability are also improved. Back care procedures such as methods of lifting are also taught. Hydrotherapy is helpful in improving general fitness and mobility.

- Clinical psychologist: A cognitive-behavioural approach may improve coping strategies, medication use and functional impairment.[21]
- Dietitian: Weight loss in those patients with excess body fat helps to reduce strain on the lumbar spine.
- Social worker: The social worker provides assistance in obtaining financial help and solving domestic problems.

## Physical treatments

- Drugs: Patients may be physically and psychologically dependent on a variety of opioid or non-opioid medications which, in general, have no role in the management of chronic back pain. The aim should be to reduce dependence on drugs through a detoxification programme. Antidepressants, however, can act centrally to alleviate pain and may improve sleep patterns.
- Epidural blockade: With or without steroids, this may break the cycle of muscular spasm by temporarily denervating the paraspinal musculature. Exercise may be facilitated by the use of continuous lumbar epidural analgesia using local anaesthetic agents of a concentration sufficient to provide analgesia with minimal motor blockade.
- Transcutaneous electrical nerve stimulation (TENS): This technique may provide a degree of pain relief in a proportion of FBSS patients by stimulation of the dorsal columns of the spinal cord, thereby gating pain.[22]
- Acupuncture, including electroacupuncture, is of unproven benefit in the management of the FBSS patient.[23]

## Surgery

### Reoperation

Salvage back surgery has inherently poor results with good outcomes variably estimated at between 25 and 80%.[24] Most studies show that success rates decrease with second and subsequent operations.[25] Poor results are associated with compensation cases, pending litigation, psychosocial problems, lack of objective preoperative findings and a short painfree interval following the original surgery.[26-28]

The only absolute indication for repeat surgery is the presence of the cauda equina syndrome.[29] Patients incapacitated by severe back pain who have failed to respond to conservative measures and have a proven root lesion may also be candidates for surgery; however, long-standing neural damage may be irreversible. In general, repeat surgery is more likely to compound than cure the problem. A psychological assessment may help to eliminate those patients in whom maladaptive behaviour might prohibit a successful outcome.

### Other surgical techniques

- Dorsal column stimulation: A surgically implanted electrode may be suitable in those patients in whom a trial of TENS provides good temporary pain relief, particularly in those with radicular pain and arachnoiditis.[30]
- Surgically implanted intrathecal catheters: These may be of benefit when other measures fail. Patient-controlled intrathecal boluses of opioids from an implanted reservoir are delivered into the subarachnoid space.
- Facet joint denervation by radiofrequency neurolysis may be indicated in the management of the patient in whom pain is attributable to the facet joints, as confirmed by prior local anaesthetic blockade.
- Neurosurgical procedures such as neurectomy, dorsal rhizotomy and stereotactic procedures have inconsistent and poor results in the treatment of chronic pain.[31]

## References

1. Flor H, Turk DC. Etiological theories and treatments for chronic back pain. 1. Somatic models and interventions. *Pain* **19:** 105–121, 1984
2. Long DM, Filtzer DL, BenDebba M, Hendler NH. Clinical features of the failed back syndrome. *J Neurosurg* **69:** 61–71, 1988
3. Finneson BE. A lumbar disc surgery predictive score card. *Spine* **3:** 86, 1978
4. Finneson BE. A lumbar disc surgery predictive score card. A retrospective evaluation. *Spine* **4:** 141, 1979
5. Burton CV, Kirkaldy-Willis WH, Yong-Hing K, Heithoff KB. Causes of failure of surgery on the lumbar spine. *Clin Orthop Rel Res* **157:** 191–199, 1981
6. Bertrand G. The 'battered' root problem. *Orthop Clin North Am* **6** (suppl): 305–310, 1975
7. Burton CV. Lumbosacral arachnoiditis. *Spine* **3:** 24, 1978
8. Bourne IHJ. Lumbosacral adhesive arachnoiditis: a review. *J R Soc Med* **83:** 262–265, 1990
9. Guyer DW, Wiltse LL, Eskay ML, Guyer BH. The long-range prognosis of arachnoiditis. *Spine* **14:** 1333–1341, 1989
10. Benoist M, Ficat C, Baraf P, Cauchoix J. Postoperative lumbar epiduroarachnoiditis: diagnostic and therapeutic aspects. *Spine* **5:** 432–436, 1980
11. Sihvonen T, Herno A, Paljarvi L, Airaksinen O, Partanen J, Tapaninaho A. Local denervation atrophy of paraspinal muscles in postoperative failed back syndrome. *Spine* **18:** 575–581, 1993
12. Waddell G, McCulloch JA, Kummel EG, Venner RM. Non-organic physical signs in low back pain. *Spine* **5:** 117–125, 1980
13. Delamarter RB, Ross JS, Masaryk TJ, Modic MT, Bohlman HH. Diagnosis of lumbar arachnoiditis by magnetic resonance imaging. *Spine* **15:** 305–310, 1990

14. Hochhauser L, Kieffer SA, Cacayorin ED, Petro GR, Teller WF. Recurrent postdisk-ectomy low back pain: MR-surgical correlation. *Am J Radiol* **151:** 755–760, 1988
15. Modic MT, Pavlicek W, Weinstein MA *et al.* Magnetic resonance imaging of intervertebral disc disease. *Radiology* **152:** 103–111, 1984
16. Lang P, Chafetz N, Genant HK, Morris JM. Lumbar spinal fusion; assessment of func-tional stability with magnetic resonance imaging. *Spine* **15:** 581–588, 1990
17. Laasonen EM, Soini J. Low back pain after lumbar fusion; surgical and computed tomo-graphic analysis. *Spine* **14:** 211–213, 1989
18. Teplick JG, Haskin ME. Intravenous contrast-enhanced CT of the post operative lumbar spine: improved identification of recurrent disc herniation, scar, arachnoiditis and diskitis. *AJNR* **143:** 845–855, 1984
19. Peters JL, Large RG. A randomised control trial evaluating in- and outpatient pain management programmes. *Pain* **41:** 283–293, 1990
20. Manniche C, Lundberg E, Christensen I, Bentzen L, Hesselsoe G. Intensive dynamic back exercises for chronic low back pain: a clinical trial. *Pain* **47:** 53–63, 1991
21. Nicholas MK, Wilson PH, Goyen J. Comparison of cognitive-behavioural group treat-ment and an alternative non-psychological treatment for chronic low back pain. *Pain* **48:** 339–347, 1992
22. Melzack R, Wall PD. Pain mechanism: a new theory. *Science* **150:** 971–979, 1965
23. Richardson PH, Vincent CA. Acupuncture for the treatment of pain: a review of evaluative research: *Pain* **24:** 15–40, 1986
24. Kim SS, Michelsen CB. Revision surgery for failed back surgery syndrome. *Spine* **17:** 957–960, 1992
25. Waddell G, Kummel EG, Lotto WN *et al.* Failed lumbar disc surgery following industrial injuries. *J Bone Joint Surg* **61:** 201–207, 1979
26. Finnegan WJ, Fenlin JM, Marrel JP, Nardini RJ, Rothman RH. Results of surgical inter-vention in the symptomatic multiply operated back patient. *J Bone Joint Surg* **61A:** 1077–1082, 1979
27. Lehman TR, LaRocca HS. Repeat lumbar surgery. *Spine* **6:** 615–619, 1981
28. Spengler DM, Freeman C, Westbrook R, Miller JW. Low back pain following multiple lumbar spine procedures. *Spine* **5:** 356–360, 1980
29. Pheasant HC, Dyck P. Failed lumbar disc surgery: cause, assessment, treatment. *Clin Orthop Rel Res* **164:** 93–109, 1982
30. DeLaPorte C, Van de Kelft E. Spinal cord stimulation in failed back surgery syndrome. *Pain* **52:** 55–61, 1993
31. Loeser JD. Neurosurgical control of chronic pain. *Arch Surg* **12:** 880–883, 1977

# 17

# Postherpetic neuralgia

**N. L. Padfield**

Postherpetic neuralgia has been variably defined as a chronic painful state persisting from 4 weeks to 6 months after crusting of lesions following infection with the herpes zoster virus.

## Aetiology

This vexing condition follows infection with the virus herpes zoster. This virus has the same DNA as the varicella virus that causes chickenpox and, not surprisingly, most patients give a previous history of exposure to chickenpox. The virus lies dormant in the dorsal root ganglia, to be reactivated by certain precipitating factors such as host immunosuppression from concurrent infection, reticuloendothelial disorders, acquired immunodeficiency syndrome (AIDS) and iatrogenic immunosuppression from chemotherapy and radiotherapy. The reported incidence of the disease varies from 1.8 to 4.5 cases per 1000 population. It is increasingly common with advancing age. For instance, an 80-year-old is 10–20 times more likely to develop postherpetic neuralgia.

## Pathophysiology of nociception

In the acute infection activation of nociceptive primary afferents by direct viral attack, and secondary changes in skin, nerve, posterior root ganglion, nerve roots, leptomeninges and the spinal cord are the most reasonable explanations. But in postherpetic neuralgia both peripheral and central mechanisms are involved. Preferential loss of large fibres occurs, which probably impairs segmental pain-modulating systems, allowing increased transmission of nociceptive information through the dorsal horn of the spinal cord. It is also known that older patients have fewer large fibres than younger ones and they tend to lose more of them because of the infection. The dysaesthetic pain experienced may arise from damaged or regenerating nociceptive afferent fibres and the lancinating pain may relate to ephaptic activation of the primary afferent nociceptive nervi nervorum investing the nerve trunk itself. The evidence for central mechanisms is postulated by the failure of proximal deafferenting procedures such as neurectomy, spinothalamic tractotomy, or thalamotomy to provide sustained relief. Noxious impulses may become established in centrally located, closed, self-perpetuating and progressively self-facilitating synaptic loops.

## Investigations

Since all the evidence points to minimizing the risk of development of postherpetic neuralgia by prompt and effective treatment of the initial infection, early diagnosis is vital.

The varicella-zoster virus may be recovered from early vesicles. Scrapings of the base of the vesicle, since the virus is cell-associated, will be more productive than the vesicular fluid and will provide cellular material containing the characteristic multinucleated giant cells. Acidophilic intranuclear inclusions can be seen in the Tzanck smear stained with haematoxylin and eosin. A punch biopsy for electron microscopy provides even more reliable data, but this is not always practical in the clinical situation.

Serological testing provides late but reliable confirmation, but since viral replication occurs early in infection, rapid detection requires an alert physician and good accessible pathology services. Sadly, the common experience of most pain clinics is to see these patients once postherpetic neuralgia has developed and thus diagnosis is established.

## Differential diagnosis

• Herpes simplex versus herpes zoster

## Clinical features

The clinical symptoms are pain, dysaesthesias, paraesthesias, allodynia and paroxysms of lancinating pain in the distribution of the nerves involved. The most common sites are the cranial nerves and the thoracic dermatomes. Involvement of the extremities is extremely rare.

In the acute phase of the infection, dermatomal erythema first appears; this is then followed by the characteristic vesicles, blebs and pustules which then crust over in the next 2–3 weeks. The vesicles are highly infectious before disappearing, usually completely, within a month. The pain of the acute eruption is usually self-limiting and gone by the time the rash has healed. However, 10% of patients progress to postherpetic neuralgia and most of these patients are older than 60 years.

## Complications

• depression/loss of lifestyle/family break-up
• loss of function/restricted mobility

# Prognosis

Prognosis improves with shortening the period of neuralgia by effective treatment, hence the need for prompt referral and initiation of treatment.[1] Prognosis improves with decreasing age of onset of neuralgia; the under 60s rarely develop chronic pain. Pain in the ophthalmic division of the trigeminal nerve can be particularly difficult to relieve compared to other sites. One-fifth of cancer patients who have had herpes zoster will get it at least once again. Lastly, the personality and psychological profile of the individual will have profound effects on the prognosis.

# Management

There is no single universally effective mode of treatment for the established condition. There really appears to have been very little significant progress in the last decade.[2] In a review of current opinion of specialists from different disciplines involved in the management of chronic neuropathic pain conditions, there was surprisingly little consensus. Most were however agreed that the main therapies detailed in this chapter were appropriate and most agreed that neuroablative procedures and strong opioids were of no value or even positively harmful.[3]

When faced with a new patient in the clinic it is often a case of trying a variety of pharmacological and physical treatments in the hope that some relief will be afforded the patient. The attitude of the pain clinician and the provision of sympathetic counselling with attention to the concomitant depression, insomnia and lack of libido will do much to alleviate the suffering of the patient.

### Pharmacological therapy

- Antiviral agents are only indicated in the chronic condition where there is the risk of reinfection, e.g. patients with Hodgkin's lymphoma or immunosuppression.
- Tricyclic antidepressants: most patients are depressed, though this may not be obvious. But more importantly, the antidepressants can sufficiently enhance descending cortical inhibition to the cortical transmission/perception of the burning neuropathic pain to provide relief. The choice of agent depends on the response of the patient.[4] In order of efficacy the author prescribes: amitriptyline 10–75 mg nocte (noradrenergic and serotoninergic), maprotiline 25–50 mg nocte (noradrenergic, but also significantly fewer antimuscarinic side-effects) and fluoxitene 20 mg nocte (serotoninergic and therefore less sedating). Amitriptyline is probably the most universally efficacious but very often it is the side-effects which dictate the ultimate choice. Occasionally the addition of a phenothiazine such as fluphenazine 2 mg nocte is beneficial if therapy with a tricyclic antidepressant alone proved ineffective.
- Anticonvulsants: If lancinating painful episodes are a feature of the pain, then treatment with anticonvulsants can be beneficial. The

author starts with carbemazepine 100 mg t.d.s. and builds up to a maximum of 400 mg t.d.s. if this can be tolerated by the patient. Often, though, patients cannot tolerate such a high dose and a ceiling is imposed at 200 mg t.d.s. Rarely, sodium valproate may be a helpful alternative at 200 mg t.d.s.; this can be increased to 400 mg t.d.s. Liver function should be checked at 6-monthly intervals.

- Simple analgesics have a very limited place in the effective relief of this condition as, unfortunately, the pain very rarely responds to simple analgesics, non-steroidal anti-inflammatory agents or opiates. This last group should be avoided as these are addictive, the problem is chronic, and the side-effects of nausea and constipation will further add to the distress of these patients who are, of course, not terminally ill.

- Topically applied local anaesthetic creams like EMLA, the 50 : 50 mixture of prilocaine and lignocaine, can be beneficial,[5] but patients often complain that it is messy and that rubbing the cream in, because of the allodynia, is the most unpleasant part.

- Capsaicin ointment, now as a 0.075% preparation, has been found to be helpful in some cases. It has been shown to reduce the amount of substance P stored/released in C-fibres but some patients find it can produce a very intense burning pain of its own accord.

- Topically applied mixtures of aspirin and diethyl ether[6] at a dosage range of 750–1500 mg in 20–30 ml diethyl ether, and aspirin/chloroform mixture[7] have been reported to be successful. However, in an earlier study indomethacin stupe was compared with aspirin/chloroform solution and found to be superior in its effect and ease of usage.[8]

In addition to direct application to the painful site there are a number of other physical treatments that have been tried with variable success.

## Physical interventions

- Local infiltration into the cutaneous area of neuralgia with steroids and local anaesthetics, especially if repeated regularly, has been reported to provide moderate to significant improvement in 64–70% of patients.

- Nerve blocks: Postmortem studies have shown that the entire sensory pathway from periphery to cortex, including sympathetic ganglia, can be involved and thus pain can be initiated anywhere in the nervous system. Consequently, nerve blocks will be diagnostic, therapeutic, prognostic and even prophylactic.

- Somatic nerve blocks with local anaesthetics may help in prognosis if a neurolytic block is being considered. Alone, the response is unpredictable and only rarely helpful, even if performed early in the development of the condition.

- Sympathetic blocks are only helpful if performed in the acute stage of the condition. Even repeated blocks, if performed more than 6 months after the initial infection, are rarely effective.

- Epidural blockade may give some benefit if the site of the injection is close to the dorsal root ganglia of the affected dermatomes. But this is not the universal experience with this technique. Occasionally, if the site of the neuralgia is suitable, i.e. thoracic dermatomes, a catheter and reservoir system can be implanted. This may be sited intrapleurally rather than epidurally to minimize systemic effects from the epidural injection. The long-term advantage is that a district nurse or other trained health care worker can give regular injections of local anaesthetic with or without the addition of steroids to a patient in the community. However, this does require education and cooperation from the community nurse and may not be a practical option for every patient.

- Neurolytic techniques: Direct neurolysis of somatic nerves should only be contemplated if a block with local anaesthetic has been shown to be beneficial and that the resulting numbness is an acceptable alternative to the neuralgic pain. This is by no means always the case: patients may complain bitterly of the resulting numbness after a neurolytic procedure, especially in ophthalmic neuralgia, for example. Neurolysis can be achieved chemically with aqueous phenol 5–10%, or alcohol 50–90%, both of which can cause considerable neuritis because of inaccurate placement of the needle with spillage on to the adjacent somatic nerve. Ammonium sulphate 10% in 1% lignocaine or amonium chloride 15% has been used for its selective effect on unmyelinated C-fibres. Its action lasts from 4 to 24 weeks. It does not cause neuritis but can leave the patient with distressing numbness. Vincristine iontophoresis has been claimed to give excellent relief.[9,10] However the technique is time-consuming as it has to be performed daily for 40 min over a period of up to 4 weeks and is messy. Consequently it has not gained universal popularity.
- Physical techniques like cryotherapy to the affected somatic nerves can give temporary relief with a low incidence of neuritis. Unfortunately, because the large fibres have usually been destroyed by the disease they do not regenerate preferentially over the C-fibres and thus this does not afford the 'cure' which can occasionally happen after cryolesioning neuromata. Even radiofrequency lesioning can be useful as the lesions can be precisely sited.
- Acupuncture can be helpful in some cases, even where destructive or invasive procedures have been tried.
- Hypnosis: Pain relief can sometimes be improved by descending cortical inhibition which 'closes the gate'. It has been reported to make the unbearable bearable by changing the pattern of pain/suffering.
- Cryotherapy has already been mentioned. Locally applied cold can be comforting, especially in uncontrolled lancinating pain. Some patients keep a packet of frozen peas handy just for this purpose! Other forms are ethyl chloride spray or the commercially available PR spray.
- Transcutaneous electrical analgesia is rarely helpful, probably because there are insufficient or no high-threshold mechanoreceptors to stimulate in order to 'close the gate', having been destroyed by the viral infection. Often patients will say it makes the neuralgic pain far worse. Taking this further, in a comparative study of the use of dorsal column stimulation in different circumstances, pain was actually aggravated by dorsal column stimulation.[11]

### Psychological support

Last but by no means least, psychological support can make a huge contribution to converting the unbearable into the bearable.

Severe depression with suicidal tendencies can be seen in 50% of patients. Anxiety and stress are often present and training the patient in stress management and relaxation techniques can help control the pain to some degree. Personality will determine a patient's ability to cope. On the one hand, a type A person who is tense, perfectionist and hard-driving will show little willingness or ability to control pain, while on the other hand a dependent personality with suppressed anger and resentment will also be poor at accepting the locus of control. Often these patients manipulate friends and family. Inappropriate attention and sympathy only exacerbate the problem by reinforcing such pain behaviour.

Counselling with emphasis on explaining the relationship between the psyche and pain with the patient and the immediate family and/or friends is very worthwhile, even though it is time-consuming, because they too have to cope with the pain their loved one is experiencing.

Since many patients are elderly and live alone, social services in the form of home helps, meals on wheels and appropriate accommodation should be optimized.

## Conclusion

In conclusion, early detection and treatment of the acute infection will be the major contribution in reducing the incidence of postherpetic neuralgia and this presents the major challenge of educating the medical community at large and not just pain clinicians.[12]

## References

1. Bowsher D. Acute herpes zoster and postherpetic neuralgia: effects of acyclovir and outcome of treatment with amitryptiline. *Br J Gen Pract* **42:** 244–246, 1992
2. Robinson PN, Fletcher N. Review article: postherpetic neuralgia. *J R Coll Gen Pract* **36:** 24–28, 1986
3. Davies HTO, Crombie IK, Macrae WA. Polarized views on treating neurogenic pain. *Pain* **54:** 341–346, 1993
4. Peter C, Watson N, Chipman M, Reed K, Evans R, Birkett N. Amitryptiline versus maprotiline in postherpetic neuralgia: a randomized, double-blind, crossover trial. *Pain* **48:** 29–36, 1992
5. Lycka BA. EMLA: A new and effective topical anaesthetic. *J Dermatol Surg Oncol* **18:** 859–862, 1992
6. De Benedittis G, Besana F, Lorenzetti A. A new topical treatment for acute herpetic neuralgia and postherpetic neuralgia: the aspirin/diethyl ether mixture. An open-label study plus a double-blind controlled clinical trial. *Pain* **48:** 383–390, 1992
7. King RB. Topical aspirin in chloroform and the relief of pain due to herpes zoster and postherpetic neuralgia. *Arch Neurol* **50:** 1046–1053, 1993
8. Morimoto M, Inamori K, Hyodo M. The effect of indomethacin stupe for postherpetic neuralgia – particularly in comparison with chloroform-aspirin solution. *Pain* (suppl 5): S1–528, 1990

9. Csilik B, Kayihar-Csilik E, Szucs A. Treatment of chronic pain syndromes with ion-tophoresis of vinca alkaloids to the skin of patients. *Neurosci Lett* **31:** 87–90, 1982

10. Tajti J, Somogyi T, Szilard J. Treatment of chronic pain syndrome with transcutaneous iontophoresis of vinca alkaloids. *Acta Med Hung* **46:** 3–12, 1989

11. Shimoji K, Hokari T, Kano T *et al.* Management of intractable pain with percutaneous epidural spinal cord stimulation: differences in pain relieving effects among diseases and sites of pain. *Anesth Analg* **77:** 110–116, 1993

12. Macrae WA, Davies HTO, Crombie IK. Pain: paradigms and treatments, guest editorial. *Pain* **49:** 289–291, 1992

# 18

# Trigeminal neuralgia

S. J. Dolin

## Anatomy of trigeminal system

The sensory nuclei of the trigeminal nuclei complex receive their input from neurons of the trigeminal gasserian ganglion in Meckel's cave in the middle cranial fossa. The peripheral processes of the ganglion are distributed via the ophthalmic, maxillary and mandibular divisions of the trigeminal nerve to those regions of the face anterior to the ears. All three divisions conduct pain from their area of distribution, although in trigeminal neuralgia the mandibular divisions is most commonly affected.

The trigeminal nuclear complex has components in the midbrain, pens, medulla and even extends down into the upper cervical segments of the spinal cord. There are three sensory nuclei and one motor nucleus. The long attenuated spinal or descending nucleus descends as far as C4 to blend with the substantia gelatinosa of the cervical cord. The spinal nucleus is the nucleus usually associated with pain conduction. The motor nucleus lies in the pens and, through reflex connections with the spinal nucleus, can produce activity of the muscles of mastication (clenching of the jaw or chattering of teeth) in response to noxious stimuli to the face.

Secondary fibres originating from the neurons of the elongated spinal nucleus cross the midline and ascend to thalamus as the trigeminal thalamic tract. On the lateral aspect of the midbrain the trigeminal thalamic fibres may be vulnerable to compromise by the firm edge of the dura mater, such as by a meningioma or by trauma.

## Pathophysiology

Trigeminal neuralgia is not a specific disease but is a symptom often caused by pathology involving the fifth cranial nerve. Surgical evidence indicates abnormal vascular cross-compression of the root entry zone of the trigeminal nerve.[1] A loop of artery has been observed to impinge upon the nerve and surgical repositioning of the artery or padding of the point of contact can result in long-term pain relief. However, the link between the compression and the generation of the pain remains speculative. In a small (1–5) percentage of cases, trigeminal neuralgia is caused by a demonstrable underlying pathology such as a tumour (in Meckel's cave or

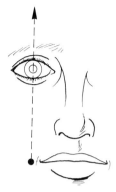

**Figure 18.1** Placement of needle for radiofrequency trigeminal ganglion thermocoagulation. The needle is placed 2–3 cm lateral to the angle of the mouth. The midpoint of the unilateral pupil can be used as a rough guide to the correct alignment in the sagittal plane.

cerebellopontine angle), aneurysm, multiple sclerosis or demyelinating peripheral neuropathies. These lesions produce destruction, irritation or demyelination of the nerve, resulting in pain. Biochemical changes seen in patients with trigeminal neuralgia include elevated substance P, and a hypoactive serotonergic system.[2] While the aetiology remains generally unknown, both central and peripheral mechanisms have been proposed.[3]

## Clinical features

- Trigeminal neuralgia (tic douloureux) presents as episodic, recurrent unilateral face pain. It is described as a sudden, high-intensity jab, or like electric shocks.
- It typically lasts only a few seconds, with repetitive bursts over a period of seconds to a few minutes, followed by a refractory period of a few minutes. Episodes may occur just occasionally or many times a day. Episodes may occur frequently over several weeks to several months followed by prolonged painfree intervals.
- It may occur in ophthalmic, maxillary or mandibular divisions but most commonly occurs in the mandibular division in the region of the lower lip and jaw. Involvement of the ophthalmic division is unusual.
- Pain is frequently triggered by trivial stimulation of the face around the nose and mouth, such as touching the face, washing, shaving, chewing and talking. Avoidance of facial stimulation by the patient is helpful in differential diagnosis. Pain relief can sometimes occur by firm pressure by the hands around but not touching the trigger point.
- Incidence per year is 2.7 : 100 000 men and 5.0 per 100 000 women. It occurs mostly in the fifth and sixth decades, but can occur in younger patients in association with multiple sclerosis, vascular anomalies and tumours.[4]
- Neurological examination of the face is nearly always normal unless there is associated underlying pathology (multiple sclerosis, vascular abnormality or tumour). Neuroradiological studies are usually normal

and are not indicated unless there is suspicion of underlying pathology. An abnormal neurological examination, including corneal reflex, warrants a neurological opinion and computed tomographic (CT) or magnetic resonance imaging (MRI) scanning.[5]

## Differential diagnosis

- Vascular abnormality, tumour or multiple sclerosis will produce episodic lancinating pain of trigeminal neuralgia but there will be an additional component of persistent aching or burning pain.[6] There may be facial sensory loss or other associated neurological deficits. In patients less than 40 years old, especially with bilateral symptoms, not previously known to have multiple sclerosis, this diagnosis should be considered.[7]
- Lesions involving the upper cervical cord may sometimes cause production of pain, or even loss of pain in the face, but will usually have manifestations of spinal cord involvement.
- Glossopharyngeal neuralgia is similar to trigeminal neuralgia except that the pain is located in the pharynx, tonsil or ear and is usually triggered by swallowing, yawning or eating.
- Atypical face pain describes face pain syndromes that cannot otherwise be classified. The pain is usually steady, diffuse, aching pain lasting

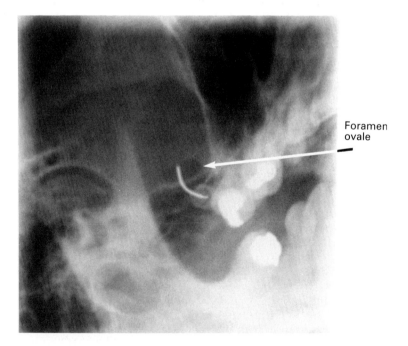

Foramen ovale

**Figure 18.2** View of foremen ovale with needle *in situ*. The foramen can be readily seen by extending the patient's neck and adjusting the angle of the image intensifier to 10° rotation and approximately 30° skew from the anteroposterior.

hours to days without paroxysms or trigger zones. It is most commonly seen in women aged 30–50.

- Postherpetic neuralgia can occur on the face and follows herpes zoster infection in the elderly. The pain is described as intense, aching, burning, with dysaesthesia.

## Treatment

### Medical treatment

Seventy per cent of patients will respond to pharmacological therapy alone. Attention must be paid to adequate dosages and combinations of drugs may be helpful.[8]

A suggested choice of drugs is to start with carbamazepine; baclofen or clonazepam may be added if carbamazepine monotherapy fails. Finally monotherapy with phenytoin, pimozide or valproic acid would be a reasonable next step.[9]

- Carbamazepine is the drug of first choice and will control the symptoms in the majority of patients.[10] A good response to carbamazepine supports the diagnosis of trigeminal neuralgia. Starting dose should be 100 mg orally twice daily, increasing by 100–200 mg every 3–4 days until pain relief is achieved or toxicity develops. A maximum dose is usually 1000–1200 mg/day, although older patients may not tolerate

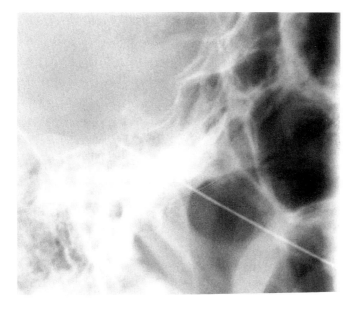

**Figure 18.3** Lateral view of skull showing needle *in situ*. The tip of the needle is inferior to the sella and should be approximately at the level of the clivus.

high doses. Carbamazepine has a short plasma half-life so needs to be given on a three- or four-times-a-day basis. A sustained-release preparation is available. After the patient has been free from pain for several weeks, attempts should be made to reduce the dose to the minimum necessary. Carbamazepine can produce bone marrow suppression and liver and renal impairment, so these should be monitored in the initial months of treatment. Sedation and ataxia are the major drawbacks with carbamazepine therapy and may require discontinuation of the drug. These side-effects can be diminished by reducing the dose. Patients may become refractory with time.

- Phenytoin once daily 300–600 mg per day. Sedation and ataxia may occur.
- Baclofen starting at 5–15 mg three times per day to a final dose of 40–80 mg per day. Sedation, ataxia and frank weakness may occur.
- Clonazepam 1–3 mg per day.[11] A therapeutic effect may be seen within 2 weeks. Sedation may occur in the elderly. Therapy should continue for at least 3–6 months.
- Valproic acid (15–30 mg/kg per day).
- Pimozide starting at 2 mg per day has been used.

### Surgical treatment

This is necessary when pharmacological therapy is ineffective or not tolerated.

- Radiofrequency (RF) trigeminal ganglion thermocoagulation can be performed by RF heating (65–75°C for 1–2 min) of an insulated needle (Radionics, 5 mm uninsulated tip) placed percutaneously through the foramen ovale into the ganglion. This is probably the procedure of choice when pharmacological therapies have failed. It is done under general anaesthesia or neuroleptanalgesia using image intensification. It is possible to stimulate (100 Hz 0.1–0.5 V) down the needle with the patient awake to determine in which division the needle is placed. General anaesthesia or sedation is needed for needle placement and for the thermocoagulation but the patient will need to be able to respond to questioning during stimulation.

  A variety of anaesthesia techniques have been used. There is a low incidence of morbidity or mortality and a high incidence of pain relief. There may be some residual sensory deficit in the face or tongue due to the procedure. It is also successful in treating trigeminal neuralgia when due to underlying pathology.[12] If needed, it can be repeated without added risk or difficulty, and may need to be repeated at intervals of 6 months–5 years.
- Injection of glycerol (0.1–0.2 ml) into the cistern of Meckel's cave through a needle placed percutaneously.[13] This is similar to RF thermocoagulation in technique. Placement can be confirmed by use of a small amount of water-soluble contrast material or electrical stimulation. Mean painfree interval has been reported to be 32 months.[14] Sensory disturbances to the face may occur with this procedure.

- Microvascular decompression of the trigeminal nerve.[1] This is a major neurosurgical operation and should probably only be considered after pharmacological and percutaneous procedures. There are associated risks, such as neurological deficit with this procedure, that do not occur with the percutaneous approach.
- Peripheral neurectomy of a branch of the trigeminal nerve to denervate the trigger area. Typically the supraorbital, infraorbital or inferior alveolar (dental) nerves are either avulsed or subjected to cryotherapy.[15] Recurrence of the pain is more common with this procedure, and repeated procedures are more difficult and less likely to succeed.

Destructive procedures of ganglion or peripheral nerves can result in a new and unpleasant dysaesthetic condition (anaesthesia dolorosa). This can be even more problematical than the original condition. It is more likely to occur if the denervation has been extensive, so care must be exercised to limit the extent of surgical procedures.

## References

1. Janetta PJ. Treatment of trigeminal neuralgia by suboccipital and transcranial operations. *Clin Neurosurg* **24:** 538–549, 1977
2. Bouckoms AJ, Poletti CH, Sweet WH, Carr D, Keith D. Trigeminal facial pain: a model of peptides and monoamines in intracerebral cerebrospinal fluid. *Agressologie* **32:** 271–274, 1991
3. Olin RJ. Etiologies of tic douloureux: trigeminal neuralgia. *Cranio* **8:** 319, 1990
4. Bullitt E, Tew JM, Boyd J. Intracranial tumours in patients with facial pain. *J Neurosurg* **64:** 865–871, 1986
5. Darlow LA, Brooks ML, Quinn PD. Magnetic resonance imaging in the diagnosis of trigeminal neuralgia. *J Oral Maxillofac Surg* **50:** 621–626, 1992
6. Cusick JF. Atypical trigeminal neuralgia. *JAMA* **245:** 2328–2329, 1981
7. Iragui VJ, Wiederholt WC, Rominie JS. Evoked potentials in trigeminal neuralgia associated with multiple sclerosis. *Arch Neurol* **43:** 444–446, 1986
8. Zakrzewska JM, Patsalos PN. Drugs used in the management of trigeminal neuralgia. *Oral Surg Oral Med Oral Pathol* **74:** 439–450, 1992
9. Green MW, Selman JE. Review article: the medical management of trigeminal neuralgia. *Headache* **31:** 588-592, 1991
10. Crill WE. Carbamazepine. *Ann Intern Med* **79:** 844–847, 1973
11. Swerdlow M, Cundill J. Anticonvulsant drugs used in the treatment of lancinating pain. A comparison. *Anaesthesia* **36:** 1129–1132, 1981
12. Sweet WH, Wespic JG. Controlled thermocoagulation of trigeminal ganglion and rootlets for differential destruction of pain fibres: Part 1. Trigeminal neuralgia. *J Neurosurg* **40:** 143–156, 1973
13. Hakanson S. Tic douloureux treated by the injection of glycerol into the retrogasserian subarachnoid space; long term results. *Acta Neurochir Suppl* **33:** 471–472, 1984
14. Fujimaki T, Fukushima T, Miyazaki S. Percutaneous retrogasserian glycerol injection in the management of trigeminal neuralgia: long-term follow-up. *J Neurosurg* **73:** 212–216, 1990
15. Quinn JH. Repetitive peripheral neurectomies for neuralgia of second and third divisions of trigeminal neuralgia. *Clin Neurosurg* **24:** 550–556, 1977

# 19

# Phantom limb pain

**J. E. Williams**

Phantom limb pain is the experience of pain within the amputated portion of the limb. Following amputation, almost all patients will experience phantom sensations such as awareness of size, position and movement, but a smaller number of patients will actually complain of pain in the phantom limb. Phantom limb pain is an extremely distressing condition which is very difficult to treat despite the use of numerous therapeutic modalities. Most success has come from attempting to treat any pain that exists prior to amputation.

## Incidence

The incidence of phantom limb pain has been reported in many different surveys as being between 2 and 97%. Early reports of the incidence were of the order of 5–10% of amputees; however these were probably gross underestimates of the true incidence because of patients' reluctance to admit pains for fear of losing credibility with their doctor. More recent reports have indicated an incidence of between 65 and 85% of amputees. One survey[1] showed that 85% of all amputees had phantom limb pain sufficiently severe to necessitate withdrawal from social and work environments for considerable periods of time each year, and they concluded that severe phantom limb pain is the 'usual condition' for amputees.

Phantom limb pain will usually improve in time. Jensen *et al.*[2] showed the incidence of pain declining from 72% of amputees immediately following surgery to 59% at 2 years. Other studies reveal an incidence of 10% at 2 years following amputation.

## Aetiology

Most amputations are either traumatic or occur as a result of systemic diseases such as diabetes or vascular occlusive disease. There is no difference in the incidence of phantom limb pain between the different causes. However, the severity and incidence of phantom limb pain are greater in patients who had poorly controlled preamputation pain and in patients with more proximal amputations.

The precise aetiology of phantom limb pain is still not clear but there are numerous different theories based on clinical and scientific studies. It is likely that after amputation change occurs throughout the nervous system from the periphery to the brain.

Proposed aetiological mechanisms include the following:

### Peripheral changes

In the cut nerve endings, painful neuromata and nerve sprouts develop which are exquisitely tender and sensitive to touch (allodynia).

### Spinal cord

Following sustained nociceptive input from a painful limb prior to amputation, morphological changes in the dorsal horn neurons and their receptive fields occur. These changes then propagate the pain response after amputation. The $N$-methyl-D-aspartate (NMDA) receptor complex may be responsible for the development of this 'memory of pain' within the cells and the subsequent changes (plasticity) in their functioning.

### Changes in the brain

These processes of memory of pain and plasticity also occur in the brain. Prolonged afferent input to the brain results in plastic changes within the cells and a development of a memory of the pain. When amputation occurs, the lack of further afferent input upsets this memory and pain is re-experienced.

## Clinical features

The patient with phantom limb pain may vary from experiencing occasional mild paraesthesiae causing minimal interference with daily life to constant severe pain disrupting normal activity and sleep. Usually the pain is described as burning, aching or cramp-like with occasional sharp, knife-like pains which may be exacerbated by periods of stress or fatigue.

## Management

Treatment of phantom limb pain is an urgent problem that should be treated as soon as possible to prevent more permanent plastic changes occurring within the nervous system. However, it is a condition that is often markedly resistant to any therapy. Sherman et al.[3] reported that only 1% of over 2000 amputees receiving treatment for phantom limb pain had lasting benefits from any of a multitude of treatments attempted.

Understandably, there is a high incidence of depression and anxiety amongst patients. Appropriate psychological and educational support should be available for patients and their family. Such support may help in reducing the incidence and severity of chronic pain.

A full medical history and physical examination should be taken from all patients. In particular, the presence of any precipitating factors should be investigated and the stump examined for skin infections, bony spurs, calluses, poorly fitting prostheses and trigger points.

## Prophylactic treatment

Bach et al.[4] reported the effectiveness of epidural bupivacaine for 3 days prior to amputation in reducing the incidence of phantom pain in the first postoperative year. They proposed that by reducing peripheral input the pain memory is abolished, resulting in fewer postoperative pain problems. However, the number of patients included in this study was small and the results have not yet been repeated in any other studies.

## Treatment of established phantom limb pain

- Physiotherapy and other conservative measures: This includes help with fitting of prostheses, transcutaneous electrical nerve stimulation, ultrasound, hot or cold pads and rest.
- Non-steroidal anti-inflammatory drugs: These are sometimes effective. A test dose of intravenous ketorolac could be tried and if effective, oral non-steroidal anti-inflammatory drugs could be started.
- Anticonvulsants and antidepressants: Carbamazepine (400–600 mg/day) has been effective in treating sharp, lancinating pains. Amitriptyline (up to 100 mg/day) is effective in many chronic pain conditions. Chlorpromazine (up to 500 mg/day) has been used, but side-effects may be prominent.
- Other drugs: Ketamine (NMDA antagonist), has been used subcutaneously with some success (0.1–0.2 mg/kg). There have been some reports of success with the use of $\beta$-blockers (propranolol 80 mg daily).
- Nerve blocks: Many different nerve blocks have been tried. Their effectiveness is based upon anecdotal reports in the literature. It is hoped that by blocking peripheral input to the central nervous system, periods of analgesia might result. Frequency of performing nerve blocks will depend on their effectiveness. The following blocks have been used:
  - trigger point injections using local anaesthetic solution
  - infiltration of local anaesthetic into painful areas
  - sympathetic nerve block (stellate ganglion block or lumbar sympathetic block); these blocks may help differentiate somatic and sympathetically mediated pain
  - regional nerve blocks (e.g. brachial or lumbar plexus)
  - neuraxial opioids, such as fentanyl 75 $\mu$g, have been used effectively in the immediate postoperative period, but their use may aggravate symptoms in the patient with established phantom limb pain.
- Invasive therapies: Invasive techniques such as cordotomy and neuroablation have been used but success rates are low. Dorsal column stimulators have been shown to be only minimally effective in some patients. Intrathecal opioid therapy via indwelling catheter may be helpful in some patients.

## Conclusion

Phantom limb pain remains a very difficult pain problem. Whenever possible, treatment should commence preoperatively in an attempt to break the memory of pain which may have become established within the nervous system over time. In established phantom limb pain, management should commence with an initial evaluation to include a full history, clinical examination and relevant investigations. Local causes of pain within the stump should be excluded. Following this, treatment with drugs and nerve blocks should be started. Throughout, it is important to recognize the importance of psychological and social factors in the overall well-being of the patient with phantom limb pain.

## References

1. Sherman RA, Sherman C. Prevalence and characteristics of chronic phantom pain among American veterans: results of a trial survey. *Am J Phys Med* **62:** 227–238, 1983
2. Jensen TS, Krebs B, Nielsen J, Rasmussen P. Immediate and long-term phantom limb pain in amputees: incidence, clinical characteristics and relationship to preamputation pain. *Pain* **21:** 267–278, 1985
3. Sherman RA, Sherman CJ, Parker L. Chronic phantom and stump pain among American veterans: results of a survey. *Pain* **18:** 83–95, 1984
4. Bach S, Noreng MF, Tjellden NU. Phantom limb pain in amputees during the first 12 months following limb amputation, after preoperative lumbar epidural blockade. *Pain* **33:** 297, 1988

## Further reading

1. Hord AH. Phantom pain. In Raj PP (ed.) *Practical Management of Pain*, St. Louis, Mosby-Year Book Inc, 1992
2. Jensen TS, Rasmussen P. Phantom pain and related phenomena after amputation. In Melzack R, Wall P (eds) *Textbook of Pain*. Churchill Livingstone, New York, 1994
3. Byas-Smith M. *Management of Acute Exacerbations of Chronic Pain Syndromes*. In Sinatra RS, Hord AH, Ginsberg B, Preble LM (eds) *Acute Pain, Mechanisms and Management*, St. Louis, Mosby-Year Book Inc, 1992

# 20

# Poststroke pain

**E. J. Roberts**

The first description of poststroke pain was by Dejerine and Roussy[1] who named it thalamic syndrome following postmortem findings in 3 patients. These patients had a characteristic clinical picture after stroke:

- slight hemiplegia
- persistent superficial hemianaesthesia and disturbances of deep sensation
- hemiataxia and astereognosis
- intractable pain
- choreoathetoid movements

At postmortem these patients were found to have a lesion localized to the external, posterior and inferior region of the thalamus which also involved the median nuclei and part of the posterior limb of the internal capsule. Dejerine and Roussy held that pain was not necessarily a constant symptom.[1]

The term thalamic syndrome is commonly used synonymously with central pain but the latter can occur after central nervous system damage at any level. Occlusive stroke of the cerebral cortex is the most common. Other less frequent causes include brainstem and cerebellar stroke and haemorrhagic stroke. The incidence of pain after stroke is 1 : 15 000. It is more likely with increasing age and when there is a partial sensory loss.

The International Association for the Study of Pain (IASP)[2] defines central pain of brain origin as 'diffuse, unilateral pain, often burning with allodynia, hypoaesthesia, hypoalgesia, hyperpathia, dysaesthesia and neurological signs of damage to structure which supply the affected region'. Thus the term poststroke pain describes pain of many different natures and intensity.

## Pathophysiology

Sensory neurons of all modalities enter the spinal cord from the periphery by the dorsal root. The pain fibres synapse with a posterior horn cell and then cross in front of the central canal and ascend cephalad in the contralateral spinothalamic tract, ending in the thalamus. This is where pain reaches the conscious level. Other sensory input also ends here via ascending reticular fibres and the posterior column. From the thalamus the stimulation reaches the higher centres, which in their turn exert a descending control over sensory input. There are direct and indirect pathways exerting a modulating influence at every level of brainstem and spinal cord, including the dorsal horn of the spinal cord, where they are thought to form part of the 'gate control' of pain mechanism.

The pain following stroke is caused by a destruction of function in this central pain pathway. There is faulty conduction and the modulating mechanisms are disrupted. It is thought that irritative mechanisms in the damaged grey matter contribute to the pain.

Tasker used electrical stimulation of the brain during stereotactic pain relief surgery to investigate this. In patients with central pain, burning and painful sensations were frequently evoked at sites both ipsi- and contra-laterally after stimulation of the mesencephalic tegmentum medial to the spinothalamic tract and the medial thalamus. In those not suffering from central pain there was almost no abnormal response to the stimulation. As the responses were not in the expected part of the body, some somato-topographic rearrangement is suspected, i.e. abnormal connections on the afferent and efferent pathways. The somatotopographic reorganization suggests that the stroke, in destroying parts of the thalamus or other higher centres, results in the redirection of afferent pathways. A deafferented part of the thalamus may acquire new afferent pathways while maintaining its normal routes to the cortex.

Tasker also found that the recording of neuronal activity was abnormal at the thalamic level in these patients with alterations in spontaneous and evoked firing rates, and abnormal responses to stimulation.

There have been few studies investigating changes following central nervous system damage but they do show that, although there is limited regeneration of neuronal tissue, those elements which remain can undergo considerable alteration which may affect their function and the processing of somatosensory information. Lesions of similar site, size and nature do not all produce the same degree of poststroke pain, if any. It appears that a threshold of neuronal activity has to be reached before pain is felt and that this varies greatly between patients and with their affect and personality.

## Clinical features

The pain onset may be immediate or long after the initial insult but the pain picture is similar in both groups. Selected patients are particularly suscept-ible to developing pain following a stroke, particularly with increasing age. The neurological lesion may present with clinically detectable sensory loss, but need not, although the involvement of somatosensory pathways and relay nuclei is necessary.

Most patients usually suffer from a constant pain, usually described as burning, numb or tingling and unlike anything normally provoked by a noxious stimulus. Some 14–50% of patients will complain of an inter-mittent or lancinating pain which may accompany the background 'steady' pain. A group of patients suffering from poststroke pain may suffer from evoked pain in response to stimuli not normally regarded as painful (allodynia). The pain may be unbearable and cause violent emotional and physical reactions. Evoked pain is usually late in onset, poorly localized and persistent. Central pain may manifest itself as facial pain and it is important to differentiate this from facial pain of trigeminal origin, as blocking the trigeminal ganglion in central pain will make it worse. A further group may suffer from sympathetic dysfunction and these present with vasomotor and trophic disorders.

The clinical picture is thus a rather depressing one, of an elderly patient with at best a constant pain and some functional loss from the stroke, which may be compounded by additional stabbing pains, evoked pain or allodynia, with or without intermittent flushing, sweating or other sympathetically mediated signs in some part of the body.

## Principles of management of poststroke pain

The three categories of poststroke pain respond to different treatments, which suggests different mechanisms for the pain:

- The steady pain is not relieved by opiates, or if there is a response it is not reversed by naloxone. It may be relieved by thiopentone, which suggests a central mechanism.
- The intermittent stabbing pain resembles nociceptive pain and may be relieved by opioids or surgery, suggesting a peripheral process.
- Evoked pain may be relieved by surgical interruption of pathways or a local anaesthetic block. Sympathetic blocks such as stellate ganglion or lumbar sympathetic block may give some temporary relief of both evoked and constant pain, as well as the obvious help with symptoms which are sympathetically mediated.

Many cases of poststroke pain are not amenable to conventional treatment and so the approach has to be somewhat empirical, whilst bearing in mind the generalizations of the previous paragraph. There is no proven method of preventing poststroke pain occurring.

### Drug treatment

A range of drugs are used, not all conventional analgesics but all involved in modifying neurotransmission.

#### Tricyclic antidepressants

These may be useful for pain described as burning and constant in nature, and for evoked allodynia pain. Amitriptyline is the usual first-choice treatment and patients may obtain relief for more than a year. Analgesia may be obtained at low doses. This group of antidepressants works by increasing the concentration of 5-hydroxytryptamine and noradrenaline in the central nervous system by blocking synaptic reuptake. They also potentiate endogenous endorphins. Treatment has to be prolonged as it may take several weeks for an effect to be achieved. The patient needs reassurance that many of the side-effects will abate with chronic use. A single night-time dose of 10–25 mg is started and can be increased after 2 weeks and again at 6 weeks to a maximum of 150 mg. It would seem to be worthwhile starting tricyclic antidepressants as soon as poststroke pain appears, because they may be more effective if used early.

### Anticonvulsants

Carbamazepine is well-recognized as a treatment for trigeminal neuralgia but may also be useful for the spontaneous shooting pains associated with poststroke pain. The dosage is the same as that for anticonvulsant therapy.

### Anti-inflammatory drugs

Poststroke pain is not generally relieved by analgesics but early use of nonsteroidal anti-inflammatory drugs may be helpful.

### Clonidine

This drug may be useful in poststroke pain, especially that which is sympathetically mediated. On introduction of the drug, sympathetic outflow is reduced. Later, it reduces the response of peripheral vessels to sympathetic outflow. Clonidine also has analgesic properties which are not reversed by naloxone and this may contribute to its usefulness. Clonidine has been used epidurally for chronic non-cancer pain and its effect is thought to be due to a postsynaptic activation of inhibitory pathways synapsing in the dorsal horn of the spinal cord.

### Opiates

Again these are not often useful but are frequently tried when other treatment has failed. The new opioid tramadol may be more effective as it has an effect on 5-hydroxytryptamine and noradrenaline uptake. Unfortunately, it has pronounced emetic properties which may preclude its use in large doses.

### Naloxone

Budd[6] reported that large doses of intravenous naloxone altered perfusion of the damaged area of the brain and afforded some analgesia. However, further studies by the Pain Research Institute at Liverpool have not reproduced these results and it seems that naloxone does not have a place in the management of poststroke pain.

## Other treatment

### Local anaesthetic blocks

These are useful in several types of pain. If the pain is well-localized, local blocks alone may afford temporary relief, but they are most often used in conjunction with a sympathetic block. Guanethidine may be given as an intravenous sympathetic block and it also has a local anaesthetic effect. The dosage is 10–20 mg using a Bier's block technique. The methods of sympathetic ganglion blockade are well-described in textbooks of local anaesthesia.

### Surgical intervention

Many surgical techniques have been tried, ranging from cordotomy through stereotactic ablation to frontal lobotomy, but with little or no success and these are not in general usage.

### Electroconvulsive therapy (ECT)

ECT has been found to be effective in other chronic pain states but a group at Oxford have shown no improvement after a 2-week course of six treatments. Deep electrical stimulation of the brain has also not been demonstrated to be a useful technique.

## Summary

Poststroke pain is a mixed group of chronic pain symptoms and as such needs careful history-taking and examination before the start of any treatment. The use of antidepressants, anticonvulsants and the judicious use of sympathetic blockade seems to be the best approach, but success with any treatment may be limited. Psychological support of the patient is of the utmost importance while treatments are tried. They will be most successful when the patient has full confidence in the practitioner.

## References

1. Dejerine, Roussy. Le syndrome thalamique. *Rev Neurol Paris* **14:** 521–532, 1906
2. Gildenberg PL. Sterotactic treatment of head and neck pain. *Res Clin Studies Headache* **5:** 102–121, 1978
3. International Association for the Study of Pain Subcommittee on Taxonomy. Classification of chronic pain syndromes and definition of pain terms. *Pain* **3** (suppl): 1986
4. Tasker RR. Identification of pain processing systems by electrical stimulation of the brain. *Hum Neurobiol* **1:** 272, 1982
5. McQuay HJ, Carroll D, Glynn CJ. Dose response for analgesic effect of amitryptiline in chronic pain. *Anaesthesia* **48:** 281–285, 1993
6. Budd K. The use of naloxone in the treatment of intractable pain. *Neuropeptides* **5:** 419–422, 1985

7. Bainton, Fox Bowsher, Wells. A double blind trial of naloxone in central post-stroke pain. *Pain* **48:** 159–162, 1992
8. Fields Dubner Corvero, Advances in pain research therapy – Proceedings of the Fourth World Congress on Pain. Raven Press, 1984
9. Lipton S. The control of chronic pain. *Curr Topics Anaesth.* Edward Arnold, 1979
10. Charlton E. *Neuropath Pain Prescribers J* **33:** 244–249, 1993

# 21

# Scar pain

N. E. Payne

Scar pain is defined as the pain felt in the scar after healing has apparently taken place. It usually presents as an extension of the early postoperative pain, and most symptoms can be related to neurological damage and subsequent neuropathic pain.

## Clinical features

Pain of this nature is characteristically of a dysaesthetic, burning nature, exhibiting allodynia and hyperpathia. An exquisitely tender spot usually represents a neuroma within the scar.[1]

## Pathophysiology

The pathophysiological mechanisms present in scar pain are not yet fully clear. Several hypotheses have been postulated. Most refer to the origins of post-traumatic pain.

- Local tissue damage releases a number of compounds like potassium ions, substance P, prostaglandins and serotonin, all of which activate the primary afferent nociceptors leading to primary hyperalgesia. It can also lead to a decreased pain threshold in the surrounding area and thus a secondary hyperalgesia and to allodynia, whereby a normally non-noxious stimulus may result in pain.
- The resultant increased peripheral nociceptor sensitivity also leads to hyperalgesia by the increased synthesis of substance P in the dorsal root ganglion, in response to peripheral inflammation and an increased synthesis of glutamate, calcitonin gene-related peptide, dynorphins and encephalins in the spinal cord, which leads to the chronicity of the pain.
- Activation of C-fibres occurs and by repeated firing in response to tissue damage may lead to 'wind-up' of N-methyl-D-aspartate receptors in the wide dynamic range (WDR) neurons. This sensitization of the WDR neurons results in hyperpathia, where there is an exaggerated response to a noxious stimulus.

- Hypoxia in the local neurons can by scar entrapment lead to damage and disorganized neuronal regeneration with ephaptic transmission, whereby there is spontaneous firing which causes typically lancinating pain.
- In addition, the sensitized nociceptors can become more sensitive to efferent sympathetic activity, resulting in sympathetically maintained pain.
- Pain from scars can become chronic because the mechanisms listed above do not resolve, and result in gene expression, as demonstrated by c-*fos* and other proto-oncogene expression in the dorsal root ganglia, the spinal cord and cortical neurons, thus leading to neurogenic pain.

There may also be a mechanical component because of cicatrization leading to intermittent nerve/muscle compression during movement. This may necessitate a physical approach like a surgical release of a band of scar tissue. Occasionally retained sutures or other materials (like mesh in hernia repairs) can cause local problems and require surgical exploration.

## Clinical features

In general the pain clinician will be asked to help where there is a neurogenic component to the scar pain. A careful history and examination must exclude or identify non-neurogenic factors.

One must ascertain:

- Is the pain constant or intermittent, as intermittent pain may suggest a mechanical component?
- Is the pain associated with a prosthesis, suture or other implanted material, because surgical exploration may be indicated?
- Is the pain cyclical (in women), as it may indicate a surgical scar endometrioma?
- Do any provoking factors like coughing or straining at stool indicate other pathology, like herniation of tissue into the scar itself?
- Is the pain affected by ambient temperature or are there associated trophic/vascular changes that would suggest a sympathetically maintained element?

Typical clinical situations where scar pain can arise:

- post-thoracotomy
- post-sternotomy
- post-Pfannenstiel incision
- post-Caesarean section
- post-inguinal hernia repair
- post-mastectomy

In one series of post-thoracotomy scar pain,[2] the pain was so bad that 1–3% of patients sought medical advice. Post-sternotomy neuralgia can commonly occur after median sternotomy for open cardiac surgery. This causes a variable pain picture due to nerve entrapment in the hypertrophied scar tissue and neuroma formation.

In one study of 54 post-sternotomy patients,[3] the pain was shown to be derived from scar-entrapped neuromata of the 4–6th intercostal nerves in the upper and mainly left interchondral spaces, since local anaesthetic block resulted in immediate relief. This could be made permanent by repeated blocks in 57.4% of the patients. Neurolytic blocks with phenol achieved relief in a further 22.2% and alcohol infiltration in a further 9%. Overall success rate was 87%. Occasionally there will be hypertrophic scarring and keloid formation (Figure 21.1).

Surgical scar endometriomata classically present as a painful surgical scar mass that increases in size or tenderness during menstruation. It may present 1–20 years following Caesarean section but also following appendicectomy, episiotomy and hysterectomy.[4] The treatment of choice for this condition is wide local excision of the scar as medical management with hormone preparations is unsatisfactory.

Another unusual cause for scar pain that is provoked by lifting or coughing is herniation into the scar.[5] This will be obvious from the history and can only be rectified surgically.

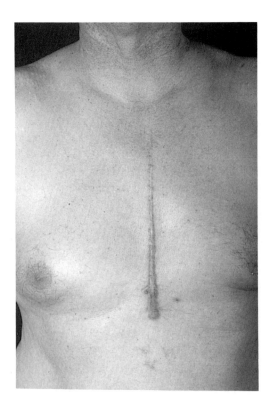

**Figure 21.1** Sternotomy keloid.

## Management

In general, neuropathic pain with no sympathetic element is difficult to treat. There is a lack of formal controlled trials assessing different modes of treatment for this condition. This means that generally there is a lack of uniformity among clinicians in their approach to these patients. There are anecdotal references in the scientific literature and a plethora of opinions!

he following management outlines an attempt to provide a rational approach to these patients and treatment devolves along three main lines – physical, pharmacological and psychological.

### Physical

The choice of treatments will usually begin with the least destructive and progress to the most destructive. This is because of the attendant risk of leaving the patient with even more severe neurogenic pain following lesioning. The treatments commonly used include the following:

- local infiltration with 0.5% bupivacaine with or without steroids (40 mg/ml methylprednisolone or 40 mg/ml triamcinolone). Pain clinicians will frequently start with bupivacaine and depot steroid preparations, although the case for steroids in such patients has yet to be proved in formal controlled clinical trials.
- local infiltration of streptomycin. The local injection of aminoglycosides has been studied more closely. In particular, streptomycin[6] has been used in the treatment of patients suffering from idiopathic facial pain, which led to trying infiltration of painful scars with it,[1] achieving some success. It is thought that the effect is achieved by reducing the excitability of peripheral nociceptors, suppressing ephaptic transmission and reducing the excitability of primary afferent nociceptors. Reduction in ephaptic transmission from sympathetic fibres to primary nociceptive afferents and modulation in the release of transmitters from primary afferent nerve terminals. Exposure to aminoglycosides may even result in cell death.

  Effect may be achieved by axonal transport of aminoglycosides to the nerve bodies in the dorsal root ganglia where protein production is altered and thus normal cellular function is impaired. Clinically streptomycin can, if given as a course of weekly infiltrations of 1 g dissolved in 1% lignocaine over 5 weeks, achieve complete resolution of neuropathic pain without causing anaesthesia. In practice, the sooner the clinician can start treatment after the development of pain, the better the likely outcome. Sometimes it is necessary to repeat the course 6 months later.

  Toxicity was a problem when large amounts of streptomycin were given parenterally, daily, for 2 months in the course of treating tuberculosis. In the outlined dosage regime it is unlikely to be a problem, but to be safe, it is advisable to have an audiogram performed initially to check on the function of the eighth cranial nerve.

The aminoglycosides can be both oto- (especially the vestibular branch) and nephrotoxic.

- Cryotherapy, especially if tender neuromas are suspected
- Infiltration of neurolytic agents phenol 6% aqueous, absolute alcohol
- Locally destructive radiofrequency lesioning
- Surgical re-exploration

Several studies have looked at cryoanalgesia for the relief of scar pain and have concluded[7–9] that the technique is useful, with a high patient acceptability and a low incidence of post-therapy sequelae. In one study of 28 patients suffering from chronic pain who had previously noted temporary relief from local anaesthetic blocks, cryogenic blocks were compared with phenol blocks of peripheral nerves and neuromas. The authors concluded that neurolytic blocks were not particularly effective, even though local anaesthetic blocks produced significant but temporary pain relief.[10] There is still no guarantee of achieving complete pain relief with these methods.

- Sympathetic nerve blocks: If it is suspected clinically that there is a sympathetically maintained element to the pain, a relevant sympathetic block with local anaesthetic should be performed. If this produces pain relief, then a permanent sympathetic block may be indicated by repeating the block with aqueous phenol 6% or absolute alcohol. But the clinician must always bear in mind the potential for producing post-denervation hypersensitivity, especially in a young patient, and that repeated sympathetic blockade may be a better option.
- Some success has been reported with infiltration of 10% solution of ammonium chloride. Although ammonium chloride can be toxic, various derivatives have been tested for local anaesthetic activity versus toxicity and there may be some promising new compounds developed.[11]
- Direct nerve stimulation using implanted electrodes has been used for post-traumatic painful peripheral neuropathies.[12] This was a small study of 19 patients followed up for an average of 11.5 months, where pain was completely relieved in 11 (58%) patients and in 4 (21%) the pain was sufficiently relieved to discontinue analgesics. The authors emphasized the importance of patient selection and implantation proximal to the area of injury.

### Pharmacological

- Opioids may not be effective because there is often a major neurogenic component to scar pain treatment. The ability to produce opiate dependence in these situations is a concern.
- Centrally acting analgesics like amitriptyline and maprotiline that enhance descending cortical inhibition via serotoninergic and noradrenergic pathways from the locus coeruleus offer the best form of therapy for continuous burning dysaesthetic pain. Both drugs have common side-effects which include dry mouth, sedation, blurred vision

and constipation. In general, maprotiline causes fewer antimuscarinic side-effects but, since the smallest size tablet is 25 mg, maprotiline will often cause considerable sedation even at the lowest dose. Amitriptyline can be started at 10 mg, but even this can cause marked sedation as well as the other side-effects.

The greatest battle the pain clinician faces is to persuade the patient that treatment needs to be continued for 6–9 months in order to help the nervous system 'heal'. The sedative effects do lessen with time, as do the other side-effects and the patient must persevere. Note that sometimes the morning sedation can be tempered by advising the patient to take the drug at 6.00 p.m. rather than on retiring for the night. Strong opioid and non-steroidal anti-inflammatory based analgesics (from the patient's viewpoint) may not actually work. Reassure the patient that they are not 'mad' and not just being treated for depression.

If there is a problem with non-compliance then the pain clinician may consider prescribing the more expensive – and often less effective – serotonin-specific reuptake inhibitors like fluoxitene which, at a dose of 20 mg, only rarely causes morning sedation. It has very few antimuscarinic side-effects and appears to be cardiovascularly stable and thus appears relatively safe in patients who have mild cardiac pathology as well.

- Anticonvulsants: Occasionally there will be lancinating pain as a component and this is thought to be due to ephaptic discharges from the damaged nerve. This can best be treated by anticonvulsant drugs such as carbemazepine at an initial dose of 100 mg t.d.s., increasing to 400 mg t.d.s., as indicated by patient response, whilst monitoring side-effects such as sedation and haematological and hepatic function. If the lancinating pain component is not controlled with carbemazepine alone, sodium valproate 200 mg t.d.s. may be substituted or even added.

  It is rare to eliminate scar pain completely by drugs alone but they are useful adjuncts to physical treatments.

**Psychological**

As with all pain, individual patients' emotional reaction will have a large bearing on their suffering. Operations that are perceived as altering body image or even mutilating, such as mastectomy/amputation, more often lead to chronic postoperative pain in the scar.

Horrific scars from burns may not demonstrate clinical hyperalgesia or hyperpathia but may lead to a patient's perception of disfigurement and negative body image which may add a substantial component to the patient's pain. Cognitive-behavioural therapy with a clinical psychologist may do a great deal to help relieve a patient's suffering.

Time is a great healer. In one study of 120 mastectomy patients, 42 (35%) developed scar pain within 3 months. Fifteen of these (13%) experienced constant scar pain. At 1 year 25 patients (23%) still had scar pain and 13 (12%) had experienced scar pain throughout the entire year, but only 2 (out of the original 15) still had constant pain.[13]

## The future

Wound healing is a complex sequence of events beginning with tissue injury, mediated by inflammation, and ending long after re-epithelialization is complete. Wound creation should aim for the minimum amount of tissue necrosis in order to prevent delays in healing. Thus, clean scalpel incisions heal far better than electrosurgically, cryosurgically or laser surgically created wounds.[14] Research and controlled clinical experience have provided a better understanding so that clinicians can influence the events of healing to reduce pain, for example, using silicone gel sheets[15] and steroids[16] in the prevention of keloid and hypertrophic scar formation.

## References

1. Gallagher J, Hamann W. Chronic neuropathic pain: aminoglycosides, peripheral somatosensory mechanisms and painful disorders. In: (Atkinson RS, Adams AP, eds) *Recent Advances in Anaesthesia and Analgesia*, vol 16. Churchill Livingstone, p. 210
2. Conacher ID. Percutaneous cryotherapy for post-thoracotomy neuralgia. *Pain* **25:** 227–228, 1986
3. Delfaque RJ, Bromley JJ. Post stemotomy neuralgia: a new pain syndrome. Comment *Anesth Analg* **69:** 692, 1989
4. Koger KE, Shatney CH, Hedge K, McClenathan JH. Surgical scar endometrioma. *Surg Gynecol Obstet* **177:** 243–246, 1993
5. Meek JC, Pollen E, Koudstaal J, Versteege C, Maesen FP. Pain in scar as an early symptom of acquired thoracic lung hernia. *Eur Respir J* **4:** 505–507, 1991
6. Stajcic Z, Juniper RP, Todorovic L. Peripheral streptomycin/lidocaine injections versus lidocaine alone in the treatment of idiopathic trigeminal neuralgia. A double-blind controlled trial. *J Cranio-Max-Fac Surg* **18:** 243–246, 1990
7. Jones MJT, Murrin KR. Intercostal block with cryotherapy. Ann R Cell Surg **69:** 261–262, 1987
8. Johannesen N, Masden G, Ahlburg P. Neurological sequelae after cryoanalgesia for thoracotomy pain relief. *Ann Chir Gynaecol* **79:** 108–109, 1990
9. Zouboulis CC, Plume P, Orfanos CE. Outcomes of cryosurgery in keloids and hypertrophic scars. A prospective trial of case series. *Arch Dermatol* **129:** 1146–1151, 1993
10. Ramamurthy S, Walsh NE, Shoenfeld L, Hoffnan J. Evaluation of neurolytic blocks using phenol and cryogenic block in the management of chronic pain. *J Pain Symptom Manage* **4:** 72–75, 1989
11. Gregan F, Novomesky P, Racanska E, Kettmann V. Synthesis and local anaesthetic activity of some derivatives of N,N-dimethyl-2-(2-alkoxyphenylcarbamoyloxy)-1, 1-dimethylammonium chlorides. *Farmaco* **47:** 327–343, 1992
12. Waisbrod H, Panhaus C, Hansen D *et al*. Direct nerve stimulation for painful peripheral neuropathies. *J Bone Joint Surg* **67B:** 470–472, 1985
13. Skov J, Kroner K, Krebs B, Hvid HM, Jorgensen HS. Pain and dysaesthesias in the mastectomy scar. *Ugeskr-Laeger* **152:** 3081–3084, 1990
14. Zitelli J. Wound healing for the clinician. *Adv Dermatol* **187:** 243–267, 1987
15. Farquhar K. Silicone gel and hypertrophic scar formation: a literature review. *Can J Occup Ther* **59:** 78–86, 1992
16. Tang YW. Intra- and postoperative steroid injections for keloids and hypertrophic scars. *Br J Plast Surg* **45:** 371–373, 1992

# 22

# Pain of unknown aetiology

**N. L. Padfield**

Commonly the pain clinician will come across a patient whose pain does not fit a known medical condition. This is perplexing for both patient and physician. Such patients have often seen many specialists and have had as many opinions as to cause, treatment and prognosis. They arrive in the clinic presenting a variety of emotions and often a considerable degree of pain behaviour. In some cases the very mystery of their condition is self-perpetuating, as the attention focused on the patient may result in secondary gain. The nature of the pain in terms of site, duration, periodicity, intensity and quality has often been long forgotten.

It is against this background that the pain clinician must return to a basic scientific evaluation of the symptoms and signs. It can be a battle of wills to prise the information from the patient, as often the patient will obstinately continue to describe symptoms in affective terms. As such interviews are time-consuming and frustrating for the clinician, it is all too easy to label the patient as mad and give up. However, the detective in us should be allowed free rein, as on the occasion of 'cracking the code' there is great satisfaction.

## History

The clinician must be satisfied as to the pathophysiology of the pain. So is it:

- nociceptive by activation of physiologically normal nociceptive nerve fibres (i.e. sharp, well-localized, etc.)
  - somatic?
  - visceral?
- neuropathic by injury to the nervous system (i.e. burning, poorly localized, etc.)?
- sympathetically maintained (i.e. with vascular and trophic changes, etc.)?
- a combination of mechanisms?

Occasionally one can be lucky and find some overlooked relevant trauma in the patient's past history, but commonly the patient will not admit or is unaware of any. Job or occupation, past or present, may give some clues – musculoskeletal strain, exposure to toxic chemicals, stress and somatization. A history of infections, especially viral flu-like illnesses, may have preceded the pain. Family history may give some pointers. Social circumstances and attitudes of immediate cohabiting family members may indicate if there is illness behaviour.

A detailed systematic enquiry into general health, allergies, medications past and present, physical treatments, i.e. physiotherapy, surgery, specific invasive pain therapies and investigations will, if not suggesting the diagnosis, often give the clinician enough information to reassure the patient that nothing serious requiring immediate rectification has been overlooked. Any previous medical illness requiring hospitalization – tuberculosis, diabetes mellitus, encephalitis, viral illnesses and streptococcal upper respiratory infections, cerebrovascular accidents – may have great relevance, though this may have escaped the patient and his or her previous medical attendants. Any history of drug abuse and any history of psychological disease must be elicited.

A detailed history of provoking and relieving factors may indicate a musculoskeletal cause but, because the sclerotomal/myotomal pain representation may mimic a number of other clinical disease entities, it is these which will have been exhaustively investigated without result. An example of this would be psoas myofasciitis mimicking renal pain or gallbladder pain. It is immensely satisfying when baffled surgical colleagues refer such patients as an act of desperation and the pain is alleviated by an appropriate local anaesthetic and steroid injection. Sadly, though, such a diagnostic and therapeutic triumph is the exception rather than the rule and if all screening tests fail to produce a satisfactory diagnosis, one is left with having to manage the patient along empirical lines.

## Common categories

Examples of commonly presenting pains of unknown origin (when history and examination along with all diagnostic tests do not produce a diagnosis/obvious cause) include:

- some types of headache
- some types of facial pain, i.e. glossodynia
- abdominal pain
- whole-limb pain
- pelvic pain
- total body pain

In such cases diagnosis is further hampered by other confusing features:

- Pain location, periodicity, character, intensity do not fit any recognizable anatomical distribution or established pathophysiological patterns.
- There may be a temporal relationship between the onset of pain and stress, caused by bereavement, for example.

- The patient may present obvious personality disorder or traits and there may be a marked discrepancy between the patient's behaviour and the severity of the pain.
- There may be other bizarre features that do not fit a typical pain syndrome. The patient may also have multiple pains in other parts of the body which may have been fully investigated without any obvious abnormality being discovered.

Whilst every effort must be made to discover the cause, it must be remembered that such exhaustive attention in terms of the clinician's time and the extent and nature of investigation will only reinforce the patient's conviction of serious illness. This is particularly so in cases of hysterical conversion. In this situation there are changes in sensory perception that do not correspond to organic nerve distribution and may be influenced by suggestion. Any anaesthesia or change of sensation that stops abruptly at the midline or that does not fit a segmental nerve supply, i.e. glove-and-stocking anaesthesia, may indicate hysteria. This impression may be reinforced by subsequent examination revealing a different area of anaesthesia or sensory deficit. If the patient still has intact stereognosis in an area of alleged anaesthesia and can also perform delicate tasks that require an intact sensorium, hysteria is a likely cause.

## Management

Whilst it is unfortunately a fairly universal experience that treatment of such patients is often followed by a poor or even adverse response, the pain clinician must make a management plan to follow. Management is often diagnostic initially and must be explained as such to the patient. Intelligible information is essential to win the confidence of your patient, without which management is doomed to failure. Management will often need to be multimodal and will include:

- anaesthetic approaches (temporary and permanent nerve blocks, epidurally administered drugs as single-shot, intermittent boluses, infusions through catheters or implanted reservoirs, etc.)
- neurostimulatory approaches (transcutaneous nerve stimulation, dorsal column stimulation)
- physical medicine approaches (physiotherapy, splinting and other surgical appliances)
- psychological approaches (training in cognitive approaches and relaxation)
- medical treatment of underlying affective disorders (depression, anxiety, schizophrenia, etc.)

Whatever modes of treatment the pain clinician follows, it is imperative not to create a rod for your back. This category of patients tends to be highly manipulative and the clinician will rue at leisure any unguarded promise as to treatment, cause or outcome. The emphasis of management must lie in encouraging patients to 'own' their pain and become responsible for coping with it. The pain clinician must be firm at the outset to make the patient understand that it is not the pain clinician's pain or problem, but exclusively the patient's. This can be a major battle but one that has to be won or else any further management is doomed to failure. The clinician must make it clear that his or her role is solely to help the patient cope with the pain problem. Realistic goals and expectations must be set from the outset.

Never promise anything that cannot be delivered in terms of response to invasive procedures and interventions or pharmacological therapy.

The use of pain diaries can be very helpful if the patient can be persuaded to cooperate. Reference to before and after treatment diaries can highlight successes by the patient in coping with the pain. The corollary is that exacerbating factors can be examined and discussed. Whatever the pain diaries show, if the patient has cooperated in their completion, the exercise is a useful education for both patient and clinician.

A typical pain diary would consist of a separate sheet for each day with divisions for each hour on the vertical axis and three divisions on the horizontal axis for pain score (visual analogue score 1–10); activity – resting, reading, walking, sleeping; and analgesic intake. Patients should be reminded that the more effort and commitment they show in completing the diaries, the better their eventual outcome.

## Common examples

### Atypical facial pain

- Half the sufferers also have headache.
- Three-quarters of such patients are female.
- Pain is often worse after therapeutic interventions – frequent nocebo response.
- Patients may express a desire for surgery and refuse psychiatric help.
- Premorbid personality is described as workaholic but when the pain intervenes they may develop anhedonia, dysphoria, insomnia, fatigue and loss of libido.

### Atypical genital pain

- Chronic pelvic pain without obvious pathology is mostly a female affliction but, rarely, males present with testicular pain.
- Patients may be convinced of serious pelvic pathology despite no obvious cause.
- In females theories include vasomotor instability with venous congestion and oedema, microscopic endometriosis or persistent hypersensitivity of pelvic viscera following parametritis.
- Onset of stress and pain appear correlated on psychological testing.
- There may be atypical anal pain (tenesmus).

**Total body pain and whole-limb pain**

This most often proves to be stress-related and responds to cognitive-behavioural training and the occasional use of psychotropic drugs, especially the antidepressants.

## Conclusion

In dealing with a patient referred with no obvious pathology despite exhaustive history-taking, physical examination and investigation, the pain clinician's chief role will be reassurance that there is nothing seriously wrong and support for the patient and family to help cope with any under-lying stress or other psychological problem. The pain clinician's attitude is paramount in the eventual success in encouraging patients to come to terms with their pain, be it real or imaginary.

23
_____

# Pain control in advanced cancer

### B. Amesbury

Pain is a common phenomenon in advanced cancer, occurring in approximately 70% of patients,[1] although as many as 25% of patients will not experience pain. However, 80% of patients with pain will have more than one pain.[2] It should be possible to achieve satisfactory pain relief in 95% or more of cases but often the figure is lower than this. In some cases the cause of the pain will not be directly due to the cancer but will be due to other disease processes. The pain of malignant disease may have physical, psychological, social and spiritual dimensions and this must be taken into consideration when planning treatments.

Palliative care refers to the area of medical practice involved in the continuing care – particularly pain and symptom control – of patients with advanced terminal diseases, particularly cancer. Palliative care also involves the psychosocial and spiritual care of patients and their families and carers and support for the bereaved.[3] As with other areas of medicine, an orderly approach should be made to each new patient beginning with a full history, and followed by examination and appropriate investigations, before a diagnosis is made and appropriate treatment is instituted. Cancer pain can be due to many causes and, therefore, an accurate diagnosis and frequent assessment of response to treatment are vital.

## Clinical features of cancer pain syndromes

- Bone metastases: for example, carcinoma of the lung, breast or prostate. These cause constant, sometimes intermittent, aching pain, often in multiple sites. Pain is worse on movement and may improve with rest. There may be tenderness over bone, e.g. a vertebra. Treat with both a non-steroidal anti-inflammatory drug (NSAID) and an analgesic according to the World Health Organization (WHO) analgesic ladder ranging from paracetamol, to weak opioid, to strong opioid.[3] Radiotherapy is also very effective in controlling bone pain.
- Invasion of hollow organ by tumour: This may occur with carcinoma of stomach or colon. There is a constant or irregular ache or spasm over the site of pain which may be worse with eating and improve with

vomiting and rest. The patient may have a distended abdomen and tender mass on examination. Treat with analgesics according to WHO analgesic ladder.

- Bowel colic or spasm: for example, carcinoma of colon. There is intermittent colicky pain with possible radiation. Pain may be worse after eating. Bowels may be disturbed. Possibly there is a distended abdomen and mass on examination. Pain may be due to constipation. Treat with analgesics (WHO analgesic ladder) and consider antispasmodics, for example, hyoscine butylbromide.

- Liver metastases or distension of liver capsule: for example, carcinoma of bowel, lung or breast. There is a constant ache or sharp pain, localized to the right upper quadrant. Hepatomegaly and tenderness on examination may be present. Treat with analgesics (WHO analgesic ladder) and dexamethasone 4–12 mg/day to reduce oedema and liver capsule distension.

- Invasion of coeliac plexus by tumour: This may occur with carcinoma of pancreas or stomach. There is a boring epigastric ache, which may radiate to the back. The patient may have local tenderness or mass. Treat with analgesics (WHO analgesic ladder) and consider coeliac plexus block.

- Bladder spasm: This occurs in carcinoma of bladder or prostate. There is intermittent colicky suprapubic pain, which may be worse on voiding urine if clots present. Suprapubic tenderness is possible. Treat the cause if possible, for example, infection or blood clots. Treat spasm with hyoscine butylbromide or oxybutynin.

- Ureteric colic: This may occur in carcinoma of ureter or bladder. There is intermittent colicky pain in the loin which may radiate to the groin. Loin tenderness is possible. Treat with hyoscine butylbromide and NSAIDs.

- Chest wall or rib pain: for example, carcinoma of lung or mesothelioma. There is a constant aching pain. The patient may have local tenderness which may be worse or stabbing in nature on breathing. Treat with NSAID and analgesic (WHO analgesic ladder). Consider intercostal nerve block, interpleural local anaesthetic or transcutaneous electrical nerve stimulation (TENS).

- Diffuse abdominal pain due to peritoneal metastases: for example, carcinoma of colon or ovary. There is a constant aching pain, and possibly sharp exacerbations. Pain may be worse on movement and there may be local tenderness or mass. Treat with analgesics (WHO analgesic ladder).

- Soft-tissue invasion: for example, carcinoma of lung or breast. Often there is an aching pain at the site of tumour and swelling if the site is superficial. Treat with analgesics (WHO analgesic ladder), NSAIDs and possibly steroids.

- Neuropathic pain, such as Pancoast's syndrome: This is a constant or intermittent stabbing or burning pain in a dermatomal distribution associated with altered sensation. Treat with analgesics (WHO analgesic ladder) and antidepressants, anticonvulsants or antiarhythmics for their pain-modifying action and consider steroids.

- Nerve compression pain: This may be caused by a retroperitoneal mass from carcinoma of ovary or colon. There is a constant aching or throbbing pain in a dermatomal distribution. Treat with analgesics (WHO analgesic ladder) and dexamethasone.
- Headache of raised intracranial pressure: This may be due to primary brain tumour or metastases. Headache may be localized or general. Reduce oedema with dexamethasone or possibly radiotherapy. Analgesia may require paracetamol or opioid.
- Epidural spinal cord compression from metastatic disease: for example, metastases from carcinoma of lung, breast or prostate. Pain is localized to the vertebral body with possible radicular pain in a dermatome and sensory changes and progressive weakness in limbs. Bladder and bowel sphincter symptoms occur late. Treat with dexamethasone and radiotherapy and consider spinal decompression.
- Painful muscle spasm: This may follow a hemiplegia secondary to a primary brain tumour. Painful spasm and muscle contractures can occur in a limb following a hemiplegia, or in the presence of a painful metastasis in a long bone. Treat with diazepam or baclofen.
- Infection of a fungating tumour: for example, carcinoma of breast. Bacterial superficial soft-tissue infection can be very painful, often when the tumour itself has not been painful. Treat with appropriate antibiotics following microbiological swab for culture and sensitivity.
- Pain related to treatment: for example, postsurgical incisional pain, postradiation mucositis or proctitis and painful peripheral neuropathy following chemotherapy. Treatment depends on the nature of the problem.

Further discussion of cancer pain syndromes is given by Portenoy.[4] Many pains in cancer patients are due to causes other than the cancer. It is important to identify these and treat accordingly.

### Common causes of non-cancer-related pain

- osteoarthritis
- simple tension headache
- constipation
- oral or oesophageal thrush
- pleurisy
- infected pressure sore
- distended bladder
- iatrogenic causes
- adverse drug reactions

## The management of cancer pain

- Accurate diagnosis of the cause of pain is essential and is obtained by taking a good history and performing an appropriate examination and investigations.
- Give the correct treatment – it may not always be an analgesic.

- Give treatment regularly, before pain returns.
- Treatment should be by mouth if possible – not injection.
- Frequent review and dose adjustments are necessary.

## The history

- The history should include full assessment of each pain including site, character, severity, precipitating and relieving factors, radiation and response to current and previous treatments. It should be determined if one or more pains are present and the same process conducted for each pain. Body or pain charts and visual analogue scales may be useful to identify painful areas and severity of pains.
- Consideration should be given to the medical history, particularly the current cancer history, for example, recently diagnosed metastatic disease. Previous problems should also be considered, such as peptic ulcer disease, arthritis and heart disease.
- Attention should be paid to psychological problems, such as depression, fear or tiredness, to social factors, such as family support, and to spiritual matters, for example, anger with God.

## Examination

The examination should be a full general examination including all the painful areas and relevant systems.

## Investigations

Plain X-rays and other radiological investigations are often the most useful. Biochemical, haematological and microbiological tests may also be helpful.

## Diagnosis

The correct diagnosis for the cause of each pain can then be made. The pain of advanced cancer has been described as 'total pain'[5] and attention to the emotional parts of the pain experience, such as anxiety, depression and insomnia, can help to achieve analgesia. The support, or otherwise, that a patient receives from his or her family and friends plays a part in the control of pain. Explanation of the cause of symptoms, reassurance about treatment and frequent follow-up all help to alleviate pain.

## Active treatments

At the time of diagnosis of the cause of pain it is important to consider active anticancer treatments as pain control measures.

- radiotherapy for the pain of bone metastases, headache from brain tumours, nerve compression pain and soft-tissue infiltration
- chemotherapy for control of small-cell lung cancer and locally advanced breast cancer

- hormone manipulation for carcinoma of breast or prostate
- prophylactic pinning of a metastasis in a long bone
- surgery for the formation of a stoma or a bypass procedure to relieve bowel obstruction
- neurosurgical decompression may have a role in spinal cord compression in addition to radiotherapy and high-dose dexamethasone

Advice from colleagues in oncology and surgery should be requested if appropriate.

## Opioid-responsive and opioid-non-responsive pain

It is possible to control most cancer pain with the use of oral analgesics either alone or with the addition of coanalgesics, for example, NSAIDs, steroids, antidepressants, anticonvulsants and antiarhythmics. However, in a small proportion of patients, particularly those with neuropathic pain, the pain does not respond well to ordinary analgesics. This has led to the distinction between opioid-responsive and opioid-non-responsive pain. In practice the side-effects of opioids may be dose-limiting despite attempts to control the side-effects. A good definition of opioid-non-responsive pain is pain that is unrelieved or poorly controlled by opioid analgesics at a dose that causes uncontrollable side-effects in spite of appropriate measures to control them.[6] Where a pain does appear to be opioid-non-responsive, the use of coanalgesics (see p. 241) is particularly important. It should then be possible to control the majority of pains in patients with cancer. As most patients have more than one pain and the pains are often at least partially responsive to opioids, most patients with advanced cancer and pain would be taking an opioid as part of their treatment.

### The World Health Organization analgesic ladder

The use of different classes of analgesic drugs has been promoted by the WHO for some years by the use of the WHO analgesic ladder.[3] This involves the progression from a

- non-opioid analgesic (for example, paracetamol) to a
- weak opioid (for example, co-proxamol) to a
- strong opioid (for example, morphine)

#### Non-opioid analgesics

For mild pain initial treatment with paracetamol is appropriate. The dose is normally 1 g 4-hourly to a maximum of 4 g/day, although a dose frequency of five times a day has been recommended.[6]

#### Weak opioids

If pain is not controlled by paracetamol, use of a weak opioid is required, this being the next step up the WHO analgesic ladder. Various weak opioids are available, for example, co-proxamol (dextropropoxyphene 32.5 mg and paracetamol 325 mg), dihydrocodeine and combinations of dihydrocodeine and paracetamol. Co-proxamol is very commonly used, the dose being two tablets 4-hourly to a maximum eight per day, although again five times a day has been recommended.[6] If analgesia is not obtained with one weak opioid, there is no benefit to be obtained by changing to another drug of the same class and a strong opioid should be used.

## Strong opioids

- Morphine is the strong opioid of choice. There are four types of preparation available for use in the UK. These are an elixir administered every 4 h, an immediate-release tablet administered every 4 h, a slow-release tablet acting over 12 h and a slow-release suspension acting over 12 h. Some centres use diamorphine elixir rather than morphine elixir.
- Morphine preparations: The morphine elixir may be prepared by the pharmacist and made to any suitable strength, and also is available as an off-the-shelf formulation that comes in two strengths of 10 mg/ 5 ml and 100 mg/5 ml. The immediate-release tablets are available in both 10 and 20 mg strengths. The slow-release tablet is available in 10, 15, 30, 60, 100 and 200 mg strengths. The slow-release suspension is available in 20, 30, 60, 100 and 200 mg strengths. Diamorphine is available only as an elixir prepared by the pharmacist at the desired concentration or a 10 mg tablet.
- Morphine metabolism: Morphine is well-absorbed from the gastro-intestinal tract, mainly in the proximal small bowel. There is extensive first-pass elimination which leads to a reduced bioavailability of oral morphine when compared with parenteral use. Morphine is metabolized in the liver to morphine-3-glucuronide and then to an active analgesic metabolite, morphine-6-glucuronide (M6G) which may account for much of the analgesic activity of the morphine.[7] M6G is excreted by the kidney and accumulates in patients with renal failure when a reduction in dose and increase in dose interval may be required.
- Administration of morphine: If possible, morphine is given by mouth at regular 4-hourly intervals and the aim of the treatment is to keep the patient painfree all the time. Patient response to treatment should be monitored frequently and the dose altered according to response. There is a direct relationship between dose and response and, with an opioid-responsive pain, no ceiling dose. The dose can range from 2.5 mg 4-hourly to 1000 mg or more 4-hourly, although very few patients will need such high doses. Most patients will need less than 200 mg in 24 h.
- Starting dose of morphine: This is 10 mg 4-hourly but the dose should be reduced to 5 mg in the elderly or those with known renal failure. Morphine elixir or immediate-release tablets are normally used initially because of the speed of onset and short duration of action. Morphine should be given 4-hourly and increases of 33–50% be made when increasing the dose, e.g. 10 to 15 mg, to 20 mg, to 30 mg, to 40 mg, to

60 mg. The patient should be reviewed frequently, particularly when treatment is initiated, for example, 2- or 4-hourly. Increases are normally made every 2–3 days but should be made more rapidly for severe pain needing rapid control. Patients may well need the regular 4-hourly dose and top-up doses of the same size as the regular dose for breakthrough pain before analgesia is achieved. The majority of patients do not need a dose of morphine in the middle of the night. However, some patients will need a 2.00 a.m. dose or benefit from a double dose (twice the regular 4-hourly dose) at bedtime. Regular, two or three times a day, assessment of pain and titration of the dose are continued until pain control is achieved. If pain continues it is important to increase the dose and not the frequency.

- Long-term treatment: Once satisfactory analgesia is achieved, many patients will be able to change to slow-release tablets given twice a day, although some patients will prefer to continue the 4-hourly elixir or tablets. Conversion to slow-release tablets is done by totalling the 24-h dose of morphine, dividing by two and giving this dose as slow-release tablets twice a day. Once stable, some patients will continue on the same morphine dose, but many will need gradual increases of the dose as their disease progresses.

### Alternatives to oral morphine

The various alternatives to morphine can be useful when the side-effects of morphine are difficult to control, such as nausea and vomiting, or when confusion and drowsiness are major problems.

- Diamorphine is used in some centres. It is a prodrug for morphine and little is detectable in the plasma after oral administration.[8] A potency ratio of 1 : 1 between oral morphine and oral diamorphine works in practice,[2,8] although some centres use a 3 : 2 ratio, i.e. 15 mg of oral morphine equivalent to 10 mg of oral diamorphine.[8]
- Phenazocine is available as 5 mg tablets, equivalent to 25 mg of morphine and given 6–8-hourly. The side-effects, particularly sedation and psychotomimetic effects, associated with phenazocine may be less than with morphine.
- Methadone is available as 5 mg tablets, equivalent to 5 mg morphine. Methadone is given 8–12-hourly (or possibly less frequently) but may accumulate when given regularly, causing drowsiness, confusion and a variable analgesic effect. Methadone may be useful in the recently described phenomenon of paradoxical pain.[9] It has been proposed that there may be an abnormal metabolism of morphine when little or no conversion of morphine-3-glucuronide to morphine-6-glucuronide occurs, leaving an excess of morphine-3-glucuronide which may have an antianalgesic effect. Replacement of morphine by methadone, which has different metabolic pathways, may be followed by effective analgesia.
- Oxycodone is an opioid prepared only as a suppository and, when given at a dose of 30 mg 6-hourly, is equivalent to oral morphine given at

20 mg 4-hourly. It may be an alternative to subcutaneous infusion of opioids.

- Fentanyl has been developed in a transdermal therapeutic system (TTS) in which the duration of action of the patches is 3 days.[10] The analgesic effects of TTS–fentanyl appear to be comparable with morphine when given at equivalent doses. TTS–fentanyl is available in four patch strengths releasing 25, 50, 75 and 100 $\mu$g/h. One study has suggested that there may be a lower incidence of constipation, nausea and vomiting, drowsiness and confusion when compared with morphine.[11]
- Tramadol is an opioid analgesic for use in moderate to severe pain which has proven to be effective in the treatment of cancer pain.[12] Its side-effect profile indicates less constipation, nausea, vomiting, drowsiness and confusion when compared with morphine. It is effective in a range between weak opioids and approximately 100 mg morphine over 24 h. The dose range of tramadol is 50–100 mg four times a day.
- Pethidine and dextromoramide have short durations of action which limit their use in patients with advanced cancer. Pentazocine is also short-acting and has a high incidence of side-effects. Buprenorphine is a partial agonist opioid and its analgesia has a ceiling effect at about 1 mg 8-hourly. For these reasons they are rarely used in palliative care.

### Side-effects of strong opioids

- Nausea or vomiting occurs in over half the patients taking oral morphine and often lasts for 3 or 4 days. It can be controlled easily with haloperidol 1.5 mg 12-hourly, which may later be stopped. Second-line treatment may be with cyclizine 50 mg 8-hourly. Not all patients will need an antiemetic and it may be appropriate, in institutional settings, not to prescribe an antiemetic with implications for increased tablet load and potential side-effects, but to wait to see if treatment is required. If nausea persists it may be due to causes other than the opioid.
- Drowsiness occurs commonly at the start of treatment with morphine but normally only lasts for a few days, although it can recur with increased doses of morphine.
- Hallucinations and confusion may occur, particularly in elderly patients. If these problems continue to be troublesome, a change to an alternative strong opioid may be necessary.
- Constipation occurs in virtually every patient and prophylactic treatment with laxatives is almost mandatory. Co-danthramer or codanthrusate or a combination of lactulose and senna are most commonly used. Rectal measures such as suppositories or enemas may also be needed.
- Occasional problems occur with a dry mouth (also consider oral *Candida*), sweating, itch and myoclonic jerks.
- Addiction to morphine is an occasional concern for the prescribing doctor or for the patient. It is not a significant practical problem, provided the treatment is given appropriately. Psychological addiction, i.e. active drug-seeking behaviour, is almost never seen in practice and an increased demand for morphine normally reflects an increased

need for analgesia. Physical dependence, i.e. the presence of a withdrawal syndrome on the removal of the drug, may develop after several months of morphine treatment, but should not be considered the same as addiction. If the requirement for opioid analgesia is removed, for example, by the use of a nerve block, the opioid can be reduced to zero over a few days, indicating little or no problem with physical dependence.[2]

- Respiratory depression is seen very rarely if morphine doses are increased with care and in response to the clinical situation. If respiratory depression does occur, the dose of morphine should be reduced and biochemical evidence of renal failure sought. The use of naloxone to reverse the effects of morphine may result in an alert patient, but one in considerable pain.

### Subcutaneous and rectal administration of opioids

The oral route is preferred for the administration of morphine but subcutaneous or rectal administration will be necessary for many patients. This may be required in cases of:

- uncontrolled vomiting
- dysphagia
- coma

Suppositories of morphine or oxycodone are available for use in this situation. The same dose of morphine is given by rectum as by mouth and at the same dose interval – 4-hourly. Oxycodone is given as a 30 mg suppository 6-hourly and this is equivalent to morphine 20 mg 4-hourly. However, rectal administration of opioids is becoming less popular with the widespread use of subcutaneous administration of opioids via portable syringe drivers. The syringe driver is used to administer the opioid, often combined with an antiemetic or sedative, as a continuous subcutaneous infusion.

The dose required for 24 h is placed in the syringe and the syringe driver delivers the drugs continuously over 24 h via a butterfly needle.

### The use of the syringe driver

- The syringe driver is a small and unobtrusive device which does not interfere with the patient's contact with his or her family in the same way that, for example, an intravenous infusion does.
- Diamorphine is normally used as the opioid of choice subcutaneously because of its greater solubility compared with morphine. There is debate about the relative potency of oral morphine and subcutaneous diamorphine. Some centres use 15 mg oral morphine, equivalent to 10 mg oral diamorphine, equivalent to 5 mg subcutaneous morphine.[2,7,8] Other centres use 10 mg oral morphine, equivalent to 10 mg oral diamorphine, which is equivalent to 5 mg subcutaneous

diamorphine. In clinical practice the patient's response to changing treatment is most important, and doses often require increasing as disease progresses.

- The administration of medication by syringe driver has changed the care of the dying patient dramatically over the last 15 years or so. Previously patients needed frequent injections of drugs, particularly analgesics and antiemetics, causing distress to patient and family and requiring a high level of input by nursing and medical staff. The syringe driver has removed these problems and improved pain symptom control considerably. The indications for the use of a syringe driver – uncontrolled vomiting, dysphagia and coma – often necessitate the use of other drugs to control nausea or vomiting and anxiety or distress.
- Nausea and vomiting may be treated by adding antiemetics, such as haloperidol (5–10 mg over 24 h), cyclizine (100–150 mg over 24 h), metoclopramide (10–40 mg over 24 h) or methotrimeprazine (25–100 mg over 24 h) to the syringe driver.
- Gastrointestinal obstruction frequency occurs in patients with intra-abdominal malignancy, and partial or complete obstruction with vomiting and colicky abdominal pain may occur. The vomiting can normally be controlled using the antiemetics as described above, administered subcutaneously via a syringe driver. Sometimes a combination is necessary, for example, haloperidol and cyclizine. The bowel stimulant action of metoclopramide may make vomiting worse in cases of bowel obstruction and is, therefore, not commonly used in such situations. Colicky pain can be controlled using hyoscine hydrobromide (20–40 mg over 24 h). An opioid analgesic will frequently also be required.
- Anxiety and distress, which are not due to treatable causes, for example, pain or distended bladder or rectum, may be controlled using midazolam (20–100 mg in 24 h) in the syringe driver.

### Coanalgesics

Coanalgesics are drugs used with, or instead of, analgesics to enhance pain control. The drugs may or may not have intrinsic analgesic activity.

- NSAIDs are frequently used for controlling pain for metastatic bone disease. Optimum doses should be used and change to an alternative NSAID considered if one is not successful. Radiotherapy may also be helpful. There is some recent evidence for improved analgesia with the use of subcutaneous ketorolac, especially in bone pain.[13] There is, however, concern about associated gastrointestinal bleeding when ketorolac is used for periods of more than 2 days. Diclofenac may also be used subcutaneously.

  There is a risk of gastric and duodenal ulceration, particularly if NSAIDs are used at the same time as steroids. Appropriate gastro-protection with an $H_2$-antagonist, proton pump inhibitor or prostaglandin analogue should be considered. NSAIDs will often be part of the treatment for advanced cancer pain as most pains have an inflammatory element and will respond to some degree to NSAIDs.

- Steroids have a place in pain control in several settings in advanced cancer. The predominant effect is due to a decrease in oedema surrounding a tumour mass. This reduces the pressure caused by the tumour mass and improves pain control. Dexamethasone is usually used because of its greater (×7) potency compared with prednisolone. This results in fewer tablets for the patient. For liver metastases dexamethasone in a dose of 4–12 mg/day should be used in conjunction with an analgesic. Soft-tissue infiltration can be controlled with NSAIDs and analgesics, with the possible addition of dexamethasone 4–12 mg/day.

  Nerve compression pain may respond to opioid and non-opioid analgesics and the addition of steroids may improve pain control. Dexamethasone may be used at 4–12 mg/day.

  Headache caused by raised intracranial pressure secondary to peritumour oedema, whether due to primary or secondary disease, responds well to dexamethasone in often quite high doses, for example, up to 24 mg/day. The lowest possible maintenance dose should be used once symptoms are controlled. Analgesics may also be necessary to control the headache.

  Steroids should be given early in the day as patients may experience insomnia due to their stimulant effect. The response to treatment should be closely monitored and doses reduced if possible. If no benefit is noted the steroids should be discontinued. Side-effects, particularly the moonface of Cushing's syndrome, and the development of or disturbance of control of diabetes may cause some problems with continued usage of steroids.

- Antidepressants, anticonvulsants and antiarhythmics for neuropathic pain: neuropathic pain is sometimes difficult to control satisfactorily. The pain is described as a burning or stabbing pain in a dermatomal distribution associated with altered sensation. Neuropathic pain may be due to invasion or compression of nerves by tumour, or may be indirectly related to the cancer, for example, a malignant neuropathy, or may be treatment-related, for example, chemotherapy-induced neuropathy.

Neuropathic pain commonly has one of three basic characters:

- continuous burning pain
- intermittent stabbing or shooting pain
- allodynia – light touch, for example, clothing, causing pain

Analgesics, often opioids, may have some effect on the pain and may be used initially but other drugs which have a pain-modifying action will often be needed. An antidepressant (for example, amitriptyline 25–150 mg at night) may be used for constant burning pain. An anticonvulsant may be appropriate for intermittent pain. The two most commonly used anticonvulsants are carbamazepine (200–800 mg/day) and sodium valproate (400–1200 mg/day). Some antiarhythmics have been useful in neuropathic pain, particularly flecainide 100 mg twice a day. Steroids may also improve the control of neuropathic pain, e.g. dexamethasone 4–12 mg/day.

- Diazepam/baclofen: Muscle relaxants may be necessary to control the uncomfortable muscle spasm which follows a painful bone metastasis or hemiplegia secondary to brain tumour.
- Antibiotics: Infection in soft tissue often leads to pain requiring antibiotics. Infection can occur as a complication of the general disease process, for example, cellulitis, and normally responds to penicillin. Infection in fungating tumours is often anaerobic and associated with unpleasant odours. A microbiological swab should be taken for culture and sensitivity and treatment commenced with oral, or more commonly topical, metronidazole and possibly flucloxacillin.
- Biphosphonates: There has recently been some evidence to support the use of biphosphonates to improve the pain of metastatic bone disease, for example, in carcinoma of the breast.[14] Biphosphonates may be given by mouth or intravenously. Further studies are needed to confirm clinical benefits and the most appropriate dosage and route of administration.

### Spinal opioids and local anaesthetics and nerve blocks

Spinal opioids and/or local anaesthetics (either intrathecal or epidural) can be used on occasions, but opinion as to the indications for use are not clear.[6] Opioid side-effects are less than with oral administration as doses are lower and better pain control has been reported in some cases. Improved analgesia may occur with the addition of local anaesthetic. Peripheral nerve blocks, such as interpleural and intercostal blocks, may also help the pain of advanced malignant disease.

Advice should be sought from specialist anaesthetists experienced in pain control using spinal drugs (see also Chapter 24).

### Transcutaneous electrical nerve stimulation

In some patients TENS may help to control the pain of advanced malignancy. TENS stimulates peripheral nerves via the intact skin using two small electrodes connected to a portable stimulator. It may help the pain of bone metastases, visceral pain or neuropathic pain. Similar benefit may also be obtained from acupuncture.

## Surgery

Orthopaedic surgery can give dramatic results when used with appropriate patients. Mobility can be improved and pain control achieved using internal fixation for patients with pathological fractures or potential fractures. Good results can also occur following surgical decompression of the spinal cord after a cord compression due to metastatic disease. Surgery for bowel obstruction often has good results in appropriately selected patients.

## Psychological support

The concept of 'total pain' encompasses psychological, social and spiritual factors as well as the physical aspects of pain.[5]

- A depressed patient will have pain which is harder to control and the use of antidepressants should be made early in a person's illness if appropriate.
- Anxieties and fears about the illness, its complications and prognosis can be addressed by honest and effective communication between patient and doctor.[15]
- Support from family and friends is vital and is much easier in an atmosphere of full knowledge and understanding of the problem presented. Collusion (hiding of knowledge) between patient and family can be very destructive and addressing it often improves the pain control as well as relationships between, for example, the patient and spouse.[15]
- On occasions patients will have great spiritual difficulties and anger with God and the involvement of ministers or chaplains may be very helpful.

## Professional support

A network of support services for patients with advanced cancer is developing throughout the UK. Many hospitals are establishing hospital-based palliative care nurse specialists, often supported by Cancer Relief Macmillan Fund (CRMF). Referral of hospital patients to these nurses is often helpful to both patient and medical and nursing staff.

Most cities and towns have local hospice services offering inpatient and home care facilities. The home care nurses, again often supported by CRMF, visit patients and families at home and provide advice on pain and symptom control to the primary care team of general practitioner and district nurse. Psychosocial support is offered to the patient and family.

Hospice medical staff and hospital consultants in palliative medicine are available for consultation and advice when necessary. Specialist anaesthetists in pain clinics are able to offer their skills and specialist knowledge and technology where appropriate.

## Conclusion

Most pain in advanced cancer can be relieved using the appropriate oral drugs. Other methods are available for difficult problems when they occur. The advice of specialist staff from hospices, specialists in palliative medicine and specialist anaesthetists in pain clinics should be sought if required.

## Terminology – opioid and opiate

The term opioid refers to all drugs, both naturally occurring and synthetic, which have morphine-like activity and are antagonized by naloxone. Opiate refers to naturally occurring drugs obtained from the poppy, such as morphine and codeine. Thus morphine is both an opioid and an opiate, while a synthetic drug such as diamorphine is only an opioid.

# References

1. Saunders C, Sykes N (eds). *The Management of Terminal Malignant Disease*, 3rd edn. London: Edward Arnold, 1993
2. Reynard CFB, Tempest S. *A Guide to Symptom Relief in Advanced Cancer*, 3rd edn. Manchester: Haigh & Hochland, 1992
3. World Health Organization. *Cancer Pain Relief and Palliative Care. Report of a WHO Expert Committee.* Geneva: World Health Organization, 1990
4. Portenoy RK. Cancer pain: pathophysiology and syndromes. *Lancet* **339:** 1026–1031, 1992
5. Twycross RG, Lack SA. *Therapeutics in Terminal Cancer*, 2nd edn. Edinburgh: Churchill Livingstone, 1990
6. Hanks GW, Justins DM. Cancer pain: management. *Lancet* **339:** 1031–1036, 1992
7. Gorman DJ. Opioid analgesics in the management of pain in patients with cancer: an update. *Palliat Med* **5:** 277–294, 1991
8. Hanks GW, Hoskin PJ. Opioid analgesics in the management of pain in patients with cancer. A review. *Palliat Med* **1:** 1–25, 1987
9. Morley JS, Watt JWG, Wells JC *et al.* Methadone in pain uncontrolled by morphine. *Lancet* **342:** 1243, 1993
10. Lehmann KA, Zech D. Transdermal fentanyl: clinical pharmacology. *J Pain Symptom Manage* **7:** S8–S16, 1992
11. The TTS-Fentanyl Multicentre Study Group. Transdermal fentanyl in cancer pain. *J Drug Dev* **6:** 93–97, 1994
12. Budd K. Tramadol; chronic pain – challenge and response. *Drugs* **47** (suppl 1): 33–38, 1994
13. Blackwell N, Bangham L, Hughes M *et al.* Subcutaneous ketorolac – a new development in pain control. *Palliat Med* **7:** 63–65, 1993
14. Patterson AHG, Powles N, Kanis AJ *et al.* Double-blind controlled trial of oral clodronate in patients with bone metastases from breast cancer. *J Clin Oncol* **11:** 59–65, 1993
15. Maguire P, Faulkner A. How to do it. Communicate with cancer patients: 2 Handling uncertainty, collusion and denial. *Pr Med J* **297:** 972–974, 1988

# Further reading

Doyle D, Hanks GW, MacDonald N (eds). *Oxford Textbook of Palliative Medicine*. Oxford: Oxford University Press, 1993

Saunders C, Sykes N (eds). *The Management of Terminal Malignant Disease*, 3rd edn. London: Edward Arnold, 1993

Twycross RG, Lack SA. *Therapeutics in Terminal Cancer*, 2nd edn. Edinburgh: Churchill Livingstone, 1990

Regnard CFB, Tempest S. *A Guide to Symptom Relief in Advanced Cancer*, 3rd edn. Manchester: Haigh & Hochland, 1992

Maguire P, Faulkner A. How to do it. Communicate with cancer patients: 1 Handling bad news and difficult questions. *Br Med J* **297:** 907–909, 1988

# 24

# Invasive techniques for pain control in advanced cancer

**S. J. Dolin**

For a small but significant number of patients who do not obtain adequate pain control through medical manoeuvres alone, the involvement of an anaesthetist may be of significant value.

## Analgesia via catheter[1]

Catheter techniques enable direct delivery of relatively small doses of analgesic drugs to their site of action. Drugs commonly used are the opioids, morphine or diamorphine, and local anaesthetics, usually bupivacaine. They may be used alone or in combination depending on the situation. Catheter techniques have proved to be very helpful in some cases of malignant pain that have not been controlled by systemic opiates and other medications mentioned in Chapter 23. They are also indicated when effective pain control can be obtained with systemic opioids but with unacceptable side-effects such as sedation, nausea and vomiting. Following a successful trial of catheter-delivered analgesia in hospital or in the hospice, catheters can be managed in the community in the long term but may require a lot of hospital–community communication.

- Epidural catheters can be placed percutaneousiy in the lumbar spine for low back, pelvis, hip or leg pain, or in the thoracic spine for pain in the abdominal wall or chest wall. They are useful when pain is bilateral. Continuous infusion of low-dose bupivacaine 0.1–0.125% 1–4 ml/h can give analgesia without sensory or motor deficit and patients can be mobile. Tolerance can occur with time but is not marked. Morphine or diamorphine starting at 5–10 mg/day can be used, either alone or in combination with bupivacaine. Side-effects can include nausea, vomiting, pruritus and urinary retention, but these are usually transient. Respiratory depression is not usually a problem as these patients have usually already been exposed to high-dose opioids. Epidural catheters can be tunnelled and exteriorized with a filter. Because of the large volumes required they are not suitable for an implanted reservoir. They can be managed at home using a continuous-infusion portable pump (e.g. Bard) with 100–250 ml bags of medications made up by pharmacy and can be changed by community nurses or even by the patient every few days. The presence of an inline antimicrobial filter adds a degree of protection against infection but must be changed regularly.

- Intrathecal catheters can be placed percutaneously in the lumbar spine and can be fed cephalad for control of pain in the thorax, abdomen or lower limbs. Face, neck or upper limb pain may warrant placement of intrathecal catheters in the cervical region. They are suitable for opioid administration. Combination of intrathecal opioids with bupivacaine (up to 2.5–5.0 mg per hour) have been shown to be effective in refractory cancer pain, without sensory or motor loss.[9] Morphine (preservative-free) or diamorphine spreads through the cerebrospinal fluid and the spinal cord effects are relatively widespread compared to epidural infusion. Side-effects include sedation, nausea, vomiting, pruritus and urinary retention but are usually transient. Suitable starting doses of morphine and diamorphine are 0.3–0.5 mg twice daily, but doses may need to be considerably higher due to drug tolerance (up to 10–25 mg per day).

  Respiratory depression is unusual as these patients have already been exposed to high-dose opioids by other routes. Intrathecal catheters can be tunnelled and exteriorized or can be connected to implanted subcutaneous ports for intermittent injection or implanted reservoirs which patients can operate themselves and will need refilling every 1–2 months (Cordis Secor). There are also electromechanical pumps with variable continuous infusion options (Medtronic).

- Intraventricular catheters:[2] Some neurosurgical centres use this technique, which may be indicated in uncontrolled head and face pain. It will require a burr hole to place the catheter. Morphine or diamorphine has been used at doses starting at 0.5–1 mg every 12–24 h. They can be suitable for an implanted subcutaneous reservoir. Reports have generally been favourable with good results and few side-effects.

- Interpleural catheters[3] can be used for continuous local anaesthetic infusions into the pleural space between the parietal and visceral pleura. It is indicated for unilateral thoracic or chest wall pain or even upper abdominal pain when systemic opioids have been ineffective. The catheter can be placed percutaneously through the posterior thoracic wall between the fourth and eighth intercostal space approximately 8–10 cm from the midline. An 18 G Tuohy with an epidural catheter is suitable. The needle is placed superior to the ribs and an audible and palpable click is observed as the needle passes through the intercostal membrane and enters the pleural space. Some means of detecting negative pressure such as a balloon or a column of fluid is useful. The catheter can be fed in up to 20 cm. A small pneumothorax may occur during catheter placement but usually resolves spontaneously or can be aspirated through the catheter. Bupivacaine 0.5% 1–5 ml/h should be sufficient. This should result in good analgesia without toxic side-effects of bupivacaine (tremor, convulsions, cardiac arrest) unless the patient develops liver failure when accumulation of bupivacaine may occur. Plasma concentrations can be measured. The catheter can be tunnelled and exteriorized and patients can manage with a portable pump (Bard) with a 100–250 ml reservoir which can be changed every few days.

- Other routes (brachial plexus/lumbar plexus). Catheter techniques for continuous local anaesthetic infusion of the brachial and lumbar plexuses have been described and may be suitable for intractable arm or leg pain which is unilateral. This technique is likely to result in some sensory and motor deficit. However, it may have an occasional place in pain management.

## Contraindications for catheter techniques

- Bleeding diathesis may result in haematoma formation with possible spinal cord or nerve root compression.
- Septicaemia in the presence of a foreign body (catheter) may well lead to abscess formation and possible neurological deficit.
- Immunosuppressed patients may be at risk of infection from indwelling catheters.
- Insulin-dependent diabetes predisposes to infection of indwelling catheters.
- Catheter techniques are inappropriate without support for their ongoing management.

## Side-effects of catheter techniques

- Side-effects of opioids delivered via epidural or intrathecal catheter: respiratory depression, nausea, vomiting, dysphoria, urinary retention and pruritus. These are unusual complaints as patients have often been exposed previously to high-dose systemic opioids. If present, these problems are usually self-limiting and can be managed by dose adjustment.
- On initiation of spinal opioid therapy, patients previously treated with systemic opioids may experience a withdrawal syndrome if systemic opioids are suddenly withdrawn.
- The incidence and significance of complications of chronically implanted catheters are unknown. Postmortem studies have revealed occasional localized fibrous reactions to epidural catheters. However, most patients did not have any significant changes.[4] Fibrosis does not seem to occur with intrathecal catheters.
- Infection is clearly one of the main concerns with indwelling catheters. This is likely to be more common with systems that need daily injecting compared to those with reservoirs that only need refilling every few weeks to months. Infections may be around the skin or in the sub-cutaneous tissues or may be more serious such as epidural infection or meningitis.[5] All infections need to be treated aggressively and may necessitate the removal of the indwelling catheter and reservoir or port.

## Neurolytlc nerve blocks

These have the advantage of being definitive techniques that, when success-ful, may obviate the need for other analgesics or the ongoing care required for catheters.

- Coeliac plexus block[6] (see Chapter 11). This is ideal for relief of malignant pain secondary to pancreatic carcinoma, retroperitoneal metastases, peritoneal carcinomatosis, colonic carcinoma, gastric carci-noma, and liver and spleen capsular distension. These conditions result in pain in the upper abdomen, back or both. The needle is placed anterior to T12–L1 vertebral bodies under fluoroscopic or com-puted tomographic guidance and 40–50 ml of 50–100% alcohol is injected. Success rates vary from 57 to 94%. Side-effects include ortho-static hypotension and diarrhoea, although these are usually mild and transient. There have been isolated reports of paraplegia following this procedure.
- Chemical lumbar sympathectomy has been used to control visceral pain caused by pelvic cancers. Pain from extensive intra-abdominal tumour spread may require a combination of coeliac plexus and lumbar sympa-thetic neurolytic blocks.
- Intrathecal neurolysis:[7] This technique has been in use for more than 50 years. Alcohol 50–100%, or phenol 4–10% dissolved in glycerol 10–100%: when injected intrathecally, absolute alcohol is hypobaric and 4–5% phenol in absolute glycerol is hyperbaric compared to cerebrospinal fluid. When alcohol is used the patient is positioned so that the dorsal roots to be blocked are in the most superior position. With phenol the patient is positioned so that the dorsal roots to be blocked are in the most dependent position. Alcohol can be painful on injection, while phenol is generally better tolerated. Success rates are in the region of 50–60%. Complications of intrathecal neurolysis are those of sphincter and motor paresis.

   Sacral rhizotomy with alcohol can be effective for perianal, perineal and genital pain associated with carcinoma of the rectum, bladder or genitalia. A lumbar puncture is done at the L5/S1 interspace and the patient positioned head-down. Absolute alcohol (100%) is injected in aliquots of 0.25 ml until a maximum of 2 ml is injected or until numb-ness rises as far as S2 on the posterior calf. The level will descend to S3 (back of thigh) several hours later. The sensory deficit must not be allowed to rise as far as S1 as the neurological deficit will be unaccept-able. While motor loss can be avoided, the effect on sphincter control is unpredictable. The ideal patient is one with both faecal and urinary diversion. Alternatively the procedure can be done with hyperbaric phenol using a head-up technique.
- Epidural neurolysis with phenol or alcohol has been introduced as an alternative to intrathecal block and is preferred for wide segmental block. The ideal application is in patients with chest wall or abdominal wall pain. Alcohol concentrations used are 30–100% and phenol 6–10%. Success is variable.

Care must be taken when considering neurolytic blocks that the pain is not deafferentation pain with established neurological deficit as deafferentation pain may well be worsened by further neurolysis.

## Ablative neurosurgery

- Nerve root section (rhizotomy): This technique, while not generally useful, can provide relief in specific situations such as infiltrations of the brachial plexus by carcinoma of the breast. Surgical rhizotomy of the dorsal roots of C5–8, which requires a laminectomy, may relieve the pain but will leave the arm without sensation.
- Percutaneous cordotomy[8] involves the interruption of the anterolateral ascending spinothalamic tract of the spinal cord which carries pain fibres from the opposite side of the body. Cordotomy is indicated in patients with unilateral pain who still have intact sphincter and motor function and a life expectancy of 6–12 months, although longer-lasting results have been reported. It can be done percutaneously at the cervical (C2) level for pain in the arm or chest wall. After correct needle position determined by stimulating via the needle with the patient awake, a lesion can be made by radiofrequency. Up to 80% success rate has been reported. A C2 cordotomy may interfere with ipsilateral phrenic nerve function on the non-painful side, leading to possible respiratory insufficiency. There will be associated loss of temperature and touch sensation on the side opposite to the lesion. Cordotomy can also be done surgically at the thoracic (T2) level for pain below the T10–T12 dermatome. It is not necessary to select an exact level but simply one sufficiently cephalad to the site of the pain. Weakness of the leg on the side of the lesion is a possibility. Bilateral cordotomy is not recommended as it results in severe autonomic and sphincter dysfunction.

## References

1. Hanks GW, Justins DM. Cancer pain management. *Lancet* **339:** 1031–1036, 1992
2. Labato RD, Madrid JL, Fatela LV, Rivas JJ, Reig E, Lamas E. Intraventricular morphine for control of pain in terminal cancer patients. *J Neurosurg* **59:** 627–633, 1983
3. Finemann SP. Longterm postthoracotomy cancer pain management with interpleural bupivacaine. *Anesth Analg* **68:** 694–697, 1989
4. Carl P, Crawford ME, Ravlo O, Bach V. Long term treatment with epidural opioids: a retrospective study comprising 150 patients treated with morphine chloride and buprenorphine. *Anaesthesia* **41:** 32–38, 1986
5. Plummer JL, Cherry DA, Cousins MJ, Gourlay GK, Onley MM, Evans KHA. Long term spinal administration of morphine in cancer and non-cancer pain: a retrospective study. *Pain* **44:** 215–220, 1991
6. Thompson GE, Moore DC, Bridenbaugh LD *et al.* Abdominal pain and alcohol coeliac plexus nerve block. *Anesth Analg* **56:** 1–5, 1977
7. Ferrer-Brechner T. Epidural and intrathecal phenol neurolysis for cancer pain: review of rationale and techniques. *Reg Anaesth* **8:** 14–20, 1981
8. Rosomoff HF, Carrall F, Brown J *et al.* Percutaneous radiofrequency cervical chordotomy technique. *J Neurosurg* **23:** 639–644, 1965
9. Sjoberg M, Applegren L, Einarsson S *et al.* Long-term intrathecal morphine and bupivacaine in refractory cancer pain. I. Results from the first series of 52 patients. *Acta Anaesthesiol Scand* **35:** 30–43, 1991

# 25

# Pain in human immunodeficiency disease

**L. Marshall**

The human immunodeficiency virus (HIV) is a lymphotrophic retrovirus which depletes helper T cells. The resulting reduction in cell-mediated immunity predisposes to specific opportunistic infections and malignancies. This constellation of diseases has been designated acquired immunodeficiency syndrome (AIDS). The interval between infections with the virus and the onset of AIDS is 10 years on average.[1]

Currently it is estimated that there are 10 million cases of HIV infection worldwide.[2]

Pain in HIV disease is common, with the prevalence increasing as the disease progresses. Various studies have shown that at least 60% of those with Centers for Disease Control (CDC) group IV disease (AIDS-defining illnesses) have significant pain.[3-5] This figure rises to 97% in those close to death.[6]

As lifespan has been increased with the use of antiretroviral agents and prophylaxis for infections, so the quality of that life has become more important. Pain is often seen as a constant reminder of disease and therefore mortality. Thus it is not only the physical aspects of the pain that must be considered, but also the psychological, social and emotional.

The range of symptoms is similar to that found in cancer; however there is more often an underlying treatable cause in HIV infection, so that a knowledge of the common causes of pain and their treatment is essential. An organic cause for the pain should always be assumed and excluded.

The commonest complaints of pain are:[7,8]

- headaches
- abdominal pain
- skin ulceration
- peripheral neuropathy
- oral cavity conditions
- odynophagia (pain on swallowing)
- arthralgia

Evaluation and treatment of pain are best understood by a review of the various body systems and how HIV manifests itself. It is important to remember that frequently a patient may have more than one pathology present.

## Neurological manifestations: headaches

This is a common problem which occurs in 10–25% of patients.[8,9] It is difficult to accurately diagnose and one must have a high index of suspicion. It is important to consider common underlying problems, such as stress, anxiety and migraine, as causes.

### Causes

- *Toxoplasma gondii*
- *Cryptococcus neoformans*
- sinusitis, including unusual organisms (e.g. *Pseudomonas*)
- *Listeria*
- HIV headache
- traditional bacterial meningitis – rare
- *Mycobacterium tuberculosis* (TB)
- primary central nervous system lymphoma
- metastatic non-Hodgkin's lymphoma
- Kaposi's sarcoma – rare

### Investigation

- Computed tomography (CT) and/or magnetic resonance imaging (MRI) may show diagnostic features such as ring-enhancing lesions in toxoplasmosis or those of lymphoma. It is also helpful to show sinusitis, especially ethmoidal. Raised intracranial pressure will need to be excluded before lumbar puncture is undertaken.
- Lumbar puncture, as well as showing non-specific changes of raised protein and cells and excluding bacterial causes, may give the diagnosis of *Cryptococcus* by Indian ink staining and the presence of cryptococcal antigen.
- Biopsy of cerebral space-occupying lesions may be required to make a definitive diagnosis in some patients.
- Serology: As almost all cases of toxoplasmosis are reactivations, the absence of *Toxoplasma* immunoglobulin G antibodies allows one to exclude the diagnosis. However, the presence of cryptococcal antigen is a significant finding.

### Treatment

- Toxoplasmosis: Sulphadiazine, pyrimethamine and folinic acid is the combination of first choice. Alternatives are dapsone with pyrimethamine, clindamycin or atovaquone.
- *Cryptococcus:* Intravenous amphotericin B in those with severe disease or oral fluconazole. This will also treat *Candida*. Both toxoplasmosis and *Cryptococcus* require lifelong prophylactic therapy.
- HIV encephalitis: Zidovudine is the drug of first choice.
- Lymphoma: Radiotherapy and chemotherapy are both used. Radiotherapy with steroids often relieves the headaches.

## Peripheral neuropathies

Various types have been described, including:

- Symmetrical, mainly sensory neuropathy which generally occurs late in the disease in those with CDC group IV illnesses. It is the most common, with a prevalence of some 25%.[10] It is thought to be due to HIV infection of the nerves itself. The commonest symptom is pain in the soles of the feet with paraesthesia. Examination shows absent ankle jerks and decreased proprioception and diagnosis is confirmed by electrophysiological testing.
- Inflammatory demyelinating polyneuropathies, both acute (Guillain–Barré syndrome) and chronic, though pain is not a major feature. Mononeuropathy multiplex and cranial nerve palsies may be features and there is a marked pleocytosis in the cerebrospinal fluid.
- Cauda equina syndrome: This inflammatory polyradiculopathy is associated with cytomegalovirus (CMV) infection and results in both sensory and motor dysfunction with sphincter involvement; pain is less often a presenting problem.
- Drug-induced neuropathy: This is similar to that previously described due to HIV itself. It has been seen with all three of the currently available antiretroviral agents, though it is more common with didanosine (ddI) and zalcitabine (ddC) and may worsen on cessation of the drug before improving.

### Treatment

While the demyelinating polyneuropathies may be self-limiting or respond to plasmapheresis, there are few effective treatments for these common and disabling conditions. Tricyclic antidepressants, carbamazepine and mexilitine have been tried with variable effect, though often opiates are needed and transcutaneous nerve stimulators give some relief.

As leg pain is the most troublesome, epidurals have been used but the results have been mixed.

## Gastrointestinal manifestations

### Oropharynx

- *Candida albicans:* Oropharyngeal candidiasis is present in 75% of patients[10] and may present as discomfort and pain but is often asymptomatic. It may be pseudomembranous, hyperplastic, erythematous or present as angular cheilosis. Typically there are white plaques visible on the buccal surfaces and palate but in the erythematous form these may be absent. Diagnosis is by microscopy and culture.
- Ulceration: Again, this is a common complaint and important as this may lead to inanition. Common causes include idiopathic aphthous ulcers, which may be very large and coalesce, herpes simplex virus (HSV), CMV, and Epstein–Barr virus (EBV). Lymphoma may present as a mass in the mouth.

- Bacterial gingivitis and dental abscesses are commonly seen, despite good oral hygiene.
- Kaposi's sarcoma is found in the oral cavity but is not often painful.

## Oesophagus

Odynophagia and dysphagia are common complaints, occurring in some 30% of patients.[11] They are a considerable cause of morbidity. Causes include:

- Candidiasis: This is the commonest cause, accounting for up to 75% of cases[11-13]. There is usually oropharyngeal candidiasis as well, though this is not essential for diagnosis.
- Ulceration caused by CMV, idiopathic aphthous ulceration, HSV and, rarely, EBV and tuberculosis.
- Kaposi's sarcoma and non-Hodgkin's lymphomas have also been described.

### Diagnosis

Endoscopic oesophagoscopy and gastroscopy is the investigation of choice as this allows gastric reflux to be excluded and biopsies to be taken for histology, microscopy and culture.

### Treatment

- Oral *Candida* usually responds to amphotericin lozenges or topical nystatin. If the response is poor or there is oesophageal disease, then fluconazole, itraconazole or ketoconazole can be used orally, with intravenous amphotericin being reserved for the most persistent cases. Maintenance therapy is often required.
- HSV ulceration should respond to acyclovir, though some resistance has now been reported. Foscarnet can be used. The ulceration due to CMV is treated with ganciclovir or foscarnet. Aphthous ulceration is often difficult to treat effectively, though soothing preparations like carmellose sodium give some relief. Carbenoxolone gel or sucralfate mouth washes are useful to encourage healing. Steroids, both topically and systemically, have been used and thalidomide in men often has a dramatic effect.

## Abdominal pain

Pain is a common complaint, reported in 30–50% of patients,[14] and is often difficult to diagnose.

- CMV colitis may lead to perforation.
- *Campylobacter* is associated with intussusception.
- CMV and cryptosporidia may cause cholecystitis and sclerosing cholangitis. The biliary tree can be a source of reinfection in those with recurrent disease.

- Pancreatitis is most commonly associated with ddI and ddC.
- Bowel obstruction may be due to lymphoma and, rarely, Kaposi's sarcoma.
- Constipation is a common cause of abdominal pain often caused by opiate therapy.

### Diagnosis and treatment

Rarely is laparotomy required for diagnosis. Sphincterotomy may be useful in those with cholangitis and coeliac plexus block may be required for intractable pain. Whilst a raised amylase helps with the diagnosis of pancreatitis, this may occur after the pain and the offending medication must be ceased immediately rather than waiting for the amylase result.

## Cramps and diarrhoea

There are many causes of these symptoms and it is important to find an organism if possible so that specific treatment can be given. An organism can be found in up to 85% of cases.[14] Diarrhoea is a major cause of weight loss and malnutrition in HIV and impinges significantly socially.

### Causes

- Bacteria
  - *Salmonella*
  - *Shigella*
  - *Campylobacter*
  - *Clostridium difficile*
  - Mycobacterium avium intracellulare (MAI)
- Parasites
  - *Giardia lamblia*
  - Cryptosporidia
  - Microsporidia (may not be pathogen)
  - *Isospora belli*
  - *Strongyloides stercoralis*
  - *Entamoeba histolytica*
- Viruses
  - CMV
  - HIV itself has been implicated

### Diagnosis

Consecutive stool cultures are important, with special staining required for some pathogens such as cryptosporidia and MAI. It may also be necessary to perform gastroduodenoscopy and colonoscopy to make the diagnosis by better sampling and biopsy.

*Treatment*

The diarrhoea usually responds to various combinations of loperamide, diphenoxylate and codeine phosphate. Occasionally stronger opiates are necessary and some patients require octreotide if the symptoms are severe. Whilst the standard treatment regimes for the various microorganisms above are effective in HIV, the course may often be protracted and relapsing and require suppressive antibiotic regimes. Cryptosporidia may respond to paromomycin in some patients but are difficult to eradicate. CMV responds to ganciclovir. *Clostridium difficile* is found in those on long-term antibiotics and is treated with vancomycin or metronidazole.

## Anorectal conditions

About one-third of homosexual patients with HIV will have anorectal conditions.[15] These include haemorrhoids, fissures, abscesses, fistulae, HSV and CMV ulceration and anorectal carcinoma. Some of these conditions can be treated conservatively but others require surgery and are a cause of much morbidity. Prophylactic acyclovir is often required in HSV and it is important to relieve any constipation which can exacerbate symptoms.

## Arthropathies

Various syndromes are recognized and joint pain as a complaint varies greatly in different series.[16,17]

- Reactive arthritis akin to Reiter's syndrome is the most common arthritis. Diarrhoea or sexually acquired infections can be the precipitating factor. There is an association with human leukocyte antigen (HLA)-B27. Presentation is often as a severe arthritis of the large joints of the legs or sacroiliitis. There may be the usual associated features of conjunctivitis, urethritis, balanitis and keratoderma blenorrhagica.
- Non-specific arthralgias and arthritis have been associated with HIV. There is no precipitating infection as in reactive arthritis, though the clinical arthritis is similar in that this is an oligoarthritis, mainly affecting the large joints of the legs or the shoulders.
- Psoriatic arthritis correlates with skin disease and this often worsens with HIV infection. This arthritis may be severe and lead to disabling deformity.
- Septic arthritis is rare but unusual organisms such as *Cryptococcus* have been found.
- Gout may also be found as a side-effect of drug treatments, e.g. pyrazinamide, or in psoriasis exacerbations and should be included in the differential diagnosis.

## Diagnosis

In reactive arthritis the underlying causative organism should be sought, either from the bowel or by specific urethral swabs and this treated if appropriate. Aspiration of the synovial fluid will aid in the diagnosis of septic arthritis and gout. The fluid is non-inflammatory in HIV-associated arthritis.

## Treatment

Non-steroidal anti-inflammatory drugs (NSAIDs) are the drugs of first choice but unfortunately reactive arthritis may not respond well to these agents. Intra-articular or systemic steroids may be required, as may other immunomodulating drugs such as methotrexate and azathioprine. These should be used with care because of their immunosuppressive action. Physiotherapy incorporating heat, splints, rest and mobilization is a helpful adjunct and patients should be referred early.

## Myopathies

Polymyositis is thought to be a direct effect of HIV infection of muscles. It is characterized by an insidious onset of proximal muscle weakness, muscle ache and associated weight loss.

Zidovudine has also been associated with a proximal myopathy, principally of the gluteal muscles. There may also be pyomyositis.

### Diagnosis and treatment

A significant rise in serum creatinine kinase occurs and the diagnosis is confirmed by electromyographic studies and biopsy. Zidovudine is ceased and immunosuppressive drugs have been used with limited success.

## Dermatological manifestations

These are the most common, though not all are painful. Common causes of painful skin conditions are:

- HSV: Ulcers are common. Long-term acyclovir may be necessary. Some acyclovir and foscarnet resistant has been reported.
- Herpes zoster virus: This may be multidermatomal. It is often a poor prognostic sign for the onset of AIDs. It requires high-dose acyclovir. Lesions may persist for months. Intractable pain may be difficult to control (see Chapter 17).
- CMV: This presents as perianal or perioral ulcers.
- Staphylococci: These are the commonest skin bacterial pathogens. It is estimated that some 50% have a staphylococcal infection during their illness.[18] They cause impetigo, cellulitis, folliculitis, pyomyositis and secondary infection of herpes, Kaposi's sarcoma and scabies.

- MAI: This is a rare cause of lymphadenitis requiring drainage.
- *Treponema pallidum.* Secondary syphilis can result in painful ulcerated lesions and should always be considered in the differential diagnosis.

The following conditions cause irritating and sometimes painful lesions.

- *Bartonella* spp.: This causes bacillary angiomatosis which may resemble Kaposi's sarcoma. It can be treated with erythromycin or doxycycline.
- *Candida:* As well as mucosal disease, *Candida* can also cause vulvo-vaginitis and balanitis.
- *Trichophyton* spp.: Tinea pedis is more common in HIV-infected individuals; nail infections are particularly troublesome. Terbinafine topically and orally is effective.
- *Cryptococcus:* Haematogenous spread occurs in 5–10% of those with disseminated disease.[18] It causes nodules, ulceration and painful plaques. Long-term prophylaxis after effective treatment is imperative.
- Scabies: This may be widespread with crusted lesions and frequent recurrence. Secondary infection is also a problem.
- Kaposi's sarcoma: These lesions are not usually painful in themselves, though those on the toes can be troublesome. They can become ulcerated and secondarily infected, however.
- Squamous cell and basal cell carcinoma: Both these lesions are more common in AIDS patients.
- Psoriasis: This condition frequently deteriorates in HIV disease and can prove refractory to standard therapy. There is a concern about the immunosuppressive qualities of phototherapy and other agents such as methotrexate.
- Reiter's syndrome: As mentioned previously, this is associated with painful arthritis as well as skin lesions.
- Drug reactions: Co-trimoxazole, which is the drug of first choice in *Pneumocystis carinii* pneumonia infection, can result in Stevens–Johnson syndrome. Foscarnet has induced painful penile ulceration in almost 30% of those undergoing induction therapy.[18] This is self-limiting.
- Thrombocytopenia may rarely cause purpura. The reduction in platelets is due to a direct action of HIV and may be the presenting symptom of HIV disease.

### General considerations in pain management in HIV disease

Pain is often poorly treated in those with HIV disease. There have been various reasons postulated for this. It may be that the underlying causes of the pain have not been fully elucidate and treated effectively. Sometimes prolongation of life at all costs has overridden the need for adequate pain relief. The patient–doctor relationship may be strained or the patient may be too unwell mentally or physically to be able to communicate the extent of the pain adequately. Also there is sometimes a reluctance to prescribe adequate doses of opiates for fear of addiction or respiratory depression.

Without the knowledge of the causes of pain and their treatments as listed above, no rational analgesia can be provided. It is worth reiterating that a treatable cause of pain should always be sought. Whilst investigating the cause, however, symptomatic relief of the pain should not be withheld.

The use of analgesic drugs should be in a stepwise manner starting with paracetamol in standard divided doses and adding other agents as required. Thus NSAIDs can be used in those with inflammatory pains and then weak opiates like codeine phosphate or dextropopoxyphene. If pain still persists then morphine can replace the previously used opiate and be increased in increments until analgesia is achieved or side-effects limit its use. This can be given orally in frequent divided doses or in slow-release formulations. Alternatively, infusion pumps may be required to achieve the desired effect. Side-effects that may need to be controlled include nausea and constipation.

Some pain does not respond well to opiate therapy and so adjuvant drugs may be required, as in peripheral neuropathy, previously described. Similarly nerve blocks can be useful where pain is not responding to seemingly adequate doses or the side-effects are intolerable. Coeliac plexus block has been used for abdominal pain which is not responding.

Care should be taken to avoid the development of pressure sores in the terminally ill. Good nursing care is essential. It is important to remember the other non-medical influences which may be contributing to the pain and deal with them early in management.

## Potential problems

The use of systemic steroids in the management of painful HIV conditions could be a problem due to their immunosuppressive effect. There is the potential to reactivate CMV and tuberculosis and thus speed the progression to AIDS. However, their use in severe infection with *Pneumocystis* has resulted in markedly increased survival. Each case should be reviewed to determine the potential benefits as opposed to the potential damage. Similarly, other immunosuppressants like azathioprine or methotrexate need to be used with care.

The use of opiates in those with a history of abuse often raises ethical problems for the attending staff. It would seem that there is no greater opiate requirement in those who had previously used intravenous drugs. Problems can arise when patients are managed at home with constant infusions of opiates with respect to how and by whom the drugs are used.

Because zidovudine undergoes glucuronidation and then renal excretion, there is concern that there may be interaction with other drugs which are metabolized in a similar fashion, including NSAIDs, paracetamol and morphine. There may be a risk of zidovudine toxicity where these agents are used together.

## Conclusion

Pain is a common symptom in HIV disease which usually has an organic cause. This cause must be elucidated so that specific treatment can be given. Whilst the investigations are being conducted, however, symptomatic analgesia should not be withheld and it is important to be aware of the patient's social, psychological and emotional state in the assessment of pain.

## Approach to pain

### Reduce noxious stimuli

- disease-specific treatments
- physical treatments
- minor analgesics

### Raise pain threshold

- care, comfort and concern
- drug therapy if appropriate, e.g. antidepressants, anxiolytics

### Reduce pain perception centrally

- opiates

### Specific pain syndrome therapies

- neuropathy
- muscle spasms
- diarrhoea/constipation

**Table 25.1** Dosages of drugs

| Drug | Dose |
| --- | --- |
| Acyclovir | 5–10 mg/kg t.d.s. i.v. |
|  | 200–400 mg 5× daily orally |
| Amphotericin B | 0.6–1.0 mg/kg daily |
| Atovaquone | 750 mg q.i.d. |
| Carbamazepine | 200 mg t.d.s. (increase slowly from 100 mg b.d.) |
| Clindamycin | 600 mg q.i.d. |
| Dapsone | 100 mg/day |
| Didanosine | 167–200 mg b.d. |
| Folinic acid | 15 mg/day |
| Fluconazole | (in cryptococcal disease) 400 mg loading then 200 mg b.d. |
|  | 50–100 mg/day for candidiasis |
| Foscarnet | 60 mg/kg t.d.s. induction then 90 mg/kg daily |
| Ganciclovir | 5 mg/kg b.d. induction then 10 mg/kg 3–5× weekly |
| Itraconazole | 100–200 mg o.d. or b.d. |
| Ketaconazole | 200–400 mg/day |
| Loperamide | 2–4 mg q.i.d. |
| Paromomycin | 500 mg q.i.d. |
| Pyrimethaamine | 25–50 mg/day |
| Sulphadiazine | 1 g q.i.d. |
| Thalidomide | 100 mg b.d. |
| Zalcitabine | 0.75 mg t.d.s. |
| Zidovudine | 250–500 mg b.d. |

# References

1. Moss AR, Bachetti P. Editorial review: Natural history of HIV infection. *AIDS* **3:** 55, 1989
2. Chin J. Global estimates of HIV infection and AIDS cases. *AIDS* **5:** S57–S61, 1991
3. Moss V. Patient characteristics, presentation and problems encountered in advanced AIDS in a hospice setting – a review. *Palliat Med* **5:** 112–116, 1991
4. Moss V. Palliative care in advanced HIV disease: presentation, problems and palliation. *AIDS* **4:** S235–S242, 1990
5. Schofferman J. Pain: diagnosis and management in the palliative care of AIDS. *J Palliat Care* **4:** 46–49, 1988
6. Singh S, Fermie P, Peters W. Symptom control for individuals with advanced HIV infection in a subacute residential unit: which symptoms need palliating? VIII International Conference on AIDS/III STD World Congress, Amsterdam, The Netherlands 19–24 July 1992, Poster Abstr. PoD 5248
7. Singer EJ, Zorilla C, Fahy-Chandon B, Chi S, Syndulko K, Tourtellotte WW. Painful symptoms reported by ambulatory HIV-infected men in a longitudinal study. *Pain* **54:** 15–19, 1993
8. Lebovits AH, Lefkowitz M, McCarthy D *et al*. The prevalence and management of pain in patients with AIDS: a review of 134 cases. *Clin J Pain* **5:** 245–248, 1989
9. Goldstein J. Headache and acquired immunodeficiency syndrome. *Neurol Clin* **8:** 947–961, 1990
10. O'Neill WM, Sherrard JS. Pain in human immunodeficiency virus disease: a review. *Pain* **54:** 3–14, 1993
11. Connolly GM, Hawkins D, Harcourt-Webster JN, Parsons PA, Husain OAN, Gazzard BG. Oesophageal symptoms, their cause, treatment and prognosis in patients with the acquired immunodeficiency syndrome. *Gut* **30:** 1033–1039, 1989
12. Bonacini M, Young T, Laine L. The causes of esophageal symptoms in human immunedeficiency virus infection. *Arch Intern Med* **151:** 1567–1572, 1991
13. Eisner MS, Smith PD. Etiology of odynophagia and dysphagia in patients with the acquired immunodeficiency syndrome (AIDS). *Gastroenterology* **98:** A446, 1990
14. Smith PD, Quinn TC, Strober W, Janoff EN, Masur H. Gastrointestinal infections in AIDS. *Ann Intern Med* **116:** 63–74, 1992
15. Wexner SD, Smithy WB, Milsom JW, Dailey TH. The surgical management of anorectal diseases in AIDS and pre-AIDS patients. *Dis Colon Rectum* **29:** 719–723, 1986
16. Hess EV, Solinger AM. Rheumatic manifestations of human immunodeficiency virus. *Arthritis Rheum* **33:** 1295–1296, 1990
17. Bennan A, Espinoza LR, Diaz JD *et al*. Rheumatic manifestations of human immunedeficiency virus infection. *Am J Med* **85:** 59–64, 1988
18. Dover JS, Johnson RA. Cutaneous manifestations of human immunodeficiency virus infection: part II. *Arch Dermatol* **127:** 1549–1558, 1991

26

# Psychological therapies in pain management

**J. M. Green**

Patients with chronic pain problems adapt in a variety of ways to the continued presence of pain. These include the development of pain behaviours, changes in physical activity level, medication use, usage of health personnel, employment and depression. There is a higher incidence of depression in chronic pain patients than in patients without pain, although only 33% are clinically depressed.[1]

## Operant conditioning and pain behaviour

In any area of life, new behaviours become established when rewards follow them. These rewards may be easy to recognize, for example, food, praise, or more subtle and difficult to identify, such as avoidance of difficult social situations, and particular kinds of desired attention. Conversely, if new behaviours are followed by negative rewards, such as discomfort, or criticism, those new behaviours will not become established. When behaviour which was previously rewarded ceases to be so, that behaviour will tend to die away or be extinguished. This will happen faster if positive rewards are replaced by negative ones.

Sometimes unexpected rewards follow new patterns of behaviour and these behaviours, which would otherwise have been temporary, become long-standing. If these behaviours are undesirable, behaviour therapy, using what is known about learning, conditioning and extinction, can be employed to alter them. This is done by eliminating the positive rewards which followed the behaviour and by rewarding or reinforcing the desired behaviour patterns instead.[2]

Fordyce described specific pain behaviour.[3,4] This starts as a normal initial response to an acute injury, so includes a reduction in general activity levels, shielding of the injured part with avoidance of certain specific movements or activities. In an acute injury this allows the body's recovery from the noxious insult. In chronic pain, this ceases to have a physiological purpose, and instead becomes destructive in effect.

So, in chronic pain, behaviour which started as a classical response to an acute injury could be followed by unexpected rewards and thus be reinforced. These may be direct or indirect. *Direct* rewards might include attention and permission to rest. *Indirect* rewards might include sanctioned avoidance of aversive agents, e.g. heavy work, stressful social encounters.

## Adaptation to pain

Pain behaviour is one example of a coping strategy. These are adaptations to minimize the impact of pain on the individual. Most pain behaviours, such as rest are negative coping strategies, involving withdrawal from the environment. Positive coping strategies would include such things as exercise. Passive or negative coping strategies are usually associated with a perception of helplessness and a greater degree of psychological and physical disability.

Beliefs also influence the ability of patients to adapt successfully to pain. Of particular importance are the locus of control and perceived self-efficacy in performing given tasks. Patients who feel they have control over the pain and over the outcome have an internal locus of control. Some patients attribute control over pain to external forces or chance. They are said to have an external locus of control, and may be less likely to use active coping strategies, to be more distressed by their pain and more depressed.[5] Patients with higher perceived ability respond better to some aspects of pain management programmes designed to increase mobility.

Over a period, pain alters the role of patients within their social group; they take a more passive part than previously, and further, by the global reduction in activity levels, pain caused by movement is increased, even for activities not initially directly affected by the pain. Thus a spiral of decreasing ability and increasing passivity may be established. Both patients and their family may perpetuate the sick role, particularly if there are hidden gains for either the patient or family members, such as less aggression from a previously dominant husband. Understanding the principles of operant conditioning allows the use of approaches designed to modify the unwanted illness behaviour.

## Psychological methods of altering pain behaviour

There are various different psychological approaches to altering behaviour in pain patients. In most cases these are used in combination. The most commonly used approaches are:

- behavioural therapy
- cognitive therapy
- cognitive-behavioural therapy
- family therapy
- pain management programmes

Other approaches less frequently used include biofeedback and hypnosis.

## Behavioural therapy

Fordyce suggested pain behaviours might be reduced through the use of behavioural therapy. The behavioural programme he described involved manipulating the environment both in the clinic and at home by involving the patient's family.

- Analgesia is changed to a time-determined (-contingent) rather than pain-contingent regime.
- A programme of exercise is initiated where rest periods are dependent on the quota (amount of exercise), not on pain.
- Attention and social feedback from the health care team and the family are focused on achievement, not on pain.
- Education about the nature of pain, particularly the gate control theory of pain,[6] is included for patients and their families.
- Relaxation training is given.

Programmes typically last for 6 weeks' inpatient stay, with the aim of a full day's activity to be attained by the end, with medication at a stable low dose or entirely eliminated.

Merskey[7] suggested that this approach was unlikely completely to remove a pain which had some organic basis, but although expensive in resources, there are improvements in drug-taking, pain complaints and activity levels, and these persist into the long term. Linton has also reviewed such programmes.[8]

## Cognitive therapy

Cognitive therapy has been written about extensively by Aaron Beck. Originally he described it as a method of shifting the thinking of patients with depression from their characteristic negative or maladaptive ones to more positive ideas.[9,10] Patients are helped to examine and challenge their thoughts and feelings, and to develop more balanced thinking. Cognitive therapy was soon extended to the treatment of other psychological disorders,[11,12] including pain management, where it is useful in patients who are not clinically depressed.

There are three types of cognitive approaches described by Mahoney and Arnkoff:[13]

- cognitive restructuring – changing negative thoughts to more positive ones
- coping skills training – techniques for stress management, including relaxation and imagery
- problem-solving

The coping skills taught, such as relaxation and imagery, are examples of active coping strategies.

## Cognitive-behavioural therapy

Cognitive-behavioural therapy combines the principles of behaviour therapy with those of cognitive therapy. Turk and Rudy[14] stated that the cognitive-behavioural perspective is based on five central assumptions:

- People actively make sense of information and do not simply react to it passively.
- Thoughts can stimulate or modify moods, alter physiological processes, influence the environment and can serve as the spur for behaviour. Conversely, mood, physiology, environmental factors and behaviour can influence thoughts.
- Behaviour is caused both by the person and by the environment.
- Individuals can learn more adaptive ways of thinking, feeling and behaving.
- People are capable of, and should be involved in, the altering of their maladaptive thoughts, feelings and behaviours.

## Biofeedback

Biofeedback is the use of increased awareness of the physiological parameters of the body, e.g. heart rate, muscle tension, to enable a patient to learn to alter these parameters. It has been used widely in the management of response to pain, particularly in the management of headaches, both migrainous and tension headaches.

To make the patient aware of a physiological parameter, the signal must be heightened, and the results fed back to the subject, usually as a visual or an auditory signal. Once the patient is aware of the parameter (e.g. muscle tension), he or she can begin to learn to modify it. The two main methods used are:

- electromyogram feedback, which gives an indication of muscle tension
- skin warmth, particularly in vascularly mediated headache

Because the subject has tangible evidence of the variable being measured, techniques to try and reverse changes, such as relaxation, are easier to learn, and immediate evidence of any success is confirmed. Relaxation techniques are usually combined with biofeedback in the clinical situation. It has also been used in other pain states, particularly those associated with increased muscle tension, for example in chronic back pain and myofascial pain.

## Family therapy

In view of what has been said about the alteration of the patient's role in chronic pain to a more passive sick role, it is obvious that the dynamic structure of the patient's family and immediate social circle will be radically altered. The altered family dynamics may tend to perpetuate the status quo, and unless the whole family understands the reasons for changes in the patient's behaviour during therapy, there may be no reinforcement of well behaviour, and inappropriate reactions to illness behaviour. It is therefore less valuable and may prove impossible to treat the patient whilst excluding the family.

It has been shown that the extinction of unwanted behaviour pattern is faster when positive rewards for desirable behaviour are used, rather than negative rewards for undesirable behaviour. A family group who is actively involved in a patient's therapy may increase the success of treatment, by acting as valued positive reinforcers of well behaviour.

The members of the family should become active participants in the rehabilitation process, in the same way that patients themselves need to become active in their treatment programme. For this, the family members need to attend sessions alongside the patient, learning the fundamental principles of cognitive-behavioural theory with the patient, as well as being present during assessments of progress.

### Hypnosis

Hypnotic techniques can be useful in pain relief. It has to be borne in mind that only 5% of the population can achieve deep trance status under hypnosis, although a further 85% may achieve a light trance or deeply relaxed state. Hypnosis is time-consuming, requires expertise on the part of the practitioner and needs reinforcement over time. There are several different approaches to pain reduction under hypnosis:

- relaxation
- direct diminution of pain
- substitution of another sensory modality which is more acceptable, e.g. warmth
- displacement in the perceived site of pain to a more peripheral body part
- dissociation, where a different location associated with pleasant experiences is imagined instead, for example, a sunny day at the beach

The efficacy of hypnosis tends to diminish with time, so to prolong this, self-hypnosis may be taught. In patients who are well-motivated this is not difficult. Failure of previously successful self-hypnotizing patients requires review and possibly further reinforcement of techniques.

### Pain management programmes

Pain management programmes have become established over the last few years as offering the most comprehensive psychological approach to the treatment of chronic pain. They are based on cognitive-behavioural principles, and are described in the next chapter. The approach described by Fordyce to behavioural therapy forms a major component of such programmes.

# References

1.  Turner JA, Romano JM. Self report screening measures for depression in chronic pain. *J Clin Psychol* **40:** 909–913, 1984

2.  Gross R. *Psychology – Science of Mind and Behaviour*, 2nd edn. Hodder & Stoughton, London, 1992

3.  Fordyce WE. A behavioural perspective on chronic pain. *Br J Clin Psychol* **21:** 313–320, 1982

4.  Fordyce WE. Behavioural science and chronic pain. *Postgrad Med J* **60:** 865–868, 1984

5.  Jensen MP, Turner JA, Romano JM, Karoly P. Coping with chronic pain: a critical review of the literature. *Pain* **47:** 249–283, 1991

6.  Melzack R, Wall PD. Pain mechanisms: a new theory. *Science* **150:** 971–979, 1965

7.  Merskey H. Psychological approaches to the treatment of chronic pain. *Postgrad Med J* **60:** 886–892, 1984

8.  Linton SJ. A critical review of behavioural treatments for chronic benign pain other than headache. *Br J Clin Psychol* **21:** 321–337, 1982

9.  Beck AT. Thinking and depression. *Arch Gen Psychol* **9:** 324–333, 1963

10. Beck AT et al. *Cognitive Therapy of Depression*. New York: Guilford Press, 1979

11. Beck AT. *Cognitive Therapy and the Emotional Disorders*. New York: International Press, 1976

12. Beck AT, Emery G. *Cognitive Therapy of Anxiety and Phobic Disorders*. Philadelphia: Center for Cognitive Therapy, 1979

13. Mahoney MJ, Arnkoff D. Cognitive and self control therapies. In: (Garfield SL, Bergin AE, eds). *Handbook of Psychotherapy and Behaviour Change*. New York: John Wiley, 1978, pp. 689–722

14. Turk DC, Rudy TE. An integrated approach to pain treatment: beyond the scalpel and syringe. In: (Tollinson CA, ed.) *Handbook of Chronic Pain Management*. Baltimore: Williams & Wilkins, 1987

# 27

# Pain management programmes

**J. M. Green and J. A. Pateman**

The prevalence of chronic pain within the community is very high. However, many people continue to function effectively in spite of the pain and never become patients. A large number of those who do present to physicians may be effectively managed by intermittent interventions and support from general practitioners. For those who fail this type of management, referral to a pain clinic may eventually ensue. Many of these patients can be successfully managed with single types of procedures or combined physical and psychological approaches within the pain clinic. A number of patients, however, do poorly in spite of this type of management, and begin to function badly in many or most areas of their lives.

Pain management programmes employ a multidisciplinary approach to such patients. The primary aim of the programme is an improvement of quality of life, rather than simply a reduction in pain, which indeed may not occur. The key features are a team approach from several specialists, aimed at education, increased overall fitness and coping abilities, and drug withdrawal. Patients are treated in groups, which provide peers who may have the same or different pain problems. Both inpatient and outpatient programmes are employed; they may be short-term, intensive courses, or occur over a longer period with more reinforcement. They are labour-intensive, and therefore expensive to run, in particular the inpatient type, and so are usually employed only for a highly selected group of patients, who have already failed other approaches.

## Type of patient

The criteria which first determine which people with chronic pain are referred to a pain clinic include the level to which the pain interferes with the person's life, their ability to learn coping strategies, and the degree of support from family and friends, as well as their premorbid personality, and the characteristics of the pain. Patients treated in the pain clinic fall into three categories:

- Treatments employed are successful and reduce pain or improve function.

- Treatments fail to reduce pain, but the patient continues to function well.
- Treatments fail and the patient also functions poorly.

This last group of patients are usually those for whom referral to a pain management programme is considered. Signs of failing function include inappropriate drug usage, crumbling family support with either antagonism or overprotection, general reduction of physical abilities, and inappropriate expectations of the future.

When the patient develops into a sick role within a family unit, secondary gains may become established for other members of the family as well as for the patient, and these become entrenched over time. The influence of the patient's family is fundamental and patient selection includes interviews with the patient's close relations, who may be involved in the treatment programme. Support from family or a significant other is an important indicator of good outcome. Reliance on drugs reduces performance, clouding cognitive faculties and reducing physical activity. Poor functional ability may further decrease as chronic inactivity, pathological interpersonal relationships and dependence on others for physical, emotional and often financial support become established.

If no intervention is made, these patients will often continue to seek a definitive diagnosis and treatment for their condition, undergoing more and more invasive interventions, with risk of further morbidity, as well as reinforcement of the sick role. This pattern may be well-established by the time of referral to a pain management programme, and have contributed to the failure of single-modality treatments.

A patient who is referred to a pain management programme is typically someone who:

- is disabled in multiple areas of his or her life
- is physically inactive
- is passive in relationships with his or her immediate family
- is isolated from other contacts
- is usually not in employment
- may also be taking multiple drug treatments

## Structure of pain management programmes

Pain management programmes vary in their structure and timetable. Features common to all include specialists from several areas working together to change the interaction between the pain and the patient fundamentally. These usually include the pain specialist, psychologist, physiotherapist, nurse specialist, and sometimes occupational therapist. The patient must be an active player in the programme, and peer interaction is important. Usually the day is divided into modules when different activities take place, including physical therapy, educational sessions and group activities. Drug withdrawal or reduction is attempted. Some programmes are specifically designed for patients with one particular pain problem, such as chronic low back pain, whereas others treat patients with a wide variety of conditions in the same group.

## Physical

These patients function below their potential physical capability because long-standing low levels of activity have affected their general health. A group physiotherapy programme increases flexibility, improves stamina and increases overall exercise tolerance. In addition, specific areas may be targeted for individuals. Pacing of activity is taught to prevent episodes of exacerbation of pain. The patient's goals need to be coordinated with the fitness programme. A gradual increase is made in activities necessary to achieve the patient's specific goals, such as sitting or walking time. Later these may be combined with group activities, such as swimming or shopping trips.

## Drug withdrawal

The most common groups of drugs taken are analgesics, anxiolytics and antidepressants. Side-effects of high-dose opioid analgesics include constipation, habituation, reduced pain tolerance, changes in mood, sleep disturbances and clouding of consciousness. The benzodiazepine group of drugs is also highly addictive, and impairs global function. Both groups become less effective after time, leading to increasing dosage. Non-opioid analgesics expose the patient to the risk of gastrointestinal ulceration, bleeding, renal impairment and hepatic and bone marrow sensitivity. Antidepressants often have anticholinergic and antihistaminic properties, causing drowsiness, constipation, and blurred vision.

Taking high doses of analgesics, long-term anxiolytics and antidepressants exposes the patient to risk of serious side-effects, is ineffective in treating pain, and further reduces the ability of the patient to function. The level of comprehension and concentration may be impaired and jeopardize the success of the whole programme. Education about drug side-effects increases compliance with drug withdrawal, and must be coordinated with the concurrent teaching of alternative coping strategies to avoid pain exacerbation and future drug dependence. Again the peer group provides valuable support. On an inpatient programme drugs may be given as a cocktail which is gradually reduced in strength. Initially, increased levels of pain may be experienced; this must be anticipated and extra support given.

## Psychological

As stated in the previous chapter, Fordyce's approach to behavioural therapy forms a large component of the psychological aspects of a pain management programme, and cognitive aspects are also important. In the maintenance of any improvements achieved, long-term coping strategies will be necessary; these can be used by the patient confidently away from the programme setting.

The principal targets are teaching goal-setting; pacing; coping strategies; education; reducing illness behaviour; and fostering group support. Goal-setting may be done as a group activity, and also provides a basis for the physical therapy programme. As an example, a patient who sets as a goal attending the opera but who can only sit for a few minutes at a time can build up sitting time as part of the physical programme. Many patients need help with setting realistic and appropriate goals, which should be re-evaluated periodically, and should include pleasurable activities as well as chores.

In attaining goals, pacing of activity becomes important. The typical activity pattern of the patient is a seesaw of under- and overactivity, with exacerbations of pain caused by overexercise resulting in periods of total rest. Often the overactivity results from frustration built up during the previous period of inactivity. In this scenario, the level of activity is determined by pain, and this is one aspect that behavioural therapy addresses. Pain level is replaced as the determinant of exercise by an exercise quota. When the initial steps are small and do not precipitate an exacerbation of pain, they can be built up stepwise, to achieve desired activities. Group support is important in a pain management programme, and in particular in an inpatient programme the peer group which forms may be very powerful. It must be remembered, however, that this peer group is temporary, and changes which are made must be sufficiently established to persist after the conclusion of the programme, when patients return to their previous environment. Coping strategies and illness behaviour have been discussed in the previous chapter, and education is discussed further below.

## Education

Education is aimed at increasing the patient's knowledge about pain, in particular the difference between acute and chronic pain. In an acutely painful condition, the purpose of the pain is to warn the individual of damage, to encourage rest of the affected part, preventing further damage and increasing healing. However, in a chronic pain condition, periods of absolute rest further increase pain when activity does occur, decrease fitness so that pain actually spreads to neighbouring parts, and lead to see-sawing levels of activity with both under- and overactivity. Many of the concepts taught are difficult to grasp initially and require both a degree of intelligence and an ability to concentrate and process information which is not clouded by high dosages of drugs.

Pacing of activity must be practised within the group. Setting of realistic goals is fundamental to an improvement in quality of life; many patients have unrealistic expectations, inappropriate to their age and condition. Acceptance that they need to learn to live *with* the pain is also a very hard concept, and for patients whose life typically revolves around medication schedules and seeking diagnosis and cure demands considerable patience and skill on the part of the professionals in the pain management programme.

## Inpatient and outpatient programmes

Inpatient programmes are high-intensity and short-duration. They may last for a few days or up to a month; they are disruptive to family life and to work if the patient is employed. The main advantage is that a powerful peer group will form, and taking patients out of the family environment initially may be necessary to enable them to alter the perception of themselves as passive sufferers. Reinforcement of concepts is most powerful, and groups at different stages of the programme with some joint sessions provide mutual reinforcement. Patient throughput is less and cost higher, as hospital standard facilities may be required, with provision for on-call medical cover, so many centres are unable to offer this type of facility.

Outpatient programmes can potentially treat a larger number of people, although over a longer time course. Changes which do occur become established within the patient's normal environment and so may be more likely to persist. However, the effects of peer pressure are less. Results are conflicting.

### Outcome

Given the high cost of pain management programmes and the current financial climate in health care, combined with the potential saving to the community from returning valuable individuals to full employment and decreasing demands on scarce health care resources, the measurement of outcomes from pain management programmes is important both to clinicians and managers.

Most patients attending a pain management programme have had multiple therapeutic attempts designed to reduce pain which have failed, so the primary goal of a pain management programme is to reduce suffering, rather than pain. Suffering can be thought of as the loss of the patient's ability to fulfil or enjoy the normal activities of daily living: work, household chores, social activities and interpersonal relationships. Reduction in levels of suffering can be measured as rates of return to work, achievement of goals, reduction in illness behaviour, increase in well behaviour, changes in medication usage, rates of presentation to physicians, or depression ratings. However, given the very heterogeneous nature of the pain population, it is easy to see that factors such as rates of return to work depend on much more than the success or failure of the treatment programme, and will vary widely between programmes.

Some authors have attempted to develop outcome measures that encompass physical, psychological and behavioural factors, to modify the bias produced by individual variables. Importantly, pain scores at presentation or discharge do not correlate with programme success. Patients' beliefs with regard to their control over the pain affect their exercise capability after the programme, as do perceived abilities. Higher self-efficacy scores are associated with higher self-reports of return to work, social activities and lower medication use at medium-term follow-up. To justify a programme, a good outcome must also be sustained, and measurement after an interval is more important than immediately after completion of a programme. Not all factors within the individual's environment are within the reach of modification by a pain management programme. Employment opportunities, long-term family support and age may modify the success of the programme. Only half of those who initially improve may maintain that improvement after a year.

## Further reading

Jensen M *et al.* Coping with chronic pain: a critical review of the literature. *Pain* **47**: 249–283, 1991

Sjogren P, Erikson J. Opioid toxicity. *Curr Opinion Anaesthesiol* **7**: 465–469

Bonica JJ. *The Management of Pain.* Philadelphia: Lea & Febiger, 1990

Nimmo WJ, Rowbotham DJ, Smith G. *Anaesthesia.* Oxford: Blackwell Scientific Publications, 1994

Williams AC, Nicholas MK *et al.* Evaluation of a cognitive behavioural programme for rehabilitating patients with chronic pain. *Br J Gen Pract* **43:** 513–518, 1993

Richardson IH, Richardson PH, Williams AC, Featherstone J, Harding VR. The effects of a cognitive behavioural pain management programme on the quality of work and employment status of severely impaired chronic pain patients. *Disabil Rehabil* **16:** 26–34, 1994

Peter J, Large R, Elkind G. Follow-up results from a randomised control trial evaluating in- and out-patient pain management programmes *Pain* **50** 41–50, 1992

28
# The future

**S. J. Dolin**

Future changes are likely to come from three directions.

## Improved delivery of chronic pain services

Pain relief is developing as a subspecialty. As it becomes recognized, this will lead to a formal structured training for pain specialists and criteria for standards of training. It will also lead to standardization of resources and facilities. There are moves to standardize codes for diagnosis and treatment which will aid national data collection about clinical need and allocation of resources.

## Early intervention and prevention

The possibility of prevention of the development of chronic pain arose with the observation that phantom limb pain may be reduced by establishing nociceptive blockade before and during amputation.[1] This led to the concept of pre-emptive analgesia: that it might be easier to prevent pain rather than to treat it. The use of preoperative and intraoperative local anaesthetics to block peripheral input and other analgesics to block nociception as a means of increasing the effcacy of postoperative analgesia has been examined. The evidence in favour of pre-emptive analgesia in acute pain has been equivocal and the validity of the concept is still being examined. To date, there have been few studies to assess the value of prevention in chronic pain, but the possibility that failure to provide adequate pain control in the early stages may contribute to the development of severe, intractable or opiate-insensitive pain is exciting and we may well see some important developments in terms of early intervention programmes in the near future.

Another possibility that must receive serious consideration from all involved with health care is whether or not early intervention and education can prevent the development of disability. This is most relevant in the area of back pain. The role of preventive educational programmes within the work situation and in the primary health care setting needs to be assessed.

Early intervention programmes involving education and physiotherapy for those with acute back pain may be able to prevent these problems becoming chronic. The epidemic of disability due to back pain crosses the bounds of health care and social services and will benefit from a very broad approach.

## Pharmacology

Over the past decade there has been an explosion in the basic scientific understanding of pain mechanisms, both for acute and more recently chronic pain. There are now multiple newly identified modulators and neurotransmitters which may be possible targets for pharmacological manipulation. Some of these are listed below:

### Factors influencing peripheral nociceptors

- immune cell factors: cytokines, enkephalins, endorphins
- neurogenic agents: neurokinins, galanin, somatostatin
- vascular agents: kinins, 5-hydroxytryptamine (5-HT), nitric oxide
- tissue injury: bradykinin, acidosis, prostanoids
- nerve growth factor
- sympathetic influences: neuropeptide Y, noradrenaline, prostanoids

### Neurotransmitters in dorsal horn of spinal cord

- glutamate
- aspartate
- substance P
- neurokinin A
- neurokinin B
- calcitonin gene-related peptide
- somatostatin

### Possible inhibitory pre- or postsynaptic influences in dorsal horn

- opioid receptors agonists at $\mu$, $\sigma$ and $\kappa$ receptor
- $\alpha_2$-adrenergic agonists
- $\gamma$-aminobutyric acid (GABA)$_A$ and GABA$_B$ receptor agonists
- 5-HT$_1$ agonists
- 5-HT$_3$ antagonists
- $N$-methyl-D-aspartate antagonists
- neurokinin antagonists

### Possible neuromodulators via interneurons in spinal cord

- cholecystokinin
- nitric oxide
- dynorphin
- glycine
- enkephalin

Which of these endogenous substances will prove most suitable for pharmacological manipulation in the future is currently speculative, but the possibilities raise great hopes for the future of the field of pain management.

## References

1. Back S, Noreng MF, Tjellden NU. Phantom limb pain in amputees during the first 12 months following limb amputation, after preoperative lumbar epidural blockade. *Pain* **33:** 297–301,1988
2. Dray A, Urban L, Dickenson A. Pharmacology of chronic pain. *Trends Pharmacol Sci* **15:** 190–197, 1994

# Invasive procedures: technical details

**N. L. Padfield**

Pain management has developed in many different directions. Those trained in this subspecialty who wish to embrace all kinds of pain problems will need to know about and become proficient in implementing increasingly invasive techniques of pain relief.[1]

This chapter will deal with four key areas:

- implantable drug delivery systems
- cryoanalgesia
- radiofrequency thermocoagulation
- electrical stimulation analgesia (including transcutaneous electrical nerve stimulation, or TENS)

## *Appendix 1*

### Implantable drug delivery systems

The conditions that respond best to this route of drug delivery are often 'end-of-the-road' situations where there has been failure of symptom control with conservative therapy. As a general caveat, a trial of a specific drug by a non-invasive route must always be undertaken before planning any implantable drug delivery system. Drugs can have more selective actions when delivered to specific targets with fewer associated systemic side-effects.

#### Indications

- malignant disease that cannot be controlled by the oral route because of untenable side-effects (intractable nausea, constipation, somnolence)
- spasticity, in association with multiple sclerosis, poststroke
- pancreatitis
- failed back
- peripheral neuropathy (caution with diabetics because of greater tendency to sepsis)

#### Drugs used or considered for the extradural/intrathecal route

- Opioid selection will depend on stability in solution (viz. morphine 70 days and diamorphine 15 days) and lipid solubility. While morphine appears to be the popular agent for cancer pain, there is evidence that a more lipid-soluble agent, sufentanil, in combination with bupivacaine is more suitable in non-cancer chronic pain such as arachnoiditis, epidural scarring and vertebral body compression fractures.[2]

- $\alpha_2$-Agonists can be used as primary analgesics or as an adjunct to morphine if the patient has developed tolerance to opioids. Clonidine is the drug most commonly used but dexmedetomidine,[3-5] which is 20 000 times more potent than clonidine, may replace it once it becomes commercially available. Epidural clonidine given as a bolus (range 300–700 $\mu$g) followed by an infusion rate of 10–50 $\mu$g/h has been used in the management of reflex sympathetic dystrophy but needs further evaluation.[6] However, a small study of 10 patients where a single dose of 150 $\mu$g administered epidurally was compared with the same dose given intravenously showed no significant difference in clinical effect between either route, but a high incidence of adverse effects was reported in both groups, even at this lower dosage.[7]

- Local anaesthetics are often used when patients become opioid-tolerant.[8,9] In one study of 52 patients with severe intractable cancer pain, doses of bupivacaine given intrathecally ranged from up to 30 mg/24 h in two-thirds of patients to up to 305 mg/24 h in the other third. In the same study the dose of intrathecal morphine was kept to 10–25 mg/24 h during the first 2 months of treatment in more than half the patients. The range of duration of infusion was from 1 to 305 days. Care must be exercised in selecting the appropriate volume and concentration in order to avoid side-effects like excessive spread, hypotension and unacceptable paraesthesiae. In a recently published study,[10] where the subject of side-effects was addressed, the authors concluded that a morphine to bupivacaine ratio of approximately 1 : 10 (0.5 mg/4.75 mg B) gave satisfactory pain control with few side-effects that would be expected to derive from intrathecal opiates but that there were cases of urinary retention, paraesthesiae and gait disturbances attributable to the bupivacaine. The median dose of morphine was 6 mg/24 h and the median daily intrathecal volume infused 10 ml/24 h. Long-term studies of opioid/local anaesthetic mixtures have demonstrated the safety and usefulness in management of cancer pain.[11]

- Baclofen is a very potent spasmolytic acting through $\gamma$-aminobutyric acid receptors but does not readily pass the blood–brain barrier. The intrathecal route is very effective at relieving muscle spasm where a bolus dose of 25–75 $\mu$g is tried and then, if a satisfactory response is obtained, it is given as a continuous infusion by a pump at a rate of 50–800 $\mu$g/24 h.[12,13] There is evidence that given this way voluntary movement can be greatly improved where it was previously hampered by greatly increased muscle tone.[14,15] Overdosage causing hypotension and drowsiness has been reported to respond to increments of 1 mg intravenous physostigmine[16] and cessation of drug administration. However, it has been reported to be insufficient to treat status epilepticus complicating overdosage and in such a case artificial ventilation and intense monitoring are mandatory.[17] Loss of consciousness can occur with doses in the range of 25–60 $\mu$g intrathecally.

- Ketamine[18] is a phencyclidine derivative and an *N*-methyl-D-aspartate (NMDA) antagonist and has been shown to have analgesic effects at an intrathecal dose range of 5–50 mg in 3 mi of 5% dextrose. However, its use is often associated with troublesome psychotropic side-effects and it is at present little used.
- Midazolam[19] has been shown to be effective preferentially by the intrathecal route rather than the epidural route. A single dose of 2 mg intrathecally has however been demonstrated to be effective for up to 1 year, so therefore it does not require to be given as a continuous infusion. In one double-blind trial of failed back syndrome patients, midazolam compared favourably with extradural Depo-Medrone and achieved a significant reduction in analgesic intake.[20]
- Octreotide[21] can be useful in the management of cancer pain by intrathecal infusion at a dose range of 5–20 $\mu$g/h. It has been found to be stable in solution for up to 28 days. It has been shown to be more effective than somatostatin and less toxic.[22]
- Calcitonin,[23,24] in a dosage of 100 IU intrathecally has been used in malignant pain[25] and postoperative pain but generally there has been little reported use because of inconsistent results and controversy over its pharmaceutical formulation.
- Non-steroidal anti-inflammatory drugs (NSAIDs): Ketorolac[26–28] has been reported as potentially useful but further clinical trials are needed. It appears to exert an effect on secondary hyperalgesia mediated by neurokinin 1 and glutamate receptors of the NMDA type.

## Equipment

- Portocath epidural system (Figure A.1)
- Cordis Secor patient-administered rechargeable reservoir (cf. patient-controlled analgesia 'on the hoof'; Figure A.2)

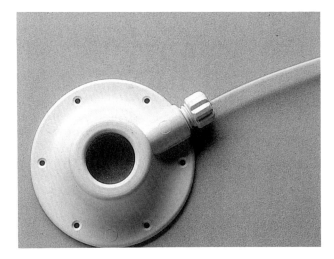

**Figure A.1** Braun Periplant Filtrosafe reservoir.

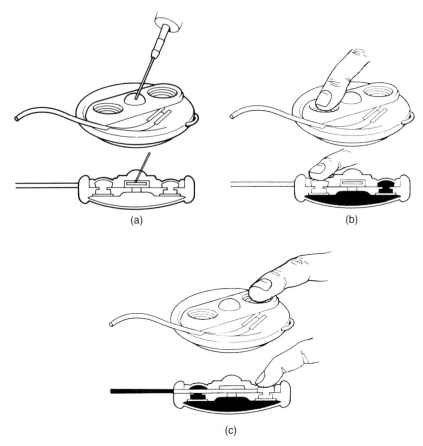

**Figure A.2** Cordis Secor 1 + 1 implantable patient-controlled reservoir. (a) The reservoir is filled via a self-sealing dome; (b) press button 1 and a single dose is transferred to the delivery button; (c) press button 2 and, whilst button 1 is filling, a single bolus is delivered.

- Synchromed – telemetrically programmed (Figure A.3)
- Anschultz – constant infusion
- Infusaid – relied on the body's heat to expand freon gas to drive the pump – very unreliable and has now been withdrawn

If opting for an implantable self-administration reservoir system one must be certain that the patient can be trusted – suicide attempts have occurred by deliberate overdosage. Siting the reservoir can be a problem in the obese since localization and then administration by depressing the reservoirs can be physically difficult.

### Routes of administration

- Temporary systems with exteriorized injection ports can be used for extradural catheters, which should be tunnelled if their use is likely to be prolonged. The procedure should be performed in clean surroundings

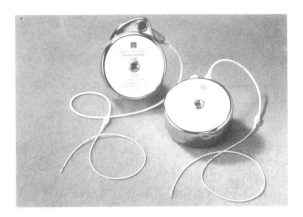

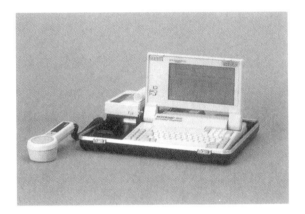

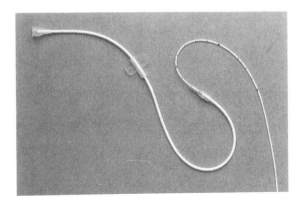

**Figure A.3** Medtronic Synchromed pump, fully implantable.

under sterile conditions. The final cutaneous exit site must be in a comfortable site for the patient, with enough catheter exposed to let the bacterial filter rest on the anterior abdominal wall. The skin exit site should be regularly examined for infection or inflammation. With a good technique of insertion and wound toilet, such a system connected to a Baxter Infusaid has been successfully used for home care management of cancer patients.[29]

- Implanted reservoirs connected to extradural catheters can be selected for prolonged administration which may be on a domiciliary, hospital or hospice situation (Figure A.4). As with the tunnelled catheters, the site of the reservoir must be comfortable for patients so that they can lie on their backs and sides without it digging into them.[30]

- Intrathecal drug delivery system: Occasionally it is desirable to infuse drugs directly into the cerebrospinal fluid. This may be done through a fine 29-gauge catheter inserted through a percutaneous introducer. This is only suitable for short-term use as there is a risk of infection or overdosage. In a study of 89 patients treated with exteriorized intrathecal catheters, despite finding bacterial colonization in 17 out of the 89 patients, none had clinical meningitis, except one who had no

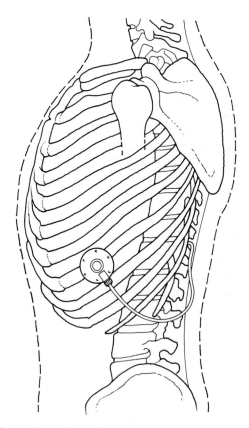

**Figure A.4** Periplant and extradural catheter *in situ*.

growth on bacterial culture of the filter. The authors concluded that, in their population, exchange of the infusion systems when empty (within 1 month) and of the antibacterial filters once a month does not appear to increase the infection risk from the opioid/bupivacaine mixtures. They also found the bupivacaine/opioid mixtures to be chemically stable within 3–10% of the original doses at 30 days.[31] All drugs, because of the small volumes involved (0.2–1 ml in the case of baclofen), should only be given by a senior nurse or doctor by this route and must be given through a bacterial filter which must have been primed with the drug given. Good pain relief can be achieved this way in the terminally ill. Postmortem studies in 15 male patients treated over 4–274 (median 81) days with morphine and bupivacaine infusion through intrathecally placed nylon catheters for relief of cancer pain had no neuropathological changes attributable either to the drugs and their preservatives, sodium metabisulphite and sodium edetate, or to the nylon catheters.[32]

### Complications of implanted drug delivery systems

- catheter – kinking, dislodgement, cerebrospinal fluid leakage (usually at catheter entry site)
- pumps – air lock, volume variation, battery leakage, power failure
- seroma
- infection, meningitis
- drugs – few are recommended to be given this way!
- Expense: There are now data[33] that there is an eventual cost-benefit because, despite the initial high cost of the equipment, the accumulated expenses are lower in comparison with other medical treatments (such as outpatient time, physiotherapy and further hospital admissions). There is also evidence that, if an intrathecal infusion is likely to be required for longer than 3 months, then a totally implanted system like the Synchromed works out cheaper in the long run, despite the higher initial cost, than an exteriorized system with an epidural catheter, bacterial inline filter and programmable pump.[34]
- recognition as implanting centre (Department of Health has issued a circular regarding supraregional specialty for any procedure performed nationally less than 1000 times per annum)

In rare instances adequate pain relief can only be obtained by the intraventricular administration of opiates. This requires placement of the catheter by a neurosurgeon and is thus beyond the scope of this book. Examples where this might be helpful are in the management of patients with terminal oral and head and neck cancers.

## Appendix 2

## Cryoanalgesia

Pain relief can be achieved by freezing nerves directly.[35] While histological studies show that epineural and endoneural circulation is disrupted, leading

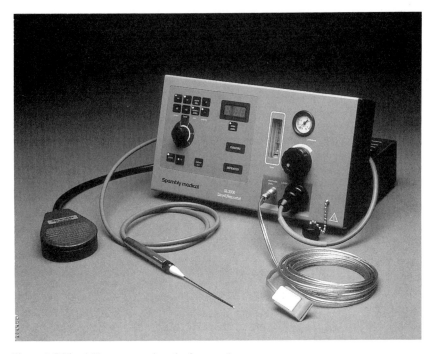

**Figure A.5** Lloyd Neurostat and probe for cryotherapy.

to severe oedema with diapedesis of polymorphonuclear cells through the vessel walls, there is a low incidence of long-term deafferentation problems since the nerve sheaths are not disrupted. Thus, the nerve axons can regenerate down the old neural tubes without scarring. Analgesia can be expected to last between 12 days and a few months and, interestingly, the analgesia can outlast the return of sensation.[36]

It is useful therefore in self-limiting conditions or in order to give the patient a 'pain holiday' for a special event (e.g. a wedding). Cryoprobes are electrically insulated up to the tip and thus the target nerves can be stimulated at 2 and 100 Hz for confirmation of accurate placement before the tip is cooled to $-60°C$ by the adiabatic expansion of nitrous oxide or carbon dioxide. The ice ball that forms after 60 s is 2–4 mm in diameter depending on the vascularity of the tissue. It can usually be performed with the help of local anaesthesia; in fact patients will often tell you how soothing the actual cryotherapy is! As a form of treatment it has its advocates[37] and its detractors.

### Indications

- neuromas
- fractured ribs (intercostal nerves)
- postherpetic neuralgia (sometimes)
- facet joint pain

- coccydynia
- scar pains

### Use of cryoprobe (Figure A.5)

- infiltration of skin surface with 1% lignocaine
- insertion of cryoprobe under image intensification
- stimulation to 100 Hz and 2 Hz for sensory confirmation and motor fibre exclusion
- injection of 1% lignocaine at site for lesion
- lesion at −60°C for 120 s
- injection of 0.5 ml of bupivacaine/Depo-Medrone mixture (10 ml 0.5% plain bupivacaine + 40 mg Depo-Medrone).

## Appendix 3

### Radiofrequency thermocoagulation

In 1974 Shealy introduced a fluoroscopically guided radiofrequency technique for facet joint denervation,[38] which has since been refined.[39] It is now currently used for the following indications.

### Indications

- facet joint disease
- trigeminal ganglion neurolysis
- dorsal root entry zone lesioning
- cordotomy
- peripheral nerve lesions
- coccydynia
- dorsal root ganglion neurolysis

The tip of a fine 23-gauge Teflon insulated flat bevelled hollow needle (Sluyter-Mehta) can be used to stimulate at 2 and 100 Hz by the insertion of the probe from the radiofrequency generator in order to locate the optimal zone for lesioning. Once located, the needle tip is then heated to 65–90°C, as measured by a thermocouple in the tip of the probe, for 60–90 s (Figure A.6). Full anaesthetic monitoring is mandatory but the patient should be awake in order to confirm accurate localization of the needle prior to lesioning.

### Use of radiofrequency lesioning

- infiltration of skin surface with 1% lignocaine
- insertion of Sluyter-Mehta needle under image intensification
- stimulation to 100 Hz and 2 Hz for sensory confirmation and motor fibre exclusion
- injection of 1% lignocaine at site for lesion

(a)

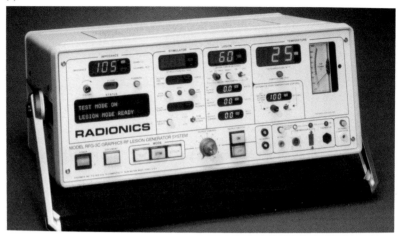

(b)

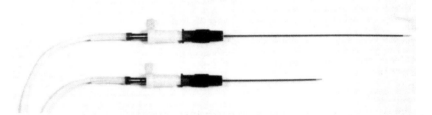

**Figure A.6** (a) Radionics radiofrequency lesion generator and (b) Sluyter-Mehta needles.

- lesion at 65–90°C for 60–90 s
- injection of 0.5 ml of bupivacaine/Depo-Medrone mixture (10 ml 0.5% plain bupivacaine + 40 mg Depo-Medrone)

If several lesions are planned, time can be saved in order to allow the local anaesthetic time to work by using two needles simultaneously and alternating localization and lesioning. Examples have already been discussed in earlier chapters – facet joint denervation for chronic low back pain arising from zygapophyseal joint pain.

## Appendix 4

### Transcutaneous nerve stimulation

Transcutaneous nerve stimulation appears to alleviate the appreciation of pain in certain circumstances where there is a peripheral nociceptive component (Figure A.7). Conversely, it does not help in central pain states and psychological pain problems.

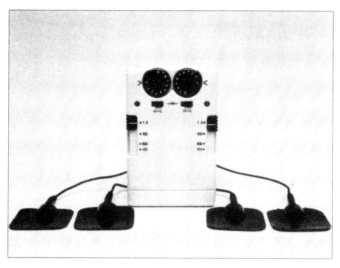

**Figure A.7** Transcutaneous nerve stimulator and pads.

### Indications

- myofascial syndromes
- peripheral nerve injuries
- phantom limb
- stump pains
- possibly in some mechanical back and neck pains

Rubber electrodes of adequate size (at least 4 cm²) to ensure low local current density (1–5 mA/cm²) are placed in the painful area with plenty of electrode gel to ensure good contact and the patient is instructed to control the amplitude and frequency of the output from a small light portable stimulator that can be worn undetected. The main advantage of this technique is that it has virtually no side-effects and it moves the locus of pain control into the patient's own hands. Even if it does not afford complete relief, it can often be very helpful in combination with physiotherapy and analgesic medication.

## Appendix 5

### Spinal cord stimulation

Stimulation of the dorsal column has been performed by direct placement of electrodes at laminectomy by neurosurgeons from the late 1960s.[40] The technique then fell into relative disrepute as the scientific basis for its action was then unexplained. In recent animal studies the vascular depressor effect induced by dorsal column stimulation was blocked by calcitonin gene-related peptide.[41] Apart from the neuromodulator involvement, analgesia appears to come from decreasing the firing of spinothalamic tract cells which are activated by small fibres. Clinical experience would suggest that stimulating the nerve axons in the dorsal columns causes antidromic antinociception and that, because of the anatomical site of the stimulation, many more nerve axons can be recruited than by more peripheral methods. Development of percutaneous techniques with a multiplicity of electrodes with four to eight stimulating sites per electrode, introduced by a modified Tuohy needle into the epidural space, has now brought this technique into the practice of pain specialists. However, there still remains a small group of patients who, because of spinal canal stenosis, epidural scarring and other physical barriers to the passage of the electrodes, require the electrodes to be placed under direct vision at laminotomy by a neurosurgeon.

### Patient selection

Before considering this expensive form of treatment, the following criteria should be satisfied:

- There is a physical basis for the complaint.
- All forms of alternative therapy have been tried.
- Psychiatric assessment has confirmed motivation and long-term commitment without major issues of secondary gain (compensation, litigation).
- The underlying pathology and topography are suitable for stimulation by the appropriate electrode system.

### Indications

- sympathetically maintained pain of one extremity[42]
  - reflex sympathetic dystrophy
  - causalgia
- peripheral deafferentation pain[43]
  - stump pain
  - intractable neuralgia, unilateral cervical or lumbosacral radiculitis
- spinal cord and peripheral root lesions
  - phantom limb
  - postherpetic neuralgia
- ischaemic pain[44,45]
  - PVD
  - diabetic neuropathy
  - intractable angina pectoris despite full medical support[46,47]
  - syndrome X (angina pectoris with normal coronary arteriograms)[48]
- pain of both upper or lower extremities
  - cervical or lumbar radiculitis
  - SMP of both arms or legs
- SMP involving both upper and lower extremities, trunk, face
- low back pain with major leg pain component
- failed back surgery syndrome without significant leg pain[49,50]

The results of 320 patients spread over a 20-year period have been published where the authors' analysis of technical and clinical prognostic factors make fascinating reading and may be useful in selecting suitable patients.[51]

## Implantable systems

- The external stimulus generator antenna and batteries transmit to a sub-cutaneous receiver (Figure A.8).
- The impulse generator and battery are buried into a subcutaneous pocket with no external apparatus.
- In use is a combination of a subcutaneous receiver which also has a pulse generator and small battery. (Once the battery has run down, this type of receiver is unable to pick up external radiofrequency stimulation.)

**Table A.1** Comparison of dorsal column stimulation systems

| Radiofrequency system + antenna | Fully implantable system |
| --- | --- |
| *Benefits* | *Benefits* |
| Power, flexibility | Patient convenience |
| Allows complete control by patient | No external attachments |
| The frequency can go to 1400 Hz | No limitations on activity |
| No surgery is required to replace the battery | |
| Power is no concern | |
| | |
| *Disadvantages* | *Disadvantages* |
| Bulky external apparatus | Battery has to be replaced surgically |
| Difficulty in operation by patient | Limited programmability |
| | Maximum frequency only up to 120 Hz |

Some patients prefer the implantable device as it does not require any heavy external apparatus which might be awkward or embarrassing. However, such systems do have to be replaced every 3–4 years depending on usage at a cost of £4000+ a time, whereas the external systems only need the batteries changed as required, which is cheaper in the long run. The combined system, whilst theoretically excellent, tends to be used as a stimulator as patients find the external system bulky and, because of the smaller battery size, it only lasts up to 18 months and therefore ends up costing the most.

## Which lead(s) should be selected?

Generally quadripolar leads are good in unilateral single-extremity pain involving one to three dermatomes; if the pain is bilateral then dual quadripolar leads are better. If the pain pattern involves four to seven dermatomes then octapolar leads should be considered, again using a dual system for bilateral pain.

(a)

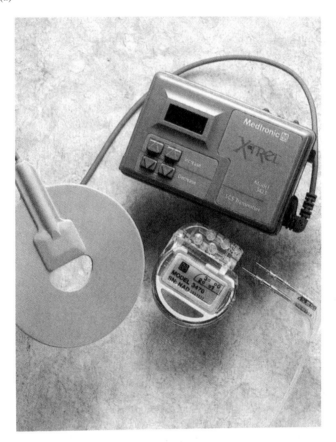

(b)

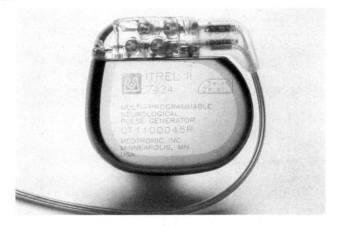

**Figure A.8** Medtronic (a) Extrel receiver/external antenna and transmitter system and (b) Itrel fully implantable Impulse generator.

## Which level?

In a study of 105 patients,[52] a database has been presented of sensory responses to electrical stimulation of the dorsal neural structures at various spine levels by epidural spinal cord stimulation. It was shown that, while some areas are relatively easy to cover with stimulation paraesthesiae (median aspect of hand, abdominal wall, anterior aspect of the thigh and the foot), others are relatively difficult (C2 root, neck, low back and the perineum). However, this is not the experience of other workers.[53]

## Implantation

- electrode placement with local anaesthesia
- trial stimulation period to confirm efficacy of dorsal column stimulation
- tunnelling the extension to the impulse generator/radio receiver (depending on which system is opted for)
- internalization of the above
- final programming which performed non-invasively and which will require the occasional revision as the tissues accommodate the implanted material

## Placement of the trial electrode

The patient is placed in the lateral position and the back is cleaned with Betadine (unless contraindicated) and draped. The catheter/electrode is then measured against the patient's back, allowing the stimulating electrodes to be 2 cm higher than the theoretical level for stimulation; the appropriate level for insertion is then marked on the skin and the catheter placed on the trolley. After infiltrating with 1% lignocaine the modified Tuohy needle is then inserted at 45° to the skin surface, the paramedian approach is favoured and the epidural space located by a combination of lateral fluoroscopy and loss of resistance to saline. The author finds it helpful to connect the Tuohy needle to a sterile burette giving set primed with normal saline and to watch for the sudden start of flow in the drip chamber once the epidural space has been entered. The guidewire is then passed all the way up the space and its progress monitored by posteroanterior fluoroscopy. Provided it does not kink or loop (usually because the needle is not sufficiently inserted and advanced into the epidural space) it is removed and the electrode(s) plus or minus stylet (depending on manufacturer) inserted and advanced to the appropriate level, which is confirmed by fluoroscopy. The proximal end is connected to an external stimulator and the electrode is then stimulated by slowly increasing the voltage until a pleasant tingling sensation is induced in the area of pain.

Once satisfactory electrode position is obtained, it is secured by suturing a winged Silastic collar, which grips the electrode by a silk ligature, to the interspinous ligament. It is then joined to an extension lead which is tunnelled laterally. The back wound is then closed with chromic catgut subcutaneously and the skin edges approximated with subcuticular Dexon. The electrode can be left exteriorized for a trial period of up to 2 weeks before it has to be removed to avoid the risk of infection. If theatre access is difficult in the intervening period before implantation or removal, the electrodes can be pulled at the exit site and then cut flush with the skin. The wires will then retract and, provided there is no infection, the electrode and remaining extension will remain sterile until the next definitive step is taken.

## Which settings?

Four parameters can be altered at the bedside:

- Electrode polarity: positive, negative and off. As a general rule, the negative electrode seems to produce greater stimulation for a given position than the positive. Electrode polarity will largely determine the anatomical site in which stimulation is experienced. By switching from one pair close together to spreading them apart to reversing the polarity of the pair and by making the case positive and the electrode(s) negative, the sites can be varied considerably without having to reposition the electrode. This can be very useful in restoring appropriate stimulation if there has been electrode shift since positioning in theatre. It does not always save the day when there has been considerable electrode migration.
- Pulse width: range 30–750 $\mu$s. By increasing the pulse width more fibres can be recruited and a wider spread of stimulation can be experienced. This is sometimes useful when certain areas seem to be difficult to reach with stimulation. A reduction in amplitude is often needed, though, as increasing the pulse width can cause the stimulation for a given amplitude to become painful.
- Frequency: 25–120 Hz for impulse generators, but can go up to 1200 Hz for antenna/radiofrequency exteriorized signal generators. Increasing the frequency can have several subjective effects. Low frequencies can feel more penetrating, even throbbing, whereas high frequencies are perceived as a constant tingling. The patient will tell you which frequency is preferred.
- Amplitude: up to 10 V. Lastly, the amplitude varies from 0 to 10 V. Patients have different sensitivities for numerous reasons. An average voltage lies in the range of 2–4 V; some very sensitive patients will find any voltage over 1.5 V unbearable, while other patients may need 6 V before they experience any stimulation. The reasons are legion, from epidural fibrosis to cord changes following trauma. It is quite usual to need to increase the amplitude at review.

## Implantation of permanent system selected

### Medtronic system

- Reopen previous median dorsal incision and gently divide tissues until silicon electrode collar and extension lead collar are located.
- Remove extension lead/collar, leaving proximal electrodes exposed.
- Prepare subcutaneous abdominal pocket tunnel up to a point in the mid axillary line and then to the median dorsal incision for connection.

### Neuromed system

- Prepare a subcutaneous pocket in abdomen then pass a hollow tunneller to mid axillary pocket, where the proximal excess lead is coiled.
- Separate and remove extension/exterior lead, leaving proximal electrode exposed.
- Gently feed the electrode down the lumen of tunneller (a 14-gauge long Abbocath is ideal) and pull the lead into the prepared abdominal pocket.
- Connect to receiver.

A few tips:

- Make sure the site is carefully chosen to allow the patient to wear a belt or waisted skirt comfortably. (It is a good idea to mark the line of the waist with a skin pencil at the preoperative visit.)
- Resist the temptation to remove any amount of subcutaneous fat to facilitate the accommodation of the impulse generator, as this can often lead to seroma or increased infection rate.
- Avoid sharp bends when implanting excess electrode or extension lead.
- Take care not to overtighten the screw connections as the delicate contacts can break or distort if overtightened.
- It is important to obliterate any potential space for haematoma formation around the implanted generator as this will weaken the signal and shorten the life of the battery.
- The patient must be nursed flat for 24 h with 'log rolling' only in order to prevent any flexion/extension of the spine and minimize any attendant electrode migration. This also allows time for a little fibrosis to help fix in the sutures and the electrode.

### Postoperative considerations

Intravenous antibiotics (e.g. cefuroxime 750 mg t.d.s.) should be administered for 72 h and then continued as an oral preparation for a further 7 days. Vancomycin is a good alternative for those patients allergic to penicillin.

The following complications have been reported:

- infection, from localized infection to meningitis
- transient paraplegia lasting about 3 months
- postoperative allodynia (touch perceived as pain)
- seroma and tenderness over the receiver or anchor site
- cerebrospinal fluid leakage
- electrode migration
- electrode failure
- receiver failure
- expanding epidural haematoma causing ascending paralysis
- sinus formation

## Deep brain stimulation

In very rare cases, deep brain stimulation may be the last resort. It has been shown in the cat to produce expression of c-*fos* immunoreactivity in the caudal medulla and upper cervical spinal cord following stimulation of the superior sagittal sinus.[54]

### Indications

- neural injury
- reflex sympathetic dystrophy
- failed back surgery syndrome
- pains whose topography is not amenable to dorsal cord stimulation
- underlying lesion has caused a loss of dorsal columns
- failure of spinal cord stimulation

As before, with dorsal column stimulation, the patient must have a suitable psychological profile.

### Sites

- sensory thalamus
- periaqueductal grey nucleus (Figure A.9)

### Complications

- 3% incidence of haemorrhage
- diplopia (when periaqueductal grey nucleus is the target)
- transient paraesthesias when the ventral basal thalamus is the target
- infection 3%, not usually in the central nervous system
- 10% malfunction of the equipment
- development of tolerance when periaqueductal grey nuclus is the target

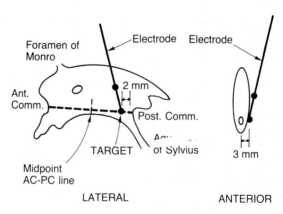

**Figure A.9** Electrode placement in reference to an outline of the third ventricle and aqueduct (Schaltenbrand-Bailey coordinates FP-10, HT-0, LT-4).

# Conclusion

There are now currently many physical methods of alleviating chronic pain. As our knowledge increases it will be easier to put the case for more invasive palliation once conservative measures have failed. Presently a lot of patients are denied implants because of cost and ignorance. As more and more data are collected from carefully selected and appropriate cases, together with a reduction in the price of the expensive implants, it is to be hoped that this effective treatment will become universally available to those who genuinely need it.

# References

1. Bedder MD. The anaesthesiologist's role in neuroaugmentative pain control techniques: spinal cord stimulation and neuraxial narcotics. In: *Progress in Anaesthesiology*, pp. 225–234, 1990
2. Hassenbusch SJ, Stanton-Hicks MD, Soukup J, Covington EC, Boland MB. Sufentanil citrate and morphine/bupivacaine as alternative agents in chronic epidural infusions for intractable non-cancer pain. *Neurosurgery* **29:** 76–81, 1991
3. Takano Y, Yaksh TL. Relative efficacy of spinal alpha-2 agonists, dexmedetomidine, clonidine and ST-91 determined in vivo by using N-ethoxycarbonyl-2-ethoxy-1,2-dihydroquinolone, an irreversible antagonist. *J Pharmacol Exp Ther* **258:** 438–436, 1991
4. Puke MJC, Weisenfeld-Hallin Z. The differential effects of morphine and the alpha-2 adrenoreceptor agonists clonidine and dexmedetomidine on the prevention and treatment of experimental neuropathic pain. *Anesth Analg* **77:** 104–109, 1993
5. Kalso EA, Pöyhiä R, Rosenberg PH. Spinal antinociception by dexmedetomidine, a highly selective alpha-2-adrenergic agonist. *Pharmacol Toxicol* **68:** 140–143, 1991
6. Rauch RL, Eisennach JC, Jackson K, Young LD, Southern NJ. Epidural clonidine treatment for refractory reflex sympathetic dystrophy. *Anesthesiology* **79:** 1163–1169, 1993
7. Carroll D, Jaddad A, King U, Wiffen P, Glynn C, McQuay H. Single-dose, randomized, double-blind, double dummy cross-over comparison of extradural and iv clonidine in chronic pain. *Br J Anaesth* **71:** 661–669, 1993
8. Van Dongen RTM, Crul BJP, De Beck M. Longterm intrathecal infusion of morphine and morphine/bupivacaine mixtures in the treatment of cancer pain: a retrospective analysis of 51 cases. *Pain* **55:** 119–123, 1993
9. Sjoberg M, Appelgren L, Einarsson S *et al.* Long-term intrathecal morphine and bupivacaine in "refractory" cancer pain. 1. Results from the first series of 52 patients. *Acta Anaesthesiol Scand* **35:** 30–43, 1991
10. Sjoberg M, Nitescu P, Appelgren L, Curelaru I. Long-term intrathecal morphine and bupivacaine in patients with refractory cancer pain. Results from a morphine:bupivacaine dose regimen of 0.5:4.75 mg/ml. *Anesthesiology* **80:** 284–297, 1994
11. Du Pen SL, Kharrasch ED, Williams A *et al.* Chronic epidural bupivacaine-opioid infusion in intractable cancer pain. *Pain* **49:** 293–300, 1992
12. Ochs G, Struppler A, Meyerson BA *et al.* Intrathecal baclofen for long-term treatment of spasticity: multi-centre study. *J Natrol Neurosurg Psychiatry* **52:** 933–939, 1989
13. Penn RD, Savoy SM, Corcos DM *et al.* Intrathecal baclofen for severe spinal spasticity. *N Engl J Med* **23:** 1517–1521, 1989
14. Latash ML, Penn RD, Corcos DM, Gottlieb GL. Effects of intrathecal baclofen on voluntary motor control in spastic paresis. *J Neurosurg* **72:** 388–392, 1990
15. Lazorthes Y, Sallerin-Caute B, Verdie J-C, Bastide R, Carillo J-P. Chronic intrathecal baclofen administration for control of severe spasticity. *J Neurosurg* **72:** 393–402, 1990

16. Mueller-Schwefe G, Penn RD. Physostigmine in the treatment of intrathecal baclofen overdose. *J Neurosurg* **71:** 273–275, 1989
17. Salturi L, Marosi MJ, Kofler M, Bauer G. Status epilepticus complicating intrathecal baclofen overdosage. *Lancet* **339:** 373–374, 1992
18. Bion JF. Intrathecal ketamine for war surgery. A preliminary study under field conditions. *Anaesthesia* **39:** 1023–1028, 1984
19. Cripps TP, Goodchild CS. Intrathecal midazolam and the stress response to upper abdominal surgery adrenocortical, glycaemic, and analgesic effects. *Clin J Pain* **4:** 125–128, 1988
20. Serrao JM, Marks RL, Morley SJ, Goodchild CS. Intrathecal midazolam for the treatment of chronic mechanical low back pain: a controlled comparison with epidural steroid in a pilot study. *Pain* **48:** 349–353, 1992
21. Penn RD, Paice J, Kroin JS. Intrathecal octreotide for cancer pain. *Lancet* **335:** 738, 1990
22. Long JB. Spinal subarachnoid injection of somatostatin causes neurological deficits and neuronal injury in rats. *Eur J Pharmacol* **149:** 287–296, 1988
23. Miralles FS, L-Soriano F, Puig MM, Perez D, Lopez-Rodriguez FM. Postoperative analgesia induced by subarachnoid lidocaine plus calcitonin. *Anesth Analg* **66:** 615–618, 1987
24. Miseria S, Torresi U, Piga A *et al*. Analgesia with epidural calcitonin in cancer patients. *Tumori* **75:** 183–184, 1989
25. Fraioli F, Fabbri A, Gnessi L, Moretti C, Santoro C, Felici M. Subarachnoid calcitonin for intolerable pain. *Lancet* **9:** 831, 1982
26. Yaksh TL, Malmberg AB. Spinal actions of NSAIDs in blocking spinally mediated hyperalgesia: the role of cyclooxygenase products. In: *Disease Therapy, Agents and Actions.* Basel: Berhausser Verlag, 1993, pp. 89–100
27. Uphouse LA, Welch SP, Ward CR, Ellis EF, Embrey JP. Antinociceptive activity of intrathecal ketorolac is blocked by the kappa-opioid receptor antagonist, norbinaltorphimine. *Eur J Pharmacol* **242:** 53–58, 1993
28. Malmberg AB, Yaksh TL. Pharmacology of the spinal action of ketorolac, morphine, ST-91, U50-488H, and L-PIA on the formalin test and an isobolographic analysis of the NSAID interaction. *Anesthesiology* **79:** 270–281, 1993
29. Ohlsson L, Rydberg T, Ede NT, Persson Y, Thulin NL. Cancer pain relief by continuous administration of epidural morphine in a hospital setting and at home. *Pain* **48:** 349–353, 1992
30. Cherry DA, Gourlay GK, Cousins JM, Cannon JB. A technique for the insertion of an implantable portal system for longterm epidural administration of opioids in the treatment of cancer pain. *Anaesth Intens Care* **13:** 145–152, 1985
31. Nitescu P, Hultman E, Appelgren L, Linder LE, Curelaru I. Bacteriology, drug stability and exchange of percutaneous delivery systems and antibacterial filters in long-term intrathecal infusion of opioid drugs and bupivacaine in "refractory" pain. *Clin J Pain* **8:** 324–327, 1992
32. Sjoberg M, Karlsson PA, Nordborg C *et al*. Neuropathological findings after long-term intrathecal infusion of morphine and bupivacaine for pain treatment in cancer patients. *Anesthesiology* **76:** 173–186, 1992
33. Bel S, Bauer BL. Dorsal column stimulation (DCS): cost to benefit analysis. *Neurochirurgica* **52:** 121–123, 1991
34. Bedder MD, Burchiel K, Larson A. Cost analysis of two implantable narcotic delivery systems. *J Pain Symptom Manage* **6:** 368–373, 1991
35. Evans PJD, Lloyd JW, Jack TM. Cryoanalgesia for intractable perineal pain. *J R Soc Med* **74:** 804–809, 1981
36. De-Coster D, Bossuyt M, Fossion E. The value of cryotherapy in the management of trigeminal neuralgia. *Acta Stomatol Belg* **90:** 87–93, 1993
37. Schuster GD. The use of cryoanalgesia in the painful facet syndrome. *J Neurol Orthop Surg* **3:** 271–274, 1982
38. Shealy CN. The role of spinal facets in back and facet pain. *Headache* **14:** 101–104, 1974

39. North RB, Han M, Zahurak M, Kidd DH. Radiofrequency lumbar facet denervation; analysis of prognostic factors. *Pain* **57:** 77–83, 1994

40. Shealy CN. Electrical inhibition of pain by stimulation of the dorsal column. *Anesth Analg* **46:** 489–491, 1967

41. Nuki Y, Kawasaki H, Taguchi T, Takasaki K, Wada A. Effects of dorsal rhizotomy on depressor response to spinal cord stimulation mediated by endogenous calcitonin gene-related peptide in the pithed rat. *J Neurosurg* **79:** 899–904, 1993

42. Robaina FJ, Dominguez M, Diaz M, Rodriguez JL, De Vera JA. Spinal cord stimulation for relief of chronic pain in vasospastic disorders of the upper limbs. *Neurosurgery* **24:** 63–67, 1989

43. Sanchez-Ledesma MJ, Garcia-March G, Diaz-Cascajo P, Gomez-Moreta J, Broseta J. Spinal cord stimulation in deafferentation pain. *Stereotact Funct Neurosurg* **53:** 40–45, 1989

44. Auginstinsson LE, Helm J, Carlsson CA, Juvegard L. Epidural electrical stimulation in severe limb ischaemia. Evidence of pain relief, increased blood flow and a possible limb-saving effect. *Ann Surg* **202:** 104–111, 1985

45. Jacobs MJHM, Jorning PJG, Joshi SR, Kitslaar PJEHM, Slaaf DW, Reneman RS. Epidural spinal cord stimulation improves microvascular blood flow in severe limb ischaemia. *Ann Surg* **207:** 179–183, 1988

46. Kujacic V, Eliasson T, Mannheimer C, Jablonskiene D, Augustinsson LE, Emanuelsson H. Assessment of the influence of spinal cord stimulation on left ventricular function in patients with severe angina pectoris: an echocardiographic study. *Eur Heart J* **14:** 1238–1245, 1993

47. Chandler MJ, Brennan TJ, Garrison DW, Kim KS, Schwartz PJ, Foreman RD. A mechanism of cardiac pain suppression by spinal cord stimulation: implications for patients with angina pectoris. *Eur Heart J* **14:** 96–105, 1993

48. Eliasson T, Albertsson P, Hardhammar P, Emanuelsson H, Augustinsson LE, Mannheimer C. Spinal cord stimulation in angina pectoris with normal coronary arteries. *Coron Artery Dis* **4:** 819–827, 1993

49. De La Forte C, Van de Kelfte E. Spinal cord stimulation in failed back surgery syndrome. *Pain* **52:** 55–61, 1993

50. Probst C. Spinal cord stimulation in 112 patients with epi/indural fibrosis following operation for lumbar disc herniation. *Acta Neurochir (Wien)* **107:** 147–151, 1990

51. North RB, Kidd DH, Zahurak M, James CS, Long DM. Spinal cord stimulation for chronic intractable pain: experience over two decades. *Neurosurgery* **32:** 384–394, 1993

52. Barolat G, Massaro F, He J, Zeme S, Ketcik B. Mapping of sensory responses to epidural stimulation of the intraspinal neural structures in man. *J Neurosurg* **78:** 233–239, 1993

53. Shimoji K, Hokari T, Kano T *et al.* Management of intractable pain with percutaneous epidural spinal cord stimulation: differences in pain relieving effects among diseases and sites of pain. *Anesth Analg* **77:** 110–116, 1993

54. Kaube K, Keay KA, Hoskin KL, Bandler R, Goadsby PJ. Expression of c-*fos*-like immunoreactivity in the caudal medulla and upper cervical spinal cord following stimulation of the superior sagittal sinus in the cat. *Brain Res* **629:** 95–102, 1993

# Index